HEALTHCARE TECHNOLOGIES SERIES 57

Medical Imaging Informatics

IET Book Series on e-Health Technologies

Book Series Editor: Professor Joel J.P.C. Rodrigues, College of Computer Science and Technology, China University of Petroleum (East China), Qingdao, China; Senac Faculty of Ceará, Fortaleza-CE, Brazil and Instituto de Telecomunicações, Portugal

Book Series Advisor: Professor Pranjal Chandra, School of Biochemical Engineering, Indian Institute of Technology (BHU), Varanasi, India

While the demographic shifts in populations display significant socio-economic challenges, they trigger opportunities for innovations in e-Health, m-Health, precision and personalized medicine, robotics, sensing, the Internet of things, cloud computing, big data, software-defined networks, and network function virtualization. Their integration is however associated with many technological, ethical, legal, social, and security issues. This book series aims to disseminate recent advances in e-health technologies to improve healthcare and people's well-being.

Could you be our next author?

Topics considered include intelligent e-Health systems, electronic health records, ICT-enabled personal health systems, mobile and cloud computing for e-Health, health monitoring, precision and personalized health, robotics for e-Health, security and privacy in e-Health, ambient assisted living, telemedicine, big data and IoT for e-Health, and more.

Proposals for coherently integrated international multi-authored edited or co-authored handbooks and research monographs will be considered for this book series. Each proposal will be reviewed by the book Series Editor with additional external reviews from independent reviewers.

To download our proposal form or find out more information about publishing with us, please visit https://www.theiet.org/publishing/publishing-with-iet-books/.

Please email your completed book proposal for the IET Book Series on e-Health Technologies to: Amber Thomas at athomas@theiet.org or author_support@theiet.org.

IET The Institution of Engineering and Technology

Medical Imaging Informatics

Machine learning, deep learning and big data analytics

Edited by
Mamoon Rashid, Vishal Goyal, Ali Kashif Bashir
and Saqib Hakak

The Institution of Engineering and Technology

Published by The Institution of Engineering and Technology, London, United Kingdom

The Institution of Engineering and Technology is registered as a Charity in England & Wales (no. 211014) and Scotland (no. SC038698).

The Institution of Engineering and Technology
Futures Place
Kings Way, Stevenage
Hertfordshire SG1 2UA, United Kingdom

www.theiet.org

British Library Cataloguing in Publication Data
A catalogue record for this product is available from the British Library

ISBN 978-1-83953-743-1 (hardback)
ISBN 978-1-83953-744-8 (PDF)

Typeset in India by MPS Limited

Cover Image: Monty Rakusen / DigitalVision via Getty Images

Contents

About the editors

Mamoon Rashid is currently working as an associate professor in the Department of Computer Engineering, Faculty of Science and Technology, Vishwakarma University, Pune, India. He also holds a position of director, Research Center of Excellence for Health Informatics, Vishwakarma University, Pune, India. He received his Ph.D. from the Department of Computer Science and Engineering, Punjabi University, Patiala, India, in the field of Medical Imaging Informatics. He has published 100+ papers indexed in SCI/SCIE journals and conferences of international repute. He also edited a book titled *Artificial Intelligence for Innovative Healthcare Informatics,* Springer, in 2022. He served as a lead guest editor for many journals indexing in Web of Science. His research interests include health informatic, medical imaging, and image processing.

Vishal Goyal is a full professor in the Department of Computer Science, Punjabi University Patiala, India, with teaching and research experience of 21+ years. He is also holding positions of co-coordinator for "Center for Artificial Intelligence and Data Science," coordinator for "Research Centre for technology Development for Differently Abled Persons," and director of the Centre for E-Learning and Teaching Excellence, Punjabi University, India. He is an approved consultant for AIU in consulting universities and colleges for accreditation rankings of NAAC, NIRF, NBA, and international linkages. He has been awarded the Young Scientist Award in 2015 by the Punjab Academy of Sciences, and two times State Award by the Government of Punjab, India. He has published 100+ research publications in various journals and conferences of national and international repute. He completed his grant projects with 10 million Indian rupees funded by various ministries of Govt. of India and has a number of projects in progress. His research areas are natural language processing, technology development for differently abled people, and machine learning.

Ali Kashif Bashir is a reader in the Department of Computing and Mathematics, Manchester Metropolitan University, UK. He is the leader of Future Networks Lab and head of Advanced Cybersecurity Testbed. He is supervising/co-supervising a number of Ph.D. students, Postdocs, and research associates. Along with his students and colleagues, he has published over 250 high-impact articles in top venues. He has obtained over £4 million external funding from UK, South Korean, Japanese, European, Asian, and Middle Eastern agencies. He is also Co-I of GM AI and GM Cyber Foundry, each having £6 million funding. He is a senior member of

IEEE, a member of 10+ IEEE technical societies, and a distinguished speaker of ACM. He has chaired several international conferences and workshops and has delivered over 40 invited and keynote talks across the globe. He also enjoys several honorary and adjunct professor positions in many countries like China, Canada, Lebanon, UAE, India, and Pakistan. He is serving as an editor-in-chief of *IEEE Technology, Policy and Ethics* and *Journal of Autonomous Intelligence*, and an editor of over 10 international journals including *Scientific Reports*, *Nature*, and *IEEE Transactions on Network Science and Engineering*.

Saqib Hakak is an assistant professor at the Canadian Institute for Cybersecurity, University of New Brunswick, Canada. He has 6+ years of industrial and academic experience. He has received a number of Gold/Silver awards in international innovation competitions and is serving as a technical committee member/reviewer of several reputed conference/journal venues. He has published 90+ papers in journals of repute. His research interests include risk management, fake news detection using AI, security and privacy concerns in IoE, applications of federated learning in IoT, and blockchain technology.

Section 1

Medical image analysis using artificial intelligence

Chapter 1

Intervention of medical images for disease prediction

Neha Singh[1], Shilpi Birla[1] and Neeraj Kumar Shukla[2]

Medical imaging is generally the first step in the detection of disease and is used to create images of part or whole body. These images are also useful for the study of anatomy and functioning by building accurate computer models of the body systems, organs, tissues, and cells. Different modalities are used for medical images like computed tomography (CT) scan, magnetic resonance imaging (MRI), ultrasound, and X-ray imaging. Medical practitioners are continuously facing challenges to interpret medical images for the prediction of different diseases. A treatment given at an early stage of many of the diseases is more effective with lesser damage. The use of data analytics techniques and machine learning algorithms offers better predictive analysis of medical images. The main challenge is the identification of the most suitable algorithms for processing medical images, build and evaluate models, and integrate clinical data in a single module. Highly accurate data-analytical tools are needed to exploit information from medical datasets, keeping in mind their peculiarities, and sparse nature of the datasets. Machine learning (ML) may provide new insights into biomedical analyses, by the development of models that can be used to predict outputs such as categorical labels, binary responses, or continuous values. This chapter presents a review of literature for brain, renal, colon, cardiovascular, and lung diseases detection and prediction using medical images. The focus is on exploring various data analytics and artificial intelligence techniques used for retrieving information from medical images for predicting diseases. This chapter aims to help researchers to identify suitable technique for disease prediction in medical images for further improvement in prediction accuracy and efficiency.

1.1 Introduction

Medical diagnosis and interpretation refer to the identification of any possible disease from observations, medical data, or images. The first step in the process is

[1]Department of ECE, Manipal University Jaipur, Jaipur, India
[2]King Khalid University, Abha, Saudi Arabia

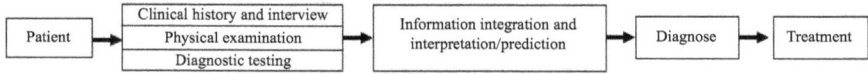

Figure 1.1   Medical diagnostic process

the study of symptoms visible by physical examination in the patient. But for more surety and possible early detection, the physical examination is followed by laboratory analysis, bio-signal analysis, and medical image analysis. If the disease is predicted at an early stage, the preventive and early treatment may be more effective with lesser damage. Figure 1.1 shows the medical diagnostic process. This chapter focuses on the acquisition of medical images using appropriate modality followed by the intervention of the captured image for disease prediction. The process of medical imaging requires to provide a safe and comfortable way of capturing the best informative diagnostic images of the body part, especially when it comes to imaging of internal body parts. These images are not only useful for medical purposes but for the study of anatomy and the functioning of organs, tissues, and cells inside the body. Human biology varies from person to person and hence when it comes to the diagnosis of a disease using some medical images, it is required to be done against a background with a wide range of normality. This needs that the medical images acquire the details precisely and the clinician judges qualitatively, the image and the corresponding data correctly. Medical practitioners are continuously facing challenges to interpret medical images for the prediction of different diseases.

The organization of this chapter is as follows: the first section briefly throws light on different image modalities used for capturing images for medical purposes. The second section provides an insight into the important image processing operations and quality assessment metrics used during pre-processing of medical images for disease prediction. The next sections to follow, review the literature for the use of different approaches on the suitable medical image for prediction of diseases for different body parts like brain, heart, kidney and colon, and eyes. Also, a review of approaches for the detection of the recent pandemic, COVID-19 is presented.

1.2   Medical imaging

Roots of medical imaging dates to the year of 1895, when X-rays were discovered by Wihelm Rontgen which opened the doors to the internal world of the physical body. With time, different frequencies from the electromagnetic (EM) spectrum were used for medical imaging. Figure 1.2 shows the evolution of medical imaging. The images are developed due to the interaction of EM waves with different internal body structures like bones, muscles, tissues, etc. Depending on the nature (density) of the interacting body structure, these waves may be absorbed, reflected, refracted, or transmitted to form medical images.

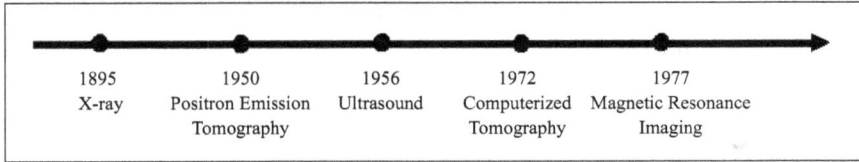

Figure 1.2 Evolution of medical imaging

Different modalities are used for medical images like X-ray imaging, computerized tomography (CT) scan, magnetic resonance imaging (MRI), ultrasound, and positron emission tomography (PET). These techniques are generally non-invasive and differ in the method of capturing the images based on the underlying technology. The organ or tissue and the disease to be studied define the imaging method [1]. For example, a CT scan is useful for bone imaging but gives poor contrast for soft tissues, which are clearly visible in MRI images [2]. This section presents an overview [3] of the medical imaging modalities.

1.2.1 X-ray

X-ray imaging is the first imaging method for studying the internal human body. It uses EM waves of short wavelength and high frequencies in the range of 10^{16}–10^{20} Hz. It is suitable for the study of bones, joints, arthritis, and tooth decay. It also finds application in the detection of diseases like pneumonia and tuberculosis in the lungs. For X-ray imaging, high-energy photons are locally focused on the body using an external source. Some photons are absorbed, while some are scattered at different angles or some pass through the body straight. The dense and hard bones in the body block the beam of X-rays and are shown as white regions in X-ray images. The nearby tissues absorb and scatter these rays based on their densities, which are reflected as gray areas in the image. The air in the lungs is displayed as black regions in X-ray images. The method is non-invasive, and the dose of X-ray and the time of its exposure to the body is controlled without any immediate health risk. However, long exposure to high-energy X-rays may damage human cells resulting in skin burns due to permanent tissue damage, hair loss, and increased possibility of causing cancer. The high energy ionizing radiations of X-rays, when absorbed by our body, may alter molecular structures. These biological effects are exploited in radiation therapy for some malignant tumors.

1.2.2 CT scan

A CT scan combines multiple cross-sectional 2D X-ray images of the body taken from different angles by a rotating X-ray source to produce a 3D image with the help of a computer. It is suitable for imaging bones, soft tissues, and blood vessels in our body to detect broken bones, tumors, blood clots, and internal bleeding. The dose of X-ray used for CT scan is higher than that used in X-ray but under controlled and safe amount. Many times, a contrast agent is introduced into the body orally or through injection to highlight specific features in the body with better contrast in the images. This contrast agent is cleared out from the body through urine.

1.2.3 MRI

MRI offers clear 3D images of soft tissues in the body like tumors, muscles, and nervous system [4]. It captures the image of the body part as if it was sliced layer by layer. Each slice can be pictured from the front, bottom, or sides as per the requirement of the expected disease. MRI has been used to test the brain, cardio-vascular diseases, gastrointestinal diseases, and many other diseases related to nerves, pancreas, kidney, uterus, ovaries, liver, and prostate. MRI also helps in evaluating cartilage injuries in joints, bone infections and tumors, and disk abnormalities in the spine. The lowest frequencies of the electromagnetic spectrum, that is, in the range of radio frequencies are used by MRI. Based on the timing of frequency used for imaging, there are two types of MRI images. T1-weighted images highlight fat tissues in the body while T2-weighted images highlight fat tissues as well as water- or fluid-based tissue in the body. Fluid-based tissues are identified by comparing T2-weighted MR images with T1-weighted images. For MRI, the body is placed in a high magnetic field which aligns the water molecules of our body (which are magnetic) in a specific direction. Short bursts of radio frequency signals are sent which disturbs the alignment of these atoms. When the EM waves are removed, the atoms move back to their original position and reemit the radio waves which are captured by the sensors. These reemitted waves are then converted to a 3D image by the computer. The energy of reemitted waves varies due to the local environment which results in contrast in the images. MRI done to capture the functioning of the brain is called functional MRI (fMRI). The flow of blood to different regions of the brain is captured for predicting any abnormality in brain functioning due to injury or Alzheimer's disease. Standard MRI cannot capture flowing blood in arteries and veins so, a contrast agent, which has magnetic properties, is injected into the bloodstream, just like for the CT scan. An MRI scan is more detailed as compared to a CT scan.

1.2.4 Ultrasound

Ultrasound [5] produces live internal images of the internal body, called sono-grams, by scanning it from outside with high-frequency sound waves of 1–5 MHz. The images are live in the sense that the movements occurring inside the body are also scanned along with the anatomy. For example, the movement of the fetus within the womb is observed along with its structure. The method is non-invasive and does not produce ionizing radiations, hence is non-hazardous to the body. Ultrasound is recommended for imaging fetus in animals and humans as it is less harmful compared to other methods. The ultrasound machine works on the prin-ciple of the Doppler effect. It uses an acoustic transducer in a handheld probe which sends high-frequency acoustic waves, some of which are absorbed while some are reflected by the tissues with different strengths depending on their characteristics.

These reflected ultrasound waves are received by the transducer in the probe. The time taken by the reflected ray to reach the transducer is used to estimate the tissue interface depth and generate an electrical voltage correspondingly. These electrical signals are digitized and sent to the processing unit to display the 2-D image on the monitor.

1.2.5   PET scan

A PET scan belongs to the class of nuclear imaging as it uses a small dose of an injectable radioactive drug called a tracer. It is useful to catch the metabolic or biochemical functions of the body organs and tissues. When injected, the tracer moves to different body organs and tissues through the blood. The signal from the tracer is then captured by a PET machine to capture a picture of the organ. PET scans are useful because the metabolic abnormalities due to many diseases in the initial stages can be detected with careful study, even before the disease itself is reflected in scans with any other modality. Cancer cells have high metabolic activity so the radioactive drug highlights them as bright points on the scan. Hence, the PET scan is very useful in not only detecting cancer at the early stage but to observe its spread, recurrence, and effect of treatment on cancer cells. These scans are combined with MRI and CT to predict brain diseases and heart diseases by observing the blood flow in different parts of these organs.

1.2.6   Artificial intelligence for improved diagnostic imaging

With technological advancements in medical imaging equipment and techniques over the years, the obtained images are expected to contain much more data than a human can analyze. Artificial intelligence (AI) plays an important part in handling such large data to identify patterns within the images to predict diseases in real-time with much more accuracy. This is possible by training the machines with a vast number of images and using AI to make the process faster, accurate, and reliable. For example, MRI scans have a direct relationship between the time of exposure and the quality of the obtained image. To accommodate a long queue of patients for MRI, a compromise on the time of exposure may be done and later AI techniques can be applied to the low-quality images obtained for better representation of the information. AI systems can characterize the abnormal findings for decision-making as not all abnormalities indicate diseases. Also, AI is used for improving the captured images.

The authors of [6] reviewed the use of AI for intravascular imaging. It uses ultrasonic frequencies which are analyzed by the intravascular ultrasonic (IVUS) data analysis system iMAP-IVUS to extract spectral parameters. Machine learning is applied to these extracted parameters to classify the plaque and identify high-risk plaques. Some other analysis systems [6] are VH-IVUS by Philips Volcano and Integrated Backscatter (IB)-IVUS by Terumo Corporation, Tokyo, Japan. The other approach for the estimation of plaque composition by IVUS analysis is based on the study of specific features in ultrasound images, for example, image texture, edges, and shadowing. AI can be useful in predicting vulnerable plaque for any future adverse events. The authors of [7] exploited the strength of AI to combine data from grayscale IVUS images with clinical and demographic data. AI is widely used in interpreting medical images too as seen in the review presented in the sections to follow for the prediction of specific diseases one by one.

1.3   Medical image processing operations

Different image modalities capture different physical quantities based on the underlying principle of operation of the machine. These captured quantities represent the internal body anatomy differently. The output is, however, represented as a digital image with some additional data. Medical images are quite different from natural images as these are required to be high-resolution images, that too usually grayscale. The underlying human body tissue responds to different imaging sources differently which results in wide variations in intensity levels within medical images. Hence, a variation in the gray level holds the major information about the tissue behavior in healthy and unhealthy conditions.

All digital images used for medical purposes are represented in digital imaging and communication in medicine (DICOM) format. This format is internationally accepted to standardize the storage, retrieval, sharing, and display of medical images captured by different modalities. A DICOM medical image contains a variable length header containing the image data. The header covers patient details like name, age, etc., image information like pixel depth and size, and some data about the imaging method [8]. DICOM supports only integers and not float-type but supports compression. This makes the medical image interoperable for different systems. Some other common image formats are neuroimaging informatics technology initiative (NIFTI), MINC, and ANALYZE. ANALYZE was introduced for multidimensional data, for example, 3D medical images but not used much nowadays. NIFTI was developed as an improvement over ANALYZE, especially for neuroimages. It uses translation and rotation to project each voxel of the 3D image on the reference frame.

Most of image acquisition methods employ electromagnetic waves which are harmful to humans, hence the images are captured with low energy doses for the short duration of exposure. This results in poor quality of raw image data with high noise content. Also, due to differences in the internal body structure of different subjects or patients, the same modality may not be able to capture the same depth of information. Therefore, data captured by machines is required to be processed for better visuals and analysis. The general image processing operations that are used to make the captured medical image clearer and easy for interpretation and prediction of disease in underlying organs are enhancement, segmentation, registration, and fusion. Additionally, image fusion to obtain a wide-angled view, image classification, and extraction of quantitative measurements using data analysis is commonly required for medical images. This section of the chapter presents an overview of these image processing operations and data analytics methods for better prediction of diseases.

The captured image undergoes enhancement which refers to the class of processing operations with the aim to improve the image either to increase the perception of objects by the observer or for further image analysis. Some examples of image enhancement processes are contrast adjustment, denoising, image sharpening, and smoothing. These processes may be pixel operations, local or global in nature. The noise and artifacts introduced in the image due to imaging machines are removed using these techniques. Human vision perceives discontinuity to identify objects, so image enhancement highlights or strengthens the edges in the image for a clearer definition of objects. On the other hand, sometimes, false edges may hinder the detection of the object of interest, so image enhancement methods are used to suppress these edges or smoothen the image. Edges are associated with sharp intensity changes (gradient) and so is noise. Hence, edge-preserving enhancement techniques [9] are generally used to denoise the image with details preserved. Improvement of contrast using thresholding, windowing, and histogram processing improves the visual quality of the images globally. Another purpose for using image enhancement is to enhance the spatial resolution of the image. However, this requires upsampling of data by interpolation.

Once the image is enhanced with expected edges preserved after denoising, the region of interest from that image is to be extracted. The processes that are required to divide the image into different parts, each having some similar characteristics, for localized analysis and better interpretation are referred to as segmentation processes. The accuracy and precision of the segmentation process is very important for diagnosis. Many times, the segmentation of medical images requires interaction with domain experts or users [9]. For example, the user may be required to interactively identify a seed point for the object of interest in the image. Following which region growing method is used for segregating the object from the background. The segmentation works on the principle of homogeneity. The region with homogeneous characteristics is identified. Some of the methods involved in the segmentation of images are edge detection, thresholding, and clustering [10].

Image registration refers to the process of transforming data from one coordinate system to the other or combining multiple images from wider coverage. Each medical imaging modality has its own purpose, advantages, and limitations. So, sometimes complimentary information captured by different modalities have to be used together for better clinical diagnosis and analysis. Combining images from different modalities is referred to as image fusion. The authors of [2] classified the source image into similar patches based on the direction of their geometrical gradient. Each of these patches is then represented using sparse representation.

1.3.1 Medical image quality assessment

Each of the above image processing operation works on different features of the image and modify the image content to suit the requirement better. However, mathematically the changes introduced due to processing need to be quantified, for which the image quality measures are useful to be understood. Most of the information about the internal body detail is stored with the variation of grayscale in the scan images. This information is sometimes overridden by noise and artifacts introduced due to imaging machines.

The most common image quality measures used for general image processing operations are Structural Similarity Index Measure (SSIM), peak signal-to-noise ratio (PSNR), and contrast-to-noise ratio (CNR). These measures require a reference image to quantify the effect of processing. Medical images differ from other natural images because the purpose of processing these images is not to obtain a beautiful image but an image with a clear and effective representation of abnormalities for accurate and quick prediction of disease. Also, the quality of the image greatly depends on the imaging method and the respective variables like radiation dose and exposure time. Image contrast, resolution (sharpness), noise, machine artifacts related to machines and humans, and distortion are other important factors [11] for medical image quality assessment. A study of image quality measures based on these factors will be significant in choosing the imaging variables during the investigation. Some full references as well as blind image quality measures for magnetic resonance (MR) images, CT, and ultrasonic images are reviewed in [12]. The major challenge for having an Image Quality Assessment (IQA) standard for medical images is that different modalities capture the body details with different characteristics and representations. Based on CNR, scan resolution, pixel size, and Shannon's information content, an image quality measure for MR images is reported in [12]. A subjective full-referenced testing measure for possibly degraded MR images is Double-Stimulus Continuous-Quality Scale (DSCQS). The MR images are expected to be degraded if they are captured fast and hence partially constructed. The possibly degraded MR images are evaluated in reference to a full k-space reconstructed image. DSCQS is less sensitive to contextual effects but is also used to evaluate ultrasound images as well as telemedicine images. Since DSCQS is a subjective measure, which may be biased, the average score obtained from different subjects is used to calculate Mean Opinion Score (MOS). The difference MOS (DMOS) is used as a measure of the quality of the image with respect to the reference image, which is very close to the objective full reference IQA measures. DSCQS also shows agreement with the perceptual difference model (PDM) which presents a map of visual difference with respect to the reference image incorporating the human visual system (HVS) components. Some no reference blind IQA measures reviewed in [12] are: Codebook Blind Image Quality measure (CBIQ), which extracts local features of the image using Gabor filters for capturing complex statistics of the images; Learning-based Blind Image Quality measure (LBIQ), which uses a statistical regression algorithm; distortion identification-based image integrity and verify evaluation (DIIVINE) index, which uses natural scene statistics; blind image notator using discrete cosine transform (DCT) statistics (BLINDS-II), which exploits the Bayesian inference model. These blind IQA measures are time consuming. A time-efficient blind measure is Blind/ referenceless image spatial quality evaluator (BRISQUE). It quantifies the distortions of test images based on luminance coefficient statistics in the spatial domain [12]. The authors stressed on using blind image quality measures that use no reference, due to the unavailability of the perfect reference image, for optimization of image acquisition and algorithm applied to these acquired images for medical diagnosis. The major limitation reported by authors in [12] is that the majority of published medical IQA measures were evaluated with artificially added distortion, rather than the actually distorted medical images.

The authors in [13] presented an experimental verification for a novel blind IQA measure. It analyzes the test image using the gradient method based on the number of isolated peaks with respect to a threshold value. As the threshold is changed, the number of isolated peaks also changes, which is represented as a curve for each image, which is used for quality assessment. The quality of X-ray, CT, and MR image depends on the dose (exposure time and energy of beam), and noise. Hence, the choice of imaging parameters for acceptable image quality is important. The authors of [13] proposed IQA measure to be used to set imaging parameters for obtaining images with acceptable CNR by quantifying the relationship between the inferior image quality rating and the impulse noise. The experiment was performed over 2,708 images of 38 patients. It is inferred that high-quality images have high maximum curvature based on the average value of isolated peaks for a lower threshold value. The authors in [14] introduced a metric for obtaining the best quality of MR images. This metric quantifies structural changes for MR images of the brain based on luminance and contrast variation as non-structural distortions together with structural distortions during the denoising process. SSIM is used to measure the structural changes. It is reported that for lower contrast and higher luminance variations during image capturing, the visual quality of the image is degraded with reducing value of SSIM.

The research for finding universal image quality measure is still advancing for medical images. The measurement without a reference is targeted and deep learning (DL) has been used for automated quality assessment. Important challenges of using DL for medical images are reported in [15]. The challenges are identified as:

- Labels for images that can be used as ground truth is difficult to be determined due to difference in opinions of different subjects.
- The number of images for all possible distinguished classes is not necessarily the same in all databases.
- Unreliable labels and unclear discrimination between classes hinder the task to classify the image.

The work in [16] applies convolutional neural networks (CNN) to assess ultrasound image quality. The accuracy is further improved by using the transfer learning strategy with CNN to overcome the limitations due to unlabeled data. The work is done on LIVE database containing 29 high-resolution reference images. Each of these images is corrupted with JPEG compression, Gaussian convolution, fast Rayleigh fading, or white noise addition to obtain a part of the final dataset for the work. Other high-resolution ultrasound images are taken from freely available websites together with the images from different departments at Tongji Hospital, with affiliation to Huazhong University of Science and Technology. The gold standard for each image in the database is taken as the average score by four doctors. The quality is assessed based on linear and Spearman's rank-order correlation coefficients that take care of the subjective score with the objective score obtained from the CNN model.

1.4   Brain disease prediction

Brain health is very essential part of overall human health as it underlies humans' ability to communicate, sense, make body balance and movements, and regulate thought, emotion, and our physiological processes. The brain is monitored and observed by scanning its sections and reading neuron activities in different parts of the brain. New technologies allow non-invasive scanning with CT, MRI, PET, and optical tomography for brain imaging. MRI is the most suitable modality for capturing brain structure and working by observing the flow of blood in the brain. The complex human brain tissue makes it difficult to read and analyze the images obtained using different modalities. The difficulty is due to the following reasons [17]:

- Internal factors
  - Fuzziness due to grayscale results in the unclear boundary between brain tissue and background
  - Local body effect
  - Uncertainty

- External factors
  - Partial volume effect
  - Migration field effect
  - Noise interference

Brain images are sometimes required to undergo different image processing operations (as discussed in Section 1.2) for better visibility and analysis. Brain MR images contain noise, artifacts, weak contrast, and weak boundaries due to complex brain structure and magnetic resonance in the equipment. The authors in [17] use the Hybrid Pyramid U-Net model for the segmentation of brain tumor in brain images with improved fuzzy clustering based on local spatial data in the image for predictive diagnosis. The authors used a fuzzy C-means algorithm which offers the advantages of dealing with inaccuracies and uncertainty of images with no requirement of setting the threshold value in advance. The authors in [18] implemented deep learning using the convolutional layer with the rectified linear unit for the classification of brain cyst based on its type, location, and size. The different classes of the cyst considered for classification are arachnoid, colloid, dermoid, epidermoid, pineal, brain abscess, and neoplastic cyst. The work uses deep neural network (DNN) classification with 150 neurons in each layer and uses the SoftMax activation function. The rectified linear unit layer in the DNN normalizes the propagating gradients and activations. The classifier is reported to provide an accuracy of 98.4%. The authors in [19] implemented a multivariate approach for the prediction of the survival of glioma patients with a robust radiomics model. Initially, 1,731 radiomics features are obtained from T2-weighted MRI for each patient, based on first-order statistics, shape and size, texture, and filter-derived feature. Of these 1,731 features, only 1,293 features, which had the intraclass correlation coefficient of 0.9, were selected for making the risk prediction model. To ensure the robustness of the model, the selected features are distributed into training and test sets in different ratios of 5:5, 3:7, 4:6, 6:4, and 7:3 repeatedly with 1,000 permutations. For each training set, features having a high correlation with overall survival were used to calculate a risk factor score, which is used to find the radiomic feature score for each test sample. Based on the median of this score, the test samples are categorized as low and high-scored samples. If the overall survival of these categories is significant, the features are chosen. About 85% of the features that were repeated in the 1,000 permutations were finally selected for the model. The model was verified with two other datasets with different compositions to ensure accuracy further by making the model unbiased with multiple databases.

1.4.1   Detection of Alzheimer

Alzheimer is a brain disease that affects memory and the functioning of the brain due to the destruction of neurons. The major cause of this disease is the deposit of proteins forming plaque around brain cells or forming tangles within the brain cells. The affected cells result in decreased messaging between them and shrinking of brain areas. Predicting Alzheimer's disease can be challenging because its symptoms often manifest over an extended period. However, when detected in its early stages, it is possible to slow down and, in some cases, even control the progression of the disease. MRI scans and data extracted from them are used for disease identification which is a tedious task and the diagnosis time can be reduced by automating the procedure using AI. The main reasons for the late realization of the disease in patients are [20]:

- Patients rarely exhibit preclinical symptoms
- No scientific evidence is there to slow the progress of the disease
- Currently used biomarkers are either expensive, invasive, or both.

The authors report that age, gender, and preclinical disease state play an important role in estimating lifetime risk and ten-year prediction of acquiring the disease of Alzheimer. The most important factor for uncertainty in the study is identified as the rate of transition between different states of the disease. The study used a multistate model based on the Markov model where the transition from one state to another depends only on the patient's present age and not on the duration, he/she has been in that state.

Different approaches of AI have been implemented for the detection and prediction of diseases based on the study of MRI images. Authors in [21] compared support vector machines (SVM), Bayes statistics, and voting feature intervals to develop a data mining model for quantifying the matching of patterns for predicting progression towards Alzheimer's disease if the patient exhibits mild cognitive impairment. Initially, a pattern of degeneration of the brain is established to differentiate between a healthy person and Alzheimer's patient. The medial temporal lobe, anterior cingulate gyrus extending towards the orbitofrontal cortex, and the subcortical thalamic-basal ganglia areas are identified as the regions which can indicate the difference between a healthy person and an Alzheimer's patient. The three classification approaches were tested to confirm the discrimination based on the selected clusters and the voting-based approach gave the best results.

The authors in [22] studied different machine learning algorithms like decision tree, random forest, SVM, XGBoost, and voting for studying the effect of various parameters for Alzheimer detection with identification of its stage. The database for the study is taken from Open Access Series of Imaging Studies (OASIS). Some of the studied parameters are sex, Mini-Mental State Examination (MMSE) score, brain volume ratio, and age. The study showed that men are more likely to get Alzheimer's disease as compared to women and brain volume is greater in the non-demented group of study. Random forest classifier showed the highest accuracy and precision but lower value of recall and F1 score as the performance parameters for the study. The authors recommended to identify and extract new features and eliminate redundant and irrelevant features for better accuracy of disease prediction from MRI scans.

The authors in [23] investigated transfer learning for CNN to classify MRI images into one of the four stages of Alzheimer: normal, early mild, late mild, and Alzheimer. The publicly available Alzheimer's disease neuroimaging initiative (ADNI) dataset is used for this work. The authors used data augmentation for achieving high accuracy using a small dataset without overfitting. Before proceeding with predicting Alzheimer, MRI images of the brain are segmented into regions indicating gray matter, white matter, and cerebrospinal fluid. The work presented in [23] focuses on gray matter and is reported to distinguish normal person and Alzheimer's patient with more than 98% accuracy. The success rate for differentiating a normal person from an early mild Alzheimer's state is 85.14% and that from a late mild Alzheimer's patient is 85.89%. The accuracy further decreases when the model tries to distinguish between different states of Alzheimer's disease.

The authors in [24] found the deep metric learning (DML) algorithm to work better as compared to CNN for categorizing the patient as healthy, having mild cognitive impairment, or having Alzheimer's disease based on an MRI of the brain. The publicly available dataset ADNI is used for this work. It is also reported that the DML algorithm improved the quality of MRI images for classification and improve the convergence of the model. DML made the MRI sharper with clear texture and better imaging effects on blood vessels in the brain MRI scan. The presented classification model is reported to show an accuracy of 0.83.

1.5   Renal and colon disease prediction

CT scan of the colon or virtual colonoscopy or CT colonoscopy is also used to study the colon and back passage or rectum. It uses specialized X-ray to study the colon for cancer and polyps as an alternative to colonoscopy. On axial 2D images, the colonic polyps are shown as soft tissue nodules with a stalk [25].

The authors in [26] compared different classifier algorithms for the prediction of chronic kidney diseases and found that a random forest classifier works best.

The other algorithms for comparison are J48 which works on the divide and conquer approach; naive Bayes which is a probability-based tool; SVM which works on the perception of decision boundaries, and k-NN which works on the relation of similarity functions with the known objects. These classifiers were compared for their performance on the basis of receiver operating characteristics (ROC), kappa statistics, root mean square error (RMSE), and mean absolute error (MAE) using data mining tool, WEKA. The database used for the work is available freely at UC Irvine Machine Learning Repository. SVM is reported to give the worst result in the detection of chronic kidney disease.

The authors in [27] investigate CT and MR images of colon cancer patients to identify the relationship between some radiomic parameters and stage of colorectal cancer. Different parameters from the tumor region are calculated from the 3D scanning and the average value over all slices is used. A least absolute shrinkage and selection operation regression model is used for 330 radiomic parameter values, computed from annotated medical image data. Ten-fold cross-validation is performed for the prediction of T-stage with the calculated radiomic parameters. The training model identified all three radiomic parameters from MR image clearly indicating that MR images hold more information than the CT images, relevant for predicting the stage of colorectal cancer.

The kidney is responsible for filtering out waste and excess fluids from the blood. Other than kidney stones, infections, and cyst cancer, chronic kidney diseases need to be diagnosed at an early stage to avoid damage to our body because if due to any major disease, the kidney function is hampered, the waste in our body builds up. Diabetes and hypertension are the major causes of renal damage. The symptoms are very late for kidney diseases. The authors of [28] studied specific parameters from three different types of MRI for distinguishing patients having diabetes with moderate chronic kidney disease (stage 3) from healthy people of the same age group and evaluated the sensitivity of the disease progression. Arterial spin labeling (ASL) perfusion MRI, blood oxygenation level-dependent (BOLD) MRI, and diffusion MRI are studied. To indicate the severity of the renal disease, various parameters of MRI are studied in association with urine protein concentration and estimated glomerular filtration rate. ASL perfusion MRI showed high sensitivity for differentiating people with healthy and unhealthy kidneys. The study also reports a high association of renal infusion with estimated glomerular filtration rate. The patients with fast progression had significantly lower perfusion and their response to furosemide in the medulla is also lower. The apparent diffusion coefficient estimated from diffusion MRI is reported to show a high correlation with histological measures of renal fibrosis. Relaxation rate is an index for BOLD MRI, which showed moderately high values for mild patients.

In some cases of serious damage or disease, the kidney is required to be completely removed. Also, it may be removed from a living donor. This process of removing a complete kidney is called complete nephrectomy. This surgery may sometimes cause surgically induced chronic kidney disease. Removal or donation of a kidney reduces the total number of nephrons. Thus, the glomerular filtration rate of the body is maintained by increased plasma flow and intraglomerular pressure on the remaining neurons. But if the remaining nephrons are unable to compensate with increased flow and pressure, it may result in induced chronic disease in the kidney. Hence, a thorough follow-up is very much required to predict any occurrence of surgically induced chronic disease in the kidney. Renal volume is a good indicator of kidney functioning which can be estimated using unenhanced CT [29]. More precisely body surface area adjusted renal volume is observed post nephrectomy. The metabolic load on each nephron may be different from subject to subject. The authors of [30] measured body surface area adjusted renal cortical volume with pre-operative CT angiography to predict the occurrence of surgically induced chronic kidney disease (CKD) after complete nephrectomy among 133 patients. The study reports that the patients who had kidney removed for a renal tumor have lower preoperative eGFR and smaller body surface area adjusted renal cortical volume after complete nephrectomy and have a higher risk of having surgically induced CKD. This study is done over a period of 6 months post-nephrectomy; however, the median time for surgically induced CKD to occur is reported to be around 6–12.7 months. Also, by 60 months improvements in the functioning of the kidney are observed after a complete nephrectomy. Hence, the authors recommended to have longer duration of study for accurate prediction.

1.6   Detection of lung diseases

Lung diseases are generally classified as airway disease, lung-tissue and lung-circulation disease. Example of lung airway disease is asthma, chronic obstructive pulmonary disease (COPD), and bronchiectasis, where the air tubes carrying oxygen and other gases in and out of the lungs are narrowed due to blockage. Lung-tissue diseases affect the structure of lung tissue, for example, inflammation in lung tissue limits the expansion of the lungs which makes it hard for the lungs to release carbon dioxide and take in oxygen. Pulmonary fibrosis is an example of lung-tissue disease. The lung-circulation diseases like pulmonary hypertension may cause clotting, scarring, or some inflammation of the blood vessels in the lungs. These diseases are also known to cause heart problems. The authors of [31] studied the trends in the occurrence of chronic respiratory diseases during the period of 1990–2017 based on data from the "Global Burden of Diseases, Injuries, and Risk Factors Study 2017" which assessed 196 countries and territories. The analysis to assess the factors for the occurrence of these diseases is made based on age, sex, region, and disease pattern together with correlations between the incidence and the World Bank income levels, sociodemographic index (SDI), and human development index (HDI) levels. COPD accounted for 54.9% of chronic respiratory diseases in 2017, as per the study. The study concluded that between the period 1990 and 2017, there has been a decrease in the occurrence of chronic respiratory diseases, COPD, pneumoconiosis, and asthma but there has been an increase in the reported cases of interstitial lung disease and pulmonary sarcoidosis during the period of study.

   X-ray, CT, and MRI are used for the detection of lung diseases. However, the type of imaging modality depends on the need for detection, staging, or follow-up. For example, chest X-rays are useful for an initial diagnostic study of pneumonia, cancer as well as pulmonary disease [32]. The study showed that the prediction of pneumonia is far better using MRI, 95% positive as compared to 27% by X-ray. CT is found useful for the detection of tumors, and pneumonia in some advanced stages. CT as well as MRI is used for lung diseases like acute pulmonary embolism, pulmonary hypertension, and pulmonary fibrosis. Pulmonary embolism refers to the condition when one of the pulmonary arteries in the lungs is blocked, generally due to blood clots that may travel from other body parts, especially from the lower legs. The gold standard for diagnosis of pulmonary embolism is CT pulmonary angiography.

The authors in [33] presented a study on the use of X-ray dark-field chest imaging technique for assessing microstructural changes in lung parenchyma of the COPD patients. The dose of radiation required for this method is only a fraction of that used in conventional X-ray and CT scan and hence can be used as a low-dose alternative for the detection of lung diseases. A dark-field chest X-ray system is developed which acquires a conventional thorax radiograph simultaneously for the 77 identified patients. The two images were assessed by five different readers. In conventional images, due to high air content, lungs appear transparent to X-ray. Darkfield images, on the other hand, provide a clear, uniform signal for the lungs. An intact alveolar structure with multiple air tissue interfaces induces strong small-angle scattering, resulting in a prominent display of the lungs and an unobstructed assessment. The ratio of forced expiratory volume in one second (FEV_1) to functional vital capacity (FVC) and Spearman correlation is used to compare the representation of lung functioning as shown by CT and darkfield images. A single-valued measurement representing darkfield signal strength for each patient is calculated as the average weighted signal levels for all readers and subregions in the image. The major challenge with the use of this technique on humans is that the patient under scanning must hold his breath for at least seven seconds, which may be an issue with patients with partial lung functioning.

1.7   Detection of cardiovascular disease

Cardiovascular disease (CVD) refers to the diseases that affect the heart and blood vessels. One of the reasons for increasing heart disease is a metabolic syndrome which refers to the occurrence of risk factors in our body which increases the chances of cardiac diseases and vascular events. Some of these risk factors are obesity, hypertension, and resistance to insulin, deposition of fats in arteries which causes the risk of blood clots. Some of the CVDs are arrhythmia, valve disease, heart failure, coronary heart disease, strokes and transient ischemic attack, peripheral arterial disease, and aortic disease. High blood pressure has been identified as a major cause of many CVDs, CKD, and dementia.

The authors in [34] present a study on the association of insulin resistance, particularly focusing on its effect on glucose and lipid metabolism in the human body, thereby resulting in the development of CVD. Figure 1.3 shows the effect of insulin resistance on blood sugar levels as compared to that of a healthy person. The

```
                    ┌─────────────┐
                    │    Food     │
                    └─────────────┘
                           │
                           ▼
                    ┌─────────────┐
                    │   Glucose   │
                    │(Blood sugar)│
                    └─────────────┘
                           │
                           ▼
                    ┌─────────────┐
                    │Rise in blood│◄──────────────────────┐
                    │ sugar level │                        │
                    └─────────────┘                        │
                           │                               │
                           ▼                               │
                    ┌─────────────┐                        │
                    │  Pancreas   │                        │
                    │ make insulin│                        │
                    └─────────────┘                        │
                           │                               │
                           ▼                               │
              ┌──────────────────────┐                    │
              │ Glucose and insulin   │                    │
              │ reach body cells      │                    │
              │ with blood            │                    │
              └──────────────────────┘                    │
               │                    │                       │
               ▼                    ▼                       │
    ┌─────────────────┐   ┌──────────────────┐             │
    │Insulin acts as  │   │ Cells resist     │             │
    │key to open cells│   │ insulin          │             │
    └─────────────────┘   └──────────────────┘             │
             │                     │                        │
             ▼                     ▼                        │
    ┌─────────────────┐   ┌──────────────────┐             │
    │Cells absorb     │   │No absorption of  │─────────────┘
    │glucose from     │   │glucose from blood│
    │blood            │   └──────────────────┘
    └─────────────────┘
      Healthy person     Person with insulin resistance
```

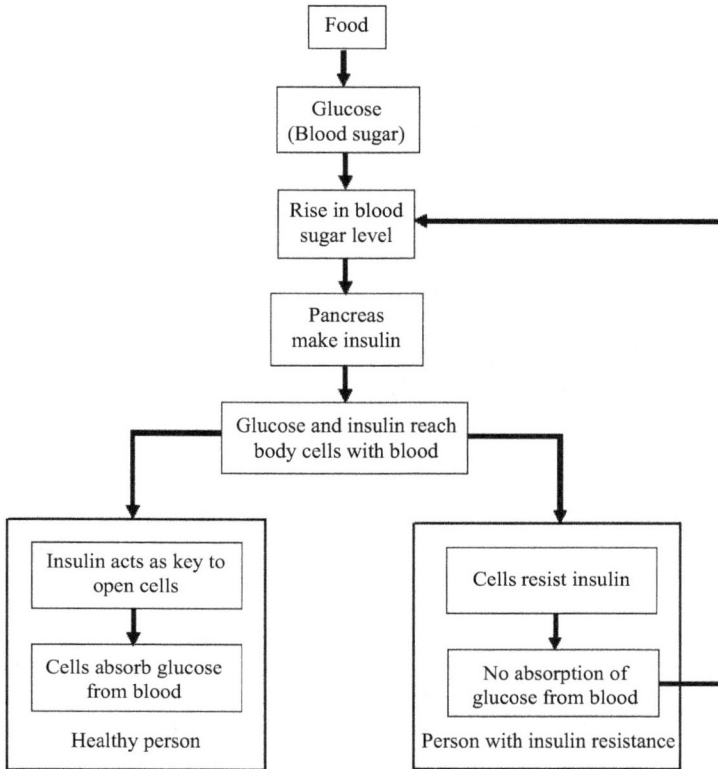

Figure 1.3   Effect of insulin resistance on blood sugar levels

blood sugar level builds up due to insulin resistance and if this level stays high over time, it may result in diabetes. High blood sugar results in inflammation which damages the inner lining of the arteries, resulting in the build-up of plaque or high cholesterol. This may obstruct blood flow to the heart and hence cause heart failure or stroke. Narrowed arteries in the lower legs cause peripheral arterial disease This makes the walls of arteries stiffer which contributes to high blood pressure. Additionally, the nerves that control the heart are damaged due to high blood sugar and inflammation.

1.8   COVID-19 detection

The sudden outbreak of COVID-19 has seen many works for accurate and real-time detection of the infection. The authors of [34] presented a survey of various AI methods used for the detection of COVID-19 patients with the help of chest X-ray and CT scans.

The authors in [35] investigated the effect of histogram equalization (HE), contrast limited adaptive histogram equalization (CLAHE), image complement, gamma correction, and balance contrast enhancement technique (BCET) on lung-segmented X-ray images for COVID-19 detection using deep CNN. The study first segmented lungs from the X-ray image followed by the evaluation of these segmented images for the classification of using seven different pretrained deep-learning networks. To equalize the number of images for infected and healthy lungs, image rotation-based augmentation technique is used. More than 98% accuracy is reported for the segmentation of the lung. Of the five investigated image enhancement methods, the Gamma correction technique proved to give the highest accuracy of more than 96% for COVID-19 detection in lung-segmented X-ray images.

The authors in [36] tested three pre-trained CNN through transfer learning to distinguish between X-ray for COVID-19 patients from that of viral pneumonia patients. The three pre-trained networks that were tested were VGG16, InceptionV3, and EfficientNetB0, of which, EfficientNetB0 is identified to give the best accuracy, sensitivity, specificity, as well as F1 scores. VGG16 is chosen due to its popularity in classification problems, InceptionV3 is chosen for its suitability for mobile applications and big data, while EfficientNetB0 is chosen for the study for its high accuracy with a reduced number of parameters. The steps followed in the study are shown in Figure 1.4. Out of 3106 images from the combined database, 806 non-augmented images are used for testing, while others are used for training after augmentation with rotation, scaling, translation, and nearest neighbor fill operations. The highest accuracy, precision, sensitivity, specificity, and F1 scores for the classification of the X-ray image into one of three classes are obtained by EfficientNetB0.

The authors in [37] analyzed chest CT scan images using deep learning, machine learning, and hybrid learning to establish the importance of other clinical, baseline, and CT features in identifying the COVID-19 stage of the patient. Important features from CT scan, and laboratory data are extracted to predict an indicative score for classification between the early stage and critical stage of COVID. The data from 255 patients was collected and used in this study. Various baseline characteristics are identified from each patient like hypertension, heart disease, diabetes, and other comorbidities. Also, some important symptoms identified in the data set are cough, fever, headache, expectoration, dyspnea, myalgia, chest and abdominal pain, temperature, pharyngeal discomfort, heart rate, blood pressure, and respiratory rate. To distinguish the early stage from the critical stage of COVID in patients, laboratory characteristics like count of white blood cells, neutrophils, monocytes, lymphocytes, C-reactive proteins, etc. are observed.

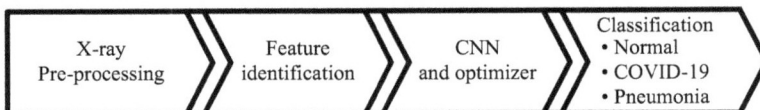

Figure 1.4   Approach used by [36]

Multiple features from the CT scans are also extracted and a CT score is calculated. These features are analyzed and together with CT score, machine learning models are implemented to calculate COVID criticality (CC) score by combining other features from laboratory data and baseline characteristics. The CC score is used by radiologists to categorize the COVID patients as early stage or severe staged. The classification is shown to be successful with a mean absolute error of 0.0165. The approach used in the paper is shown in Figure 1.5.

COVID-19 has resulted in many serious side effects as well as deaths. Hence not only the detection of COVID-19 was highly studied by researchers but its progression mortality due to COVID-19 is predicted by [38]. The authors developed an automated survival prediction model using deep learning on CT images of the chest. The authors used the U-Net pre-trained to segment lung region from the CT images as given in [39] for predicting the COVID patient survival with idiopathic pulmonary fibrosis. The U-net is trained to classify the CT images of the chest to indicate the pattern as normal or one of the four lung disease patterns namely, ground-glass opacity, reticulation, consolidation, and honeycombing. The output of the classifier was verified with the ground-truth label provided by an experienced observer.

1.9   Predictions of eye diseases

Many eye diseases are predicted and studied from the retina as it is accessible non-invasively. Also, the retina is a highly active and metabolic tissue that is also used as a marker for cognitive performance and brain health [40]. The images of the retina in the eye are called retinal fundus images which are helpful in the study of surface nerves and deep nerves near the retina. The fundus images of eyes were used for 511 women to examine the link between retinopathy and cognitive decline in women in [40]. To assess the cognitive effect, modified Mini-Mental State Examination (3MSE) was used with a study of white matter hyperintensities and lacunar infarcts in the basal ganglia. The study made it evident that retinopathy is an early marker of neurological degradations. Retinal nerves are very much like brain vessels hence observations made for retinal nerves can be used for brain nerves as well [41]. These images are used for detecting damage to the organs due to vascular diseases. The retinal images show differences in retinal nerves for sex and age. The prediction of disease is very important to have early warnings and

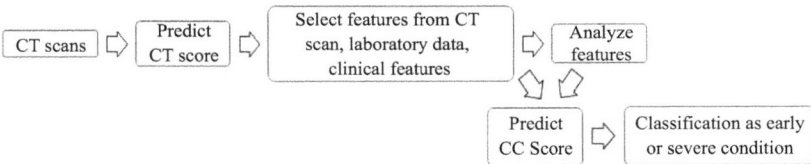

Figure 1.5   Approach used by [37]

thus, plan strategy for disease treatment in advance, especially brain diseases. Predictions based on ocular images can be used to pre-screen patients with severe diseases who can benefit from advanced testing. The paper [41] reports a CNN-based age and sex determination model on the Korean database of retinal images. Separate CNNs are used for age and sex prediction. Furthermore, it is shown that after 60 years of age, the accuracy of predictions made from these images reduces significantly when the person is healthy or is suffering from hypertension, diabetes, and smoking. Thus, the study concluded that the aging process may saturate at the age of about 60 years when observed in retinal fundus images. The study, however, does not consider the duration of any vascular disease or existence of any ocular disease.

The prediction of eye disease is also done with the retinal images. The authors of [42] worked on the idea that the distribution of training data on different datasets is more reliable for out-of-distribution generalization by CNN. Hence, they use seven datasets with feature alignment after data augmentation, while preserving optic nerve and important nerve in the images for glaucoma detection. Data augmentation is done by transforming the dataset by operations such as cropping, resizing, mirroring, and color dropping while preserving the content for glaucoma prediction but with minimum mutual information between the versions. This is expected to use more generic knowledge for training the prediction model.

Another technique for ocular imaging uses slit-lamp. The author of [43] predicts the progression of ophthalmic diseases by analyzing the temporal relationship of features from images obtained from slit-lamp. Long short-term memory (LSTM) algorithm is applied to the features extracted from the medical image using CNN. Six models were created using combinations of AlexNet, GoogleNet, and ResNet with LSTM and Recurrent Neural Network. Each of the models is trained on five ocular images to test the prediction output with the sixth image in the database. It is shown that the LSTM-based models gave higher accuracy as compared to models based on RNN and the combination of AlexNet with LSTM gave the highest accuracy as compared to other linear classifiers.

1.10   Conclusion

Medical images used in the detection and prediction of different diseases are captured by different modalities governed by different underlying principles. This chapter presents an overview of different image-capturing techniques for medical reasons followed by general image-processing operations performed for better visibility and extraction of information. Thereafter, a review is presented for the use of different medical images for brain disease, renal and colon disease, lung disease, cardiovascular disease, eye disease, and COVID-19 prediction. The choice of imaging modality depends on the disease, and the area of body to be scanned. Analyzing medical images with AI to extract maximum information from the image has been proven useful for saving time and predicting diseases for better management and care of the patient. The general approach for using AI for disease prediction involves extraction of all the effective features and using them to build models for the proper evaluation and analysis of the disease. AI is also useful for radiologists to obtain better images with optimal positioning of the machine and optimal settings for the scan based on various factors like area, and disease of focus. Another approach for integrating AI in medical imaging is to use it for improving the low-quality images obtained with lower dose of exposure to radiations.

The major challenges for disease prediction from medical images are the development of more generic image analysis techniques which is adaptable for some specific clinical tasks efficiently. The second major challenge is to establish ground truth for the classification model validation. Third, the current prediction models are mostly developed based on the available database which hinders the development of a prediction model that works on heterogeneous image data.

Most of the studies presented in the literature for predicting diseases based on medical images simply present an approach. However, for judging the real-time applicability, external validation with an independent study population is very much required. The developed approaches for the prediction of diseases from medical images are mainly guided by the available datasets and not clinical relevance.

The future of disease prediction expects a minimum user interaction required by algorithms to construct patient-specific models and predict multiple diseases from a minimum number of medical scans.

References

[1] National Academies of Sciences, Engineering, and Medicine. *Improving Diagnosis in Health Care*, Washington, DC: The National Academies Press, 2015.

[2] J.J. Zong and T.S. Qiu, "Medical image fusion based on sparse representation of classified image patches," *Biomedical Signal Processing and Control*, vol. 34, pp. 195–205, 2017.

[3] R. Bourne, *Fundamentals of Digital Imaging in Medicine*, Springer London, 2010.

[4] C. Liu, D. Jiao, and Z. Liu, "Artificial Intelligence (AI)-aided disease prediction," *Bio-Integration*, vol. 1, pp. 130–136, 2020.

[5] A.A. Umar and S.M. Atabo, "A review of imaging techniques in scientific research/clinical diagnosis," *MOJ Anatomy & Physiology*, vol. 6, no. 5, pp. 175–183, 2019.

[6] R. Fedewa, R. Puri, E. Fleischman, *et al.*, "Artificial intelligence in intracoronary imaging," *Current Cardiology Reports*, vol. 22, pp. 1–15, 2020.

[7] L. Zhang, A. Wahle, Z. Chen, J. J. Lopez, T. Kovarnik, and M. Sonka, "Predicting locations of high-risk plaques in coronary arteries in patients receiving statin therapy," *IEEE Transactions on Medical Imaging*, vol. 37, pp. 151–161, 2018.

[8]   M. Larobina and L. Murino, "Medical image file formats," *Journal of Digital Imaging*, vol. 27, pp. 200–206, 2014.

[9]   K. D. Toennies, *Guide to Medical Image Analysis - Methods and Algorithms*, Springer London, 2012.

[10]   Y. Mohamed, Y. Abdallah, and T. Alqahtani, "Research in medical imaging using image processing techniques," in: *Medical Imaging - Principles and Applications*, IntechOpen, 2019, pp. 1–16.

[11]   Y. Ding, "Medical image quality assessment," in: *Visual Quality Assessment for Natural and Medical Image*, 2018, pp. 215–264.

[12]   L. S. Chow and R. Paramesran, "Review of medical image quality assessment," *Biomedical Signal Processing and Control*, vol. 27, pp. 145–154, 2016.

[13]   M. Bielecka, A. Bielecki, R. Obuchowicz, and A. Piórkowski, "Universal measure for medical image quality evaluation based on gradient approach," in: *ICCS 2020*, Amsterdam, 2020.

[14]   M. Punga, S. Moldovanu, and L. Moraru, "Structural similarity analysis for brain MR image quality assessment," in: *TIM 2013 Physics Conference*, Timisoara, Romania, 2014.

[15]   J.J. Ma, U. Nakarmi, C.Y.S. Kin, *et al.*, "Diagnostic image quality assessment and classification in medical imaging: opportunities and challenges," in: *International Symposium Biomedical Imaging*, Iowa, USA, 2020.

[16]   S. Zhang, Y. Wang, J. Jiang, J. Dong, W. Yi, and W. Hou, "CNN-based medical ultrasound image quality assessment," *Complexity*, vol. 2021, pp. 1–9, 2021.

[17]   A.S. Belhe, J.A. Pagariya, V.V. Ganthade, M. Rashid, and P.S. Uravane, "An efficient deep learning based approach for the detection of brain tumors," in: *2022 5th International Conference on Contemporary Computing and Informatics (IC3I)*, Uttar Pradesh, India, 2022, pp. 417–421, doi:10.1109/IC3I56241.2022.10073209.

[18]   L. Kouhalvandi, L. Matekovits, and I. Peter, "Deep learning and its benefits in prediction of patients through medical images," in: *IEEE/ACM Conference on Connected Health: Applications, Systems and Engineering Technologies*, Washington, DC, USA, 2021.

[19]   G. Li, L. Li, Y. Li, *et al.*, "An MRI radiomics approach to predict survival and tumour-infiltrating macrophages in gliomas," *Brain*, vol. 145, pp. 1151–1161, 2022.

[20]   R. Brookmeyer and N. Abdalla, "Estimation of lifetime risks of Alzheimer's disease dementia using biomarkers for preclinical disease," *Alzheimer's & Dementia*, pp. 981–988, 2018.

[21]   C. Plant, S.J. Tejpel, A. Oswald, *et al.*, "Automated detection of brain atrophy patterns based on MRI for the prediction of Alzheimer's disease," *Neuroimage*, vol. 50, pp. 162–174, 2010.

[22]   C. Kavitha, V. Mani, S.R. Srividhya, O.I. Khalaf, and C.A.T. Romero, "Early-stage Alzheimer's disease prediction using machine learning models," *Frontiers in Public Health*, vol. 10, pp. 1–13, 2022.

[23]   A. Mehmood, S. yang, Z. Feng, *et al.*, "A transfer learning approach for early diagnosis of Alzheimer's disease on MRI images," *Neuroscience*, vol. 460, pp. 43–52, 2021.

[24]   X. Bi, W. Liu, H. Liu, and Q. Shang, "Artificial intelligence-based MRI images for brain in prediction of Alzheimer's disease," *Journal of Healthcare Engineering*, vol. 2021, pp. 1–7, 2021.

[25]   W. Schima and T. Mang, "CT colonography in cancer detection: methods and results," *Cancer Imaging*, vol. 4, pp. 33–41, 2004.

[26]   N. Kumar and S. Khatri, "Implementing WEKA for medical data classification and early disease prediction," in: *Third IEEE International Conference on "Computational Intelligence and Communication Technology" (IEEE-CICT 2017)*, Ghaziabad, India, 2017.

[27]   Y. Dou, X. Tang, Y. Liu, and Z. Gong, "T stage prediction of colorectal tumor based on multiparametric functional images," *Translational Cancer Research*, vol. 9, pp. 522–528, 2020.

[28]   P.V. Prasad, L.-P. Li, J.M. Thacker, W. Li, B. Hack, O. Kohn, and S.M. Sprague, "Cortical perfusion and tubular function as evaluated by magnetic resonance imaging correlates with annual loss in renal function in moderate chronic kidney disease," *American Journal of Nephrology*, vol. 49, pp. 114–124, 2019.

[29]   S. Gupta, A.H. Singh, A. Shabbir, P.F. Hahn, G. Harris, and D. Sahani, "Assessing renal parenchymal volume on unenhanced CT as a marker for predicting renal function in patients with chronic kidney disease," *Academic Radiology*, vol. 19, pp. 654–660, 2012.

[30]   S.-H. You, D.J. Sung, K.-S. Yang, *et al.*, "Predicting the development of surgically induced chronic kidney disease after total nephrectomy using body surface area–adjusted renal cortical volume on CT angiography," *Genitourinary Imaging*, vol. 212, pp. 32–40, 2019.

[31]   M. Xie, X. Liu, X. Cao, M. Guo, and X. Li, "Trends in prevalence and incidence of chronic respiratory diseases from 1990 to 2017," *Respiratory Research*, vol. 21, pp. 1–13, 2020.

[32]   M.O. Wielpütz, C.P. Heußel, F.J.F.H. Herth, and H.-U. Kauczor, "Radiological diagnosis in lung disease: factoring treatment options into the choice of diagnostic modality," *Deutsches Arzteblatt International*, vol. 111, pp. 181–187, 2014.

[33]   K. Willer, A.A. Fingerl, W. Noichl, *et al.*, "X-ray dark-field chest imaging for detection and quantification of emphysema in patients with chronic obstructive pulmonary disease: a diagnostic accuracy study," *The Lancet Digital Health*, vol. 3, pp. 733–744, 2021.

[34]   V. Ormazabal, S. Nair, O. Elfeky, C. Aguayo, C. Salomon, and F.A. Zuñiga, "Association between insulin resistance and the development of cardiovascular disease," *Cardiovascular Diabetology*, vol. 17, no. 122, pp. 1–14, 2018.

[35]   M.D.C. Abelaira, F.C. Abelaira, A. Ruano-Ravina, and A. Fernández-Villar, "Use of conventional chest imaging and artificial intelligence in COVID-19 infection. A review of the literature," *OpenRespiratoryArchives*, vol. 3, pp. 1–6, 2021.

[36] K. Santosh, R. Nagar, S. Bhatnagar, *et al.*, "Chest X ray and cough sample based deep learning framework for accurate diagnosis of COVID-19," *Computers and Electrical Engineering*, vol. 103, pp. 108391, 2022.

[37] G. Hemant, M. Awais, A.K. Bashir, *et al.*, "AI-enabled radiologist in the loop: novel AI-based framework to augment radiologist performance for COVID-19 chest CT medical image annotation and classification from pneumonia," *Neural Computing and Applications*, vol. 35, pp. 1–19, 2022.

[38] K. Indrajeet, S.S. Alshamrani, A. Kumar, *et al.*, "Deep learning approach for analysis and characterization of COVID-19," *Computers, Materials and Continua*, vol. 70, no. 1, pp. 451–468, 2021.

[39] J. Nishant, D. Prashar, M. Rashid, *et al.*, "Deep learning approach for discovery of in silico drugs for combating COVID-19," *Journal of Healthcare Engineering*, vol. 2021, pp. 1–13, 2021.

[40] T. Uemura, C. Watari, J.J. Näppi, T. Hironaka, H. Kim, and H. Yoshida, "U-radiomics for predicting survival of patients with idiopathic pulmonary fibrosis," in: *Proceedings Volume 11314, Medical Imaging-Computer Aided Diagnosis*, Houston, Texas, US, 2020.

[41] M. Haan, M. Espeland, B. Klein, *et al.*, "Cognitive function and retinal and ischemic brain changes: the women's health initiative," *Neurology*, vol. 78, pp. 942–949, 2012.

[42] Y. Kim, K.J. Noh, S.J. Byun, *et al.*, "Effects of hypertension, diabetes, and smoking on age and sex prediction from retinal fundus images," *Scientific Reports*, vol. 10, pp. 1–14, 2020.

[43] C. Zhou, J. Ye, J. Wang, *et al.*, "Improving the generalization of glaucoma detection on fundus images via feature alignment between augmented views," *Biomedical Optics Express*, vol. 13, no. 4, pp. 1–17, 2022.

Chapter 2

Breast cancer detection in pathological imaging using deep learning methods

Bharati Ainapure[1] and Reshma Pise[1]

Breast cancer is a disease that affects many women globally and is associated with a significant fatality rate. Worldwide nearly 12% of women are affected by breast cancer and the number is still increasing. To enhance breast cancer detection and patient survival rates, early and accurate identification of the disease is essential. Hence, there is a need for diagnostic models based on medical imaging which will help medical practitioners in diagnosing and treating the patients with minimum error and greater accuracy. Artificial intelligence (AI) and machine learning (ML) techniques can be used in medical imagining detecting complex relationship between different data elements so that disease detection and prognosis can be made easy. Deep learning (DL) techniques can be used to detect the most influencing features from images so that most serious diseases such as breast cancer can be treated in-time. In this chapter, a systematic evaluation of prior work based on breast cancer identification and prognosis using images like mammography, MRI, etc. along with DL and ML is carried out. Based on this the work proposes a design of three advanced DL methods: convolution neural network, ResNet, and U-Net to classify breast cancer mammography images. The models were trained to identify histopathology images into to two classes: malignant and benign. The method is implemented in two steps. The first step comprises of data selection and pre-processing and, in the second step, the implementation of three networks and performance measurement of each network. The results indicate U-net model outperformed by achieving 97.12% of accuracy compared to other networks.

2.1 Introduction

Breast cancer is a very common and life-threatening disease affecting the women's health. If it is not identified and treated in the early stage then the result will be the death of the patient. Breast cancer is one of the leading causes of death among women worldwide and is one of the most deadly diseases faced by women [1]. Breast cancer detection is challenging and women sometimes do not realize the

[1]Department of Computer Engineering, Vishwakarma University, Pune, India

symptoms in the early stages of breast cancer which increases the rate of risk and death rate also. There is left and right breast in the human body and breast cancer can start from any part of the breast like lobules, nipple, stoma, ducts, blood vessel, and lymph vessel. Worldwide nearly 12% of women are affected by breast cancer and the number is still increasing. According to the International Agency for Research on Cancer (IARC), in 2020, there were 2.3 million new breast cancer patients globally and 685,000 deaths from this and it is expected that by 2040, there will be an increase of 40% breast cancer cases in women [2,3]. Early treatment of this disease is supported by two factors: the type of cancer and in which stage it is. According to expert doctors, the cause of breast cancer is abnormal cell growth in breast. These cells later spread in meta size and spread up to lymph nodes and other parts of the body in severe cases [4]. To prevent and stop any further consequences, it becomes necessary that cancer must be diagnosed as early as possible. As soon as the doctor detects the tumor in the breast, he/she tries to find whether that tumor is malignant or benign. Malignant tumors are cancerous and can spread to other parts of the breast, in the worst case can spread to other body parts. Though, multiple breast cancer diagnostic methods are in practice such as biopsy, and imaging-based techniques like mammogram, ultrasound, bone scan, positron emission tomography (PET) scan, breast magnetic resonance imaging (MRI), computed tomography (CT) scan, and newer one breast tomosynthesis (3D mammography) [5–7] but early detection and treatment is a challenge for physicians.

The deficiency of prognosis models based on medical imaging results in difficulty for doctors to prepare a treatment plan that may increase the patient survival chance. Hence, there is a need for computerized diagnostic models based on medical imaging which will help medical practitioners in diagnosing and treating the patient with minimum error and greater accuracy [1,8,9]. The machine learning (ML), artificial intelligence (AI), and deep learning (DL)-based algorithms are used to perform the tasks like clustering, classification, anomaly detection, prediction, recommendation, ranking and system automization, etc. Such algorithms integrated into computerized systems can provide lots of opportunities for healthcare organizations in medical image analysis [10]. First, it allows healthcare workers to focus more on patient care rather than spending time on information gathering. Second, the diagnostic accuracy given by the algorithm will help them in breast cancer prediction and its stage. The models can also help medical practitioners in planning the precise treatment which can reduce treatment side effects [11]. The involvement of such computerized systems with prediction algorithms in health care can reduce the possibility of human errors, especially in process automization.

There are many breast cancer awareness drives being organized across the world so that women get educated about this and be free to open up about their problems with breast cancer. Therefore, this chapter is based on employing machine learning algorithms, to aid breast cancer detection process.

This chapter is further organized into four sections. The systematic review of the previous study has been carried out in Section 2.2. Section 2.3 describes dataset selection, preprocessing, and detailed implementation of the proposed models. The experimental setup and results of each model is discussed in

Section 2.4. The conclusion of the chapter is given in Section 2.5 followed by references.

2.2   Literature review

Discussion on previous work done by many researchers related to breast cancer detection based on image datasets is presented in the literature section. The literature first presents the work done using basic ML algorithms to predict breast cancer and then focuses on advanced techniques such as DL and transfer learning approaches used to detect breast cancer using medical imaging.

In the past, AI and ML algorithms were designed and used to analyze medical records. Today medical image data is analyzed more intelligently and efficiently with the help of tools that are recommended by advanced ML algorithms [12]. The digitized world has made image data collection and storage very approachable and at low cost. In modernized hospitals, you can see that servers like machines are collecting and sharing information including medical images. Such data can be used to train an AI and ML algorithm to create a better decision-making system [13]. Once the training of the algorithm is completed, a new patient record will be given as input and breast cancer-like disease diagnosis can be obtained automatically from the previously solved examples. Trained AI and ML models can help healthcare workers to make accurate and quick decisions about breast cancer disease diagnosis [14,15]. These algorithms can also help the inexperienced and trainee medical students to diagnose the problem attached to breast cancer patients.

As this work focuses on breast cancer detection using medical image data, around 80 number of the most recently published papers related to breast cancer diagnosis and detection using AI-ML, and DL algorithms were searched and referred. This work has obtained articles from journals and conferences indexed by the Scopus database and excluded the non-referred articles. The top databases that this work used are MDPI, IEEE Springer, ScienceDirect, and PubMed. The distribution of papers among these databases is shown in Figure 2.1. The literature is made more comprehensive from these databases using the Boolean operator. The search was carried out on each of the databases using keywords [16] "Machine learning" AND "AI", "DL" AND "Image" AND "Diagnose" AND "Detect" as shown in Table 2.1.

Figure 2.2 depicts publications on breast cancer studies using images increased around 2020 and 2022. From the search, this work limits the number of papers to eighty by only including articles using breast cancer image databases. The breast cancer image types such as MRI, CT scan, mammography, ultrasound, radiography, and breast tomosynthesis were taken into consideration for this study. The work focuses on the detection of breast cancer using AI, ML, and DL techniques and applied the following criteria for paper inclusion in this study: (1) paper language to be English; (2) breast cancer detection and treatment using imaging; (3) AI, ML, and DL techniques; (4) only biomedical engineering or medical publications that are relevant to the subject; (5) only conferences and journals publications.

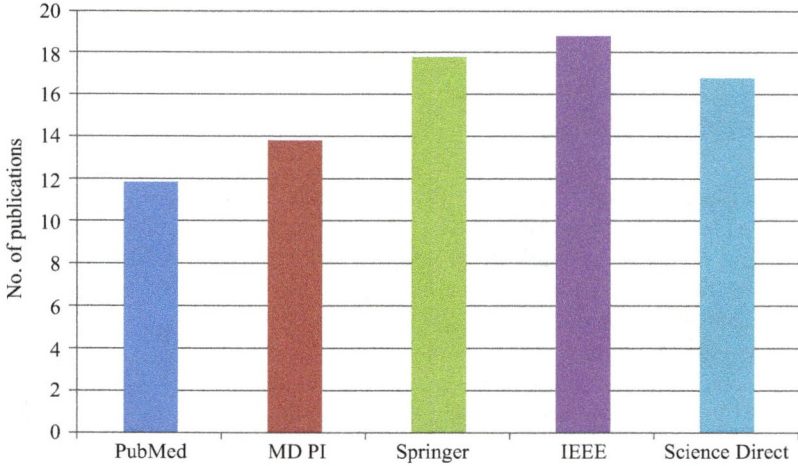

Figure 2.1   Chapter-relevant literature based on keywords

Table 2.1   Keyword search on Scopus-indexed sources

Time period	Keyword used
Jan 2010–Dec 2022	ML, AL, and DL Medical image (e.g., MRI) Diagnose, detect

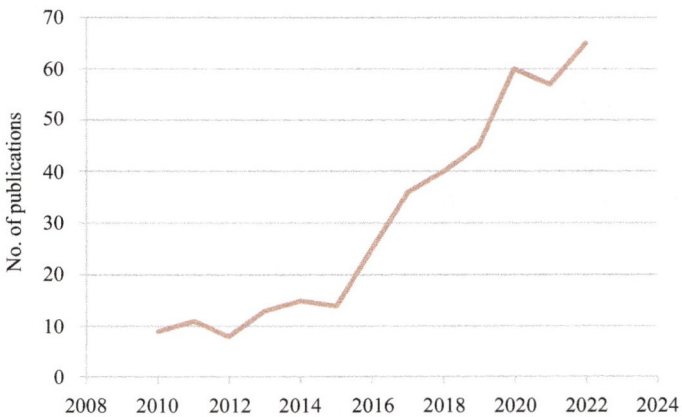

Figure 2.2   Publications on breast cancer study using images

Pre-trained DL models such as EfficientNetb0, Residual Network (ResNet)-50, and Inception-v3 [17] were used to categorize the image dataset containing breast cancer into two classes: malignant and benign. This work automatically detects the whether the tumor is malignant or not by extracting deep multi-resolution convolutional features (BoDMCF) from histopathological images. Global average pooling is used in the network to obtain the features and then the classification of breast cancer tumor is done using the support vector machine (SVM) algorithm. Images used comprises four resolutions ($40\times$, $100\times$, $200\times$, and $400\times$). The model achieved an accuracy of 99.92% in prediction [18].

Breast tumor detection in histopathology photos is carried out using DL in [19]. Authors called this network hybrid-dilated DL. The dilated technique present in the network processes the image features. These features are then sent to the AlexNet to identify the tiny objects and thin borders using the kernel model. The model overfitting was prevented using data augmentation. This technique attained an AUC performance of 96.15%.

Mammography images were used to detect the breast cancer in [20–27]. Authors used ML algorithms like K-nearest neighbor (KNN), SVM, Euclidian distance regression and segmentation, principle component analysis (PCA), artificial neural network (ANN), backpropagation neural network (BPNN), and radial basis function neural network (RBFNN) to detect the breast cancer from images. Features from images were extracted and models were trained to identify malignant and non-malignant cells from mammogram images. Performances of the models were measured using specificity, F1-score, accuracy, ROC, sensitivity, and mean square error.

Convolution neural network (CNN) and gated recurrent unit (GRU) are combined to prepare a model, which will detect breast cancer invasive ductal carcinoma (IDC) tumor. The model was able to classify IDC into two categories: $(-)$ negative and $(+)$ positive. The dataset consisted of $2,040\times$ by $1,536\times$ size pathology images extracted from the Kaggle site. The dataset size was balanced using synthetic minority oversampling technique (SMOTE) to avoid model overfitting. Experiments were carried out on Intel Core i7 processor. The model was able to achieve 86% accuracy [27].

The GoogleNet, AlexNet, and Visual Geometry Group (VGG) are DL models used in [28] to detect breast cancer in mammography images. The shallow and deep features from images were extracted using these DL networks. The network comprises three layers: fully connected, convolution and pooling. A 3×3 filter was applied in the convolution layer to extract the features. Rectified linear unit (ReLu) activation function was used in between the convolution and the pooling layer to activate neurons. Finally, the softmax function is used to categorize the image into malignant and benign type. The model showed 98.06% performance accuracy in the classification task.

Deep CNN (DCNN) was developed to detect breast cancer from MRI images [29]. The network comprises two parts: breast mass detection and region segmentation. The breast region segmentation was detected using U-Net++. In the convolution layer, 3×3 filter is used. Max pooling was applied for feature extraction.

A ReLu activation function is used in between convolution and max pooling. Binary cross-entropy loss was calculated during model validation. The model was able to achieve a 95% specificity rate.

The advanced machine learning technique particle swarm optimized wavelet neural network (PSOWNN) is used to detect breast cancer from mammography screening images [30]. Images were pre-processed using PCA and region of interest techniques. The authors used backpropagation and a feed-forward network to train the model. The network consisted of convolution, pooling and fully connected layers. During training, the network was given input images, the forward pass step is performed, at the final output layer error is calculated which is corrected using the backpropagation step. This is iteratively carried out to complete the training process. The model achieved 95.2% accuracy.

The ML model was created based on deep neural network with support value to classify histopathology images into two categories: malignant and benign [31]. The image dataset was enhanced by applying pre-processing and augmentation techniques. Feature extraction was carried out to know the values of textural, entropy, and geometrical values from the images. The Histo-sigmoid fuzzy clustering is used to know the numerical value distribution of the images. The model achieved a 97.21% accuracy.

Further more detailed literature along with a comparison of present work is explained in Table 2.2.

2.3   ML and DL techniques in medical domain

AI technologies are extensively used in healthcare service for effective clinical assessment and early and accurate detection and treatment. Doctors assess the illness as per their understanding, practice and clinical symptoms. Timely and precise analysis and prognosis are very critical for effective treatment and recovery of disease. The machine learning and DL techniques in AI have made it possible for doctors to make faster and more precise clinical diagnoses based on the symptoms and clinical features and treat the patients satisfactorily. These techniques process complex and vast volume of data and extract clinically important features about the health condition. This could be really valuable in refining the awareness of physicians.

Figure 2.3 shows the common steps performed in training an ML/DL model for prediction task such as disease diagnosis. In the first step, significant relevant data (i.e., clinical data or scan images) is collected. The data is cleaned and pre-processed. The dataset is split into two sets – train and test. The training set is input to train an ML model or deep neural network to estimate the outcome based on the significant features extracted from the training data. The test dataset is used to assess the performance of the model in terms of metrics such as precision, loss, error [38,39]. Based on the performance result, the next phase will involve selecting a different model altogether or including more input features to enhance the performance of the model.

Table 2.2   Literature details of existing work

Reference	Image dataset description	Machine learning classifier used	Performance
[32]	MRIs of 141 breast cancer patients	CNN with three layers: one fully connected, four max pooling and 10 convolution layers	Accuracy: 87.7%; Specificity: 95.1; Sensitivity: 73.9%
[33]	21,537 dynamic contrast-enhanced magnetic resonance imaging (DCE-MRI) images from 13,463 breast cancer-affected patients	Deep neural network model to predict the probability of malignancy at breast level from an input image	AUROC: 92.4% AUPRC: 72% Partial AUROC: 90% Sensitivity: 0.765 Specificity: 90%
[34]	7,909 microscopic histopathological images were collected from 82 patients. Out of these images, dataset consists of 2,480 benign and 5,429 malignant images. Two different sizes of images: 700 × 460 or 700 × 456 pixels	CNN to classify images into: malignant and benign. ReLu activation function at the inner layer and Softmax activation at the output layer are used to activate the neurons	Normal Precision: 88% Recall: 90% F1-score: 89% Cancer Precision: 91% Recall: 90% F1-score: 90%
[35]	Publically available datasets: INbreast, MIAS, and CBIS-DDSM	Modified entropy whale optimization algorithm. Algorithm simulated using pre-trained networks MobilenetV2 and Nasnet Mobile	Sensitivity: 99% F1-score: 99.16% Precision: 99.33% AUC: 1 Accuracy: 99.80%
[36]	INbeastTotal 49 images (23 benign and 26 cancer)	Shallow convolution network to render the images and then DCNN to extract features and produce class labels: malignant and non-cancer	Accuracy: 90% AUC: 92%
[37]	736 (426 benign + 310 malignant) mammography images from 344 breast cancer patients	Model is built in two stages: feature learning using CNN and then classification using SVM. The result included two classes: yes and no	AUC: 70%

DL models based on ANN have led to cutting-edge innovations in computer vision, voice recognition, and health science. DL, a form of machine learning algorithm, is motivated by the working of biological neural networks. It is a multi-layer network of computing units termed neurons operating in parallel to simulate certain cognitive tasks of humans. As shown in Figure 2.4, the network comprises (a) an input layer, (b) one or multiple hidden layers, and (c) an output layer.

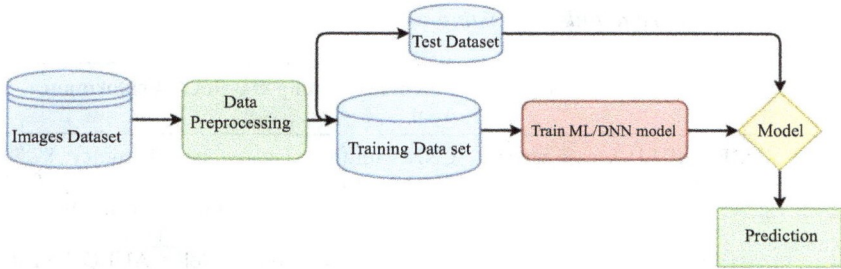

Figure 2.3   Phases in ML model development

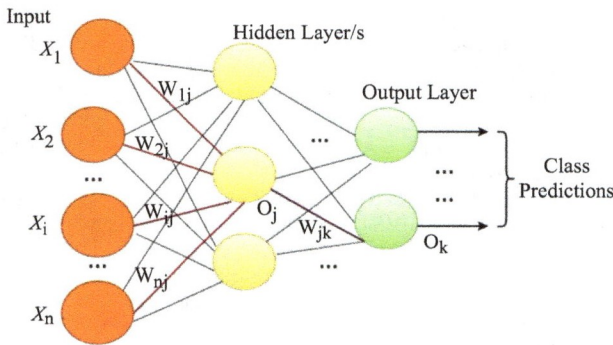

Figure 2.4   Deep neural networks

The input layer is fed with the independent variables or inputs. The neural network consists of a multiple number of hidden layers. The neurons in a layer are connected with neurons in the adjacent layer [38].

Each neuron is assigned a numeric weight "w." The ith neuron of the jth layer has a weight represented by $w_{i,j}$. The weight and an activation function determine the output of the neuron (Figure 2.5). The network is trained by presenting a large number of input instances to the input layer neurons. Each input instance is represented as a vector $X = \{x_1, x_2, ...x_n\}$ of "n" features and target class Ci. The neurons in each layer multiply the weight with the input and produce an output, which will be fed as an input to the next layer neuron. The neurons apply a non-linear activation function such as sigmoid, TanH, ReLu, and Softmax [38,40].

The neural networks are trained with an algorithm named backpropagation (backward propagation of errors), which is the standard method for training ANNs

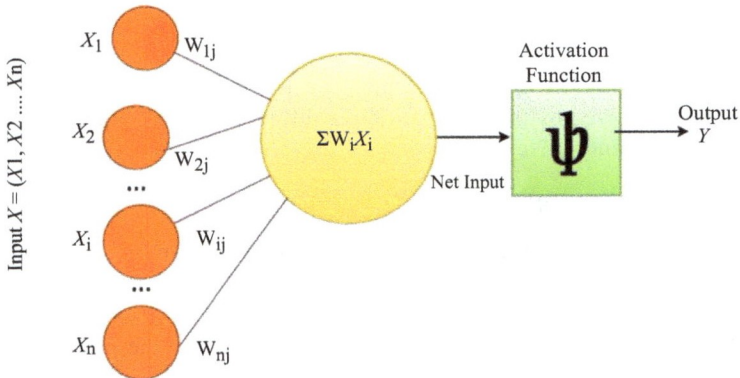

Figure 2.5   Neuron activation

for pattern recognition task. The learning algorithm iteratively fine-tunes the network's weights to reduce the prediction error and yield the expected output for an input [41,42].

The main objective of the training is to reduce the prediction error, which is the difference between the predicted and the expected output:

1. The neurons' weights are set to small random values
2. The input layer is fed with training samples. If there is an error, the algorithm adjusts the weights values.
3. The backpropagation process computes the gradient of the error function as a derivative with respect to neuron's weights. The calculation continues backwards through the network.
4. Backward pass: New weights are computed using the derived functions.
5. Forward pass is performed with the recent weights
6. The backward and forward passes are repeated until the error becomes near or equal to zero.

Digital mammography is an important and common method used in the detection, monitoring as well as assessment of treatment of breast cancer. Machine learning and especially DL techniques have been applied to effectively classify mammography images into benign and malignant classes. DCNN can extract features from input data by itself. It is an end-to-end solution for image classification tasks [43,44].

The DCNN model is trained with a large database of mammography images to extract high-level representations and identify benign and malignant cases [45,46]. This will aid professional radiologists to improve the accuracy of screening mammography.

2.4   Proposed methodology

The proposed methodology is presented in the next four subsections: data description is followed by the design of three different DL models based on CNN, residual network, and U-Net.

2.4.1   Data description

The dataset consists of breast cancer pathology images taken from the Kaggle site [47]. These images are of type invasive ductal carcinoma (IDC) cancer. These include 162 whole-mount slide images scanned at 40× size. From these, 10,110 having IDC −ve and +ve images were extracted for the purpose of model training and testing. The original images of size 50 × 50 were further reduced to 32 × 32 without altering the class labels.

This was achieved by using the image cropping technique in Python. Figure 2.6 shows sample images of malignant and benign sets.

The dataset includes three types of pathology images: original pathology images, cropped images, and Region of Interest (RoI) images. The distribution of these images is shown in Figure 2.7.

2.4.2   CNN

DL is an advanced machine learning technique that includes several types of models, such as recurrent neural networks, long short-term memory (LSTM) networks, and bi-directional LSMTs. Such networks are used to solve very complex real-life problems. One of the most popularly used DL models for the medical image classification is CNN. CNNs are part of deep neural network used for features extraction and classification of medical images [48]. These networks reduce the human effort by detecting the different features from images automatically.

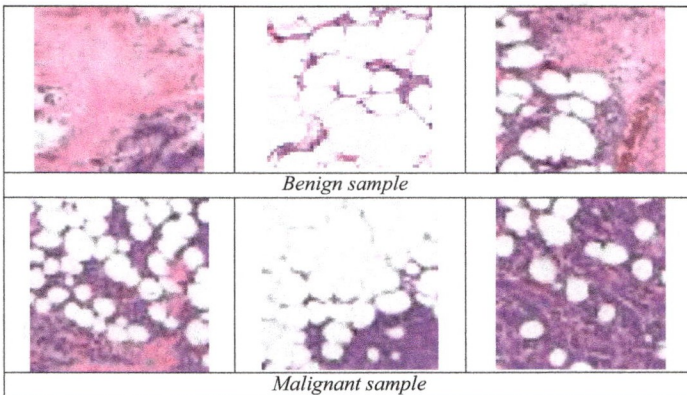

Benign sample

Malignant sample

Figure 2.6   Sample dataset images

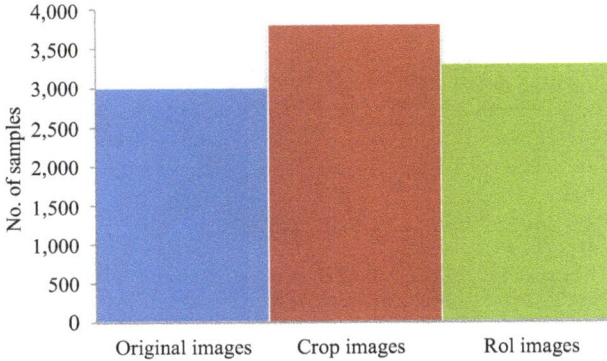

Figure 2.7   Distribution of three types of pathology images in dataset

CNN comprises five main components: Conv layer, pooling layer, an activation function, dropout layer, and flattened layer [49,50].

The convolution layer is the very first layer in the network. It is used to extract feature from the dataset of breast cancer images. Convolution is a mathematical function performed between the kernel and an input image. The kernel represents a filter of size $n \times n$. The filter is slide over the entire input image to produce the third function which will help to extract the features of images. Mathematically this is represented as follows:

$$g(x,y) = h(x,y) * f(x,y) \tag{2.1}$$

where $h(x,y)$ is filter or kernel. The output of the convolution layer is a feature map. This extracts information about noise, edges, sharpness, etc. present in the image. This output is forwarded as an input to the other layer to learn other features from the image. The Conv layer also ensures an intact relationship between pixels [51].

The next layer in the network is the pooling layer. This layer helps to decrease the computational cost of the network by reducing the size of the convolved features [49]. This layer mainly focuses on decreasing the connections between the number of layers and tries to work independently on each feature map to reduce the network cost without affecting the quality. There are different types of pooling to be applied depending on the network. In general, this layer acts as a bridge to convolution and fully connected (FC) layer. The fully connected layer, which is usually, placed before the outer layer comprises weights and biases. These weights and biases are used to connect several neurons in different layers in the network. Before the input image goes to fully connected layer, the image has to pass through the flattened layer. In the flattened layer, input images are converted into one dimension input vector. This produces a single long feature vector. Now this layer is connected to fully connected layer to carry out classification task.

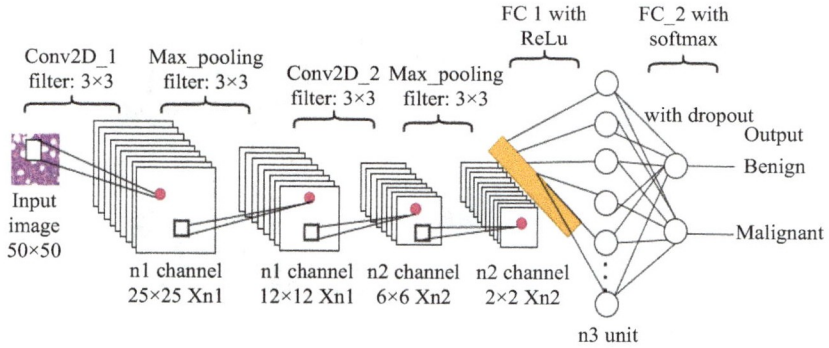

Figure 2.8   Proposed CNN model

The features that were extracted from previous layers, get connected with to fully connected layer, there is a possibility that overfitting may occur during training. This will create a negative impact on the model. To avoid the overfitting drop out layer is used. In this layer, some of the neurons are dropped which results in a reduction in the size of the model. Neurons are dropped during training and this will prevent model overfitting and also improve the performance. In the network activation, functions are used to fire the neurons to do some task. These functions help the networks to learn the kind of relationship present between variables. This will help the network to identify which information is to be forwarded and which is not to the next layers. There are various activation functions in practice, but mostly ReLu and softmax are used due to their popularity [52]. For example, in binary classification problems, softmax function is used.

In the proposed work, as shown in Figure 2.8, the DCNN model is created to classify breast cancer images into the following: benign and malignant. The network consists of the convolution layer, max pooling, flattened layer, fully connected network layer, and two activation functions: ReLu and softmax. The input image of size $50 \times 50 \times 1$ is fed into the network. Kernel of size 3×3 is used in the convolution layer to extract the features. Fully connected layer at output uses a dropout function to minimize the computational cost of the network during training. In the first fully connected layer, ReLu activation is used, and in the second FC, softmax is used. The model was trained using 25 epochs. For every epoch model loss, accuracy and validation loss were calculated. At the 25th, the epoch model achieved an accuracy of 96.81%.

2.4.3   U-Net

U-net is a U-shaped CNN architecture published in the year 2015. This network is useful in finding the RoI from medical image [53]. RoI of an image can be found by applying segmentation in U-net. U-Net consists of two identical parts: one at the

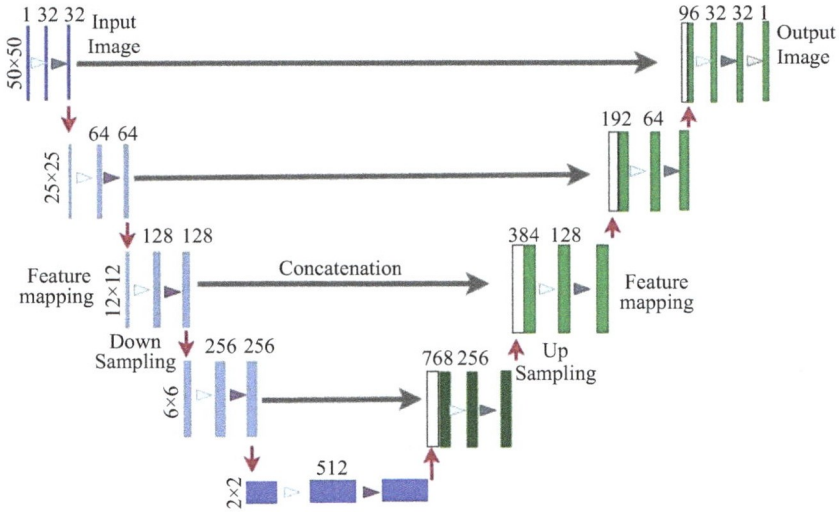

Figure 2.9   Proposed U-net architecture

left and the other on the right side. The left part of the architecture is called contracting. This includes downsampling layers. Each layer present in the model includes a common process of convolution that consists of two convolution layers and one max pooling layer. The right part of the network is the expansive part includes upsampling layers. Each of these layers comprises two transposed convolution layers and one max pooling layer [54]. In the proposed network, five upsampling and downsampling layers are proposed so that breast cancer images can be classified into the following: malignant and benign. The number of layers can be increased or decreased based on the input image size.

There are also skip connections established between corresponding downsampling layers to upsampling layers to concatenate the present layers. This will minimize the significant loss that occurred from the previous layer when the transformation is done. The final convolution layer will produce the desired output [55,56]. This layer has two filters. In each of the convolution layers, ReLu activation function is used. The training process of the U-net is stabilized as shown in Figure 2.9. At the bottom of the U-net, a sliding window like block can be seen, used in training, consisting of both upsampling and downsampling layers. This comprises two convolution layers.

2.4.4   ResNet

Image classification can be performed with better accuracy using deeper CNN. The deeper the networks, the better the results. But at a certain depth, the network accuracy starts degrading. The network introduces a gradient vanishing problem. The gradient used to calculate the loss function will reduce to zero after a certain number of iterations because of the chain rule applied to the network depth. The weights that are used to update the network will not get updated and learning will never happen at this stage. When the network stops learning ultimately the accuracy of the model will decrease. To overcome this problem, ResNets were introduced in the year 2015. ResNets are deep residual networks used for computer vision and medical image processing [57].

These networks allow one or more intermediate layers to skip during training. Such layers are called identity shortcut connections. Therefore, thousands of layers can be used to train the model without affecting the performance. The skip connection is the core technique used in residual blocks of ResNet. Due to skip connections, the image size at the output layer will vary, i.e. the input value 'x' is multiplied by weights and some bias is added to it, as shown below:

$$O(x) = f(w * x + b) \qquad (2.2)$$

When this O(x) is passed through the activation function, the net output will be

$$Y(x) = h(O(x)) \qquad (2.3)$$

With ResNet, the output can be computed as follows:

$$h(x) = h(x) + x \qquad (2.4)$$

The above output can have a problem, especially in the convolution and the pooling layer, when the size of input images varies from that of the output image size. To overcome this problem, in ResNet, skip connection pads of extra zeros increase the dimension of the image. This can be done using projection methods in which one more 1×1 convolution layer is added to the input [58,59]. Hence, (2.4) changes to the following:

$$h(x) = f(x) + w.x \qquad (2.5)$$

ResNet achieves the following objectives: (1) it maps the input image to an output image with a variable size, accommodating both shallow and deep networks; (2) it adds an identity layer, which is a 1×1 convolution layer, without compromising network performance; and (3) it ensures that the input image and output image are equal in size, despite potential variations. This technique is known as residual block and the same is shown in Figure 2.10.

Variants of ResNet like ResNet18, ResNet50 [60], ResNet 101 [61], etc. are used in practice to perform medical image segmentation and prediction. In the proposed work, ResNet18 is used [62–64]. This is shallow architecture and achieves fast training without compromising performance. In this architecture, two residual blocks in four stages are implemented. Each such block contains two convolution layers, one convolution layer is connected immediately after the input and the other is connected at the end to represent a fully connected layer. These layers are supported by pooling and the ReLu activation function. The convolution layer introduced at the beginning has 5×5 filters. The residual block has a 3×3 convolution layer followed by batch normalization. The skip connection can be

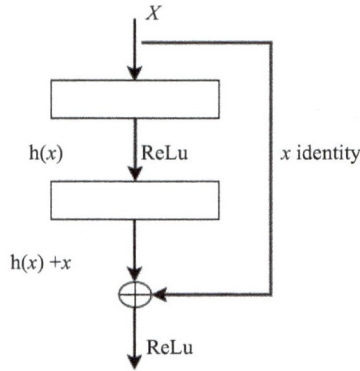

Figure 2.10   Residual block in ResNet

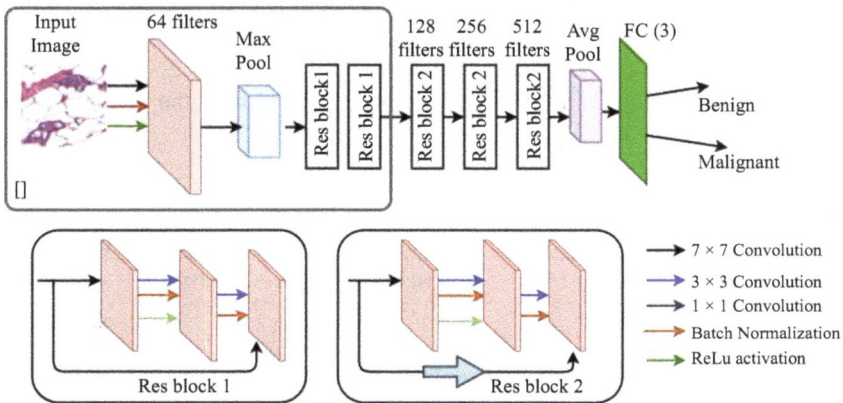

Figure 2.11   Proposed ResNet architecture

established by skipping one or two convolution layers and connecting directly with the final ReLu activation function. The model is trained for 25 epochs. Adam optimizer is used with a learning rate of 0.01. The network architecture is shown in Figure 2.11. The proposed architecture classifies the breast cancer pathology images into two classes: benign and malignant [65].

2.5   Results and discussion

Three different models were trained to classify benign and malignant images using CNN, ResNet, and U-Net. These models were implemented using Google Colab platform [66]. The dataset was split into training and testing with a ratio of 80:20. The performance of the models was evaluated using standard metrics such as precision, recall, F1-score, and accuracy [67]. True positive (TP) value defines malignant cancer images defined as malignant ones by the model. True negative (TN) is the number of benign images identified as benign by the model. False positive (FP) is the benign cancer images predicted as malignant by the model. False negative (FN) is the malignant cancer images predicted as benign by the model. The following equations are used to compute the performance of the models.

$$\text{Accuracy} = (\text{true malignant images} + \text{true benign images})/(\text{true malignant}$$
$$+ \text{ true benign} + \text{false benign} + \text{false malignant}) \quad (2.6)$$

$$\text{Recall} = (\text{true malignant})/(\text{true malignant} + \text{false benign}) \quad (2.7)$$

$$\text{Precision} = (\text{true malignant})/(\text{true malignant} + \text{false malignant}) \quad (2.8)$$

$$\text{F} - 1\text{score} = 2 * (\text{precission} * \text{recall})/(\text{precision} + \text{recall}) \quad (2.9)$$

Table 2.3 presents the performance of each of the models. It shows that U-net has performed better as compared to other models.

Figure 2.12 shows training and testing accuracy achieved using ResNet model. It can be observed that even though the model was trained for 25 epochs, the test accuracy started falling down after 20 epochs. Therefore the model stopped learning.

Table 2.3   Performance measures for CNN, ResNet, and U-Unet

Methods used	Accuracy (%)	Recall (%)	Precision (%)	F1-score (%)
CNN	95.61	94.82	94.82	94.82
ResNet	96.87	96.56	96.67	96.15
U-Net	97.12	96.78	97.43	97.34

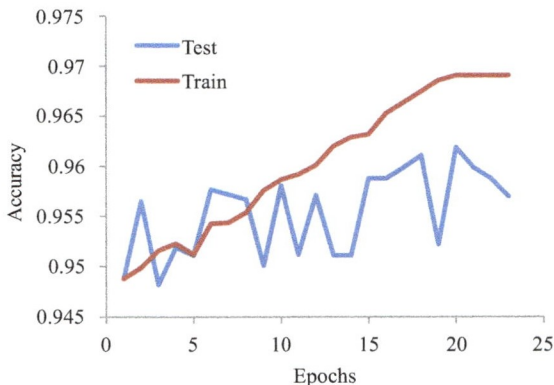

Figure 2.12   Network performance during training and testing

2.6   Conclusion

The chapter proposed three DL-based classification methods to classify mammography images. All the proposed models used binary classification method to categorize the images into benign and malignant categories. Dataset images were extracted from whole mount slide images scanned at $40\times$ size. Further there were three types of images (original, RoI, and cropped) were included to build more robust models. DL techniques used include CNN, ResNet, and U-Net. All these networks were well trained to identify RoI of the image using various techniques in each of the networks so that classification becomes accurate. Models were evaluated using standard metrics such as accuracy, F1-score, recall, and precision. CNN was able to achieve a performance of 95.61% accuracy, 94.82% recall, 94.84% precision, and 94.82% F1-score values. ResNet was able to achieve 96.86% accuracy, 96.56% recall, 96.67% precision, and 96.15% F1-score. Similarly the U-Net was able to achieve 97.12% accuracy, 96.79 % recall, 97.43% precision, and 97.34% F1-score. It can be observed from the model evaluation that uses of DL-based pre-trained networks have leveraged the classification performance. In the future: (1) model validation can be concluded with human experts; (2) performance of breast cancer image classification can be improved by applying several other emerging CNN models.

References

[1]   S. Bhise, S. Bepari, S. Gadekar, *et al.*, "Breast cancer detection using machine learning techniques," *Int. J. Eng. Res. Technol.*, vol. 10, no. 07, pp. 98–103, 2021.

[2]   "Breast cancer." https://www.who.int/news-room/fact-sheets/detail/breast-cancer [Accessed: 16-Dec-2022].

[3]   M. Arnold, E. Morgan, H. Rumgay, *et al.*, "Current and future burden of breast cancer: global statistics for 2020 and 2040," *The Breast*, vol. 66, pp. 15–23, 2022.

[4]   A. Simon and K. Robb, "Cancer: breast," In *Cambridge Handbook of Psychology, Health and Medicine, 2nd ed.*, 2014. https://www.ncbi.nlm.nih.gov/books/NBK482286/ [Accessed: 31-Dec-2022].

[5]   "Breast Cancer Early Detection and Diagnosis | How To Detect Breast Cancer." https://www.cancer.org/cancer/breast-cancer/screening-tests-and-early-detection.html [Accessed: 16-Dec-2022].

[6]   N. M. ud din, R. A. Dar, M. Rasool, and A. Assad, "Breast cancer detection using deep learning: datasets, methods, and challenges ahead," *Comput. Biol. Med.*, vol. 149, p. 106073, 2022.

[7]   A. Janowczyk and A. Madabhushi, "Deep learning for digital pathology image analysis: a comprehensive tutorial with selected use cases," *J. Pathol. Inform.*, vol. 7, no. 1, p. 26, 2016.

[8]   M. S. Ali, M. S. Miah, J. Haque, M. M. Rahman, and M. K. Islam, "An enhanced technique of skin cancer classification using deep convolutional

neural network with transfer learning models," *Mach. Learn. Appl.*, vol. 5, p. 100036, 2021.

[9]   S. S. Yadav and S. M. Jadhav, "Deep convolutional neural network based medical image classification for disease diagnosis," *J. Big Data*, vol. 6, no. 1, p. 113, 2019.

[10]   Y. Amethiya, P. Pipariya, S. Patel, and M. Shah, "Comparative analysis of breast cancer detection using machine learning and biosensors," *Intell. Med.*, vol. 2, no. 2, pp. 69–81, 2022.

[11]   S. J. S. Gardezi, A. Elazab, B. Lei, and T. Wang, "Breast cancer detection and diagnosis using mammographic data: systematic review," *J. Med. Internet Res.*, vol. 21, no. 7, 2019.

[12]   L. Balkenende, J. Teuwen, and R. M. Mann, "Application of deep learning in breast cancer imaging," *Semin. Nucl. Med.*, vol. 52, no. 5, pp. 584–596, 2022.

[13]   S. Pranshu, A. Goyal, M. A. Bivi, S. K. Singh, and M. Rashid, "Segmentation of nucleus and cytoplasm from H&E-stained follicular lymphoma," *Electronics*, vol. 12, no. 3, p. 651, 2023.

[14]   A. B. Nassif, M. A. Talib, Q. Nasir, Y. Afadar, and O. Elgendy, "Breast cancer detection using artificial intelligence techniques: a systematic literature review," *Artif. Intell. Med.*, vol. 127, 2022.

[15]   A. Akselrod-Ballin, M. Chorev, Y. Shoshan, *et al.*, "Predicting breast cancer by applying deep learning to linked health records and mammograms," *Radiology*, vol. 292, no. 2, pp. 331–342, 2019.

[16]   S. Gaurav, M. Rashid, R. Singh, A. Gehlot, and N. Sharma, "Breast cancer detection in mammogram images using machine learning methods and CLAHE algorithm," In *2022 5th International Conference on Contemporary Computing and Informatics (IC3I)*, pp. 1187–1192. IEEE, 2022.

[17]   K. Wang, B. K. Patel, L. Wang, T. Wu, B. Zheng, and J. Li, "A dual-mode deep transfer learning (D2TL) system for breast cancer detection using contrast enhanced digital mammograms," *IISE Trans. Healthc. Syst. Eng.*, vol. 9, no. 4, pp. 357–370, 2019.

[18]   D. Clement, E. Agu, J. Obayemi, S. Adeshina, and W. Soboyejo, "Breast cancer tumor classification using a bag of deep multi-resolution convolutional features," *Informatics,* vol. 9, no. 4, p. 91, 2022.

[19]   T. H. H. Aldhyani, R. Nair, E. Alzain, H. Alkahtani, and D. Koundal, "Deep learning model for the detection of real time breast cancer images using improved dilation-based method," *Diagnostics*, vol. 12, no. 10, p. 2505, 2022.

[20]   P. Sonar, U. Bhosle, and C. Choudhury, "Mammography classification using modified hybrid SVM-KNN," In *Proceedings of IEEE International Conference on Signal Processing and Communication, ICSPC 2017*, vol. 2018, pp. 305–311, 2018.

[21]   A. Rampun, P. J. Morrow, B. W. Scotney, and J. Winder, "Fully automated breast boundary and pectoral muscle segmentation in mammograms," *Artif. Intell. Med.*, vol. 79, pp. 28–41, 2017.

[22]   K. Amanpreet, M. Rashid, A. K. Bashir, and S. A. Parah, "Detection of breast cancer masses in mammogram images with watershed segmentation and machine learning approach," *In Artificial Intelligence for Innovative Healthcare Informatics*, pp. 35–60. Cham: Springer International Publishing, 2022.

[23]   C. C. Jen and S. S. Yu, "Automatic detection of abnormal mammograms in mammographic images," *Expert Syst. Appl.*, vol. 42, no. 6, pp. 3048–3055, 2015.

[24]   F. Sadoughi, Z. Kazemy, F. Hamedan, L. Owji, M. Rahmanikatigari, and T. T. Azadboni, "Artificial intelligence methods for the diagnosis of breast cancer by image processing: a review," *Breast Cancer Targets Ther.*, vol. 10, pp. 219–230, 2018.

[25]   S. Saini and R. Vijay, "Optimization of artificial neural network breast cancer detection system based on image registration techniques," *Int. J. Comput. Appl.*, vol. 105, no. 14, pp. 975–8887, 2014.

[26]   V. B. Bora, A. G. Kothari, and A. G. Keskar, "Robust automatic pectoral muscle segmentation from mammograms using texture gradient and Euclidean distance regression," *J. Digit. Imaging*, vol. 29, no. 1, pp. 115–125, 2016.

[27]   M. Pratiwi, Alexander, J. Harefa, and S. Nanda, "Mammograms classification using gray-level co-occurrence matrix and radial basis function neural network," In *International Conference on Computer Science and Computational Intelligence (ICCSCI 2015), Procedia Computer Science*, 2015, vol. 59, pp. 83–91.

[28]   N. A. Samee, G. Atteia, S. Meshoul, M. A. Al-antari, and Y. M. Kadah, "Deep learning cascaded feature selection framework for breast cancer classification: hybrid CNN with univariate-based approach," *Mathematics*, vol. 10, no. 19, p. 3631, 2022.

[29]   H. Jiao, X. Jiang, Z. Pang, X. Lin, Y. Huang, and L. Li, "Deep convolutional neural networks-based automatic breast segmentation and mass detection in DCE-MRI," *Comput. Math. Methods Med.*, vol. 2020, 2020.

[30]   A. Nomani, Y. Ansari, M. H. Nasirpour, A. Masoumian, E. S. Pour, and A. Valizadeh, "PSOWNNs-CNN: a computational radiology for breast cancer diagnosis improvement based on image processing using machine learning methods," *Comput. Intell. Neurosci.*, vol. 2022, 2022.

[31]   A. R. Vaka, B. Soni, and S. R. K., "Breast cancer detection by leveraging machine learning," *ICT Express*, vol. 6, no. 4, pp. 320–324, 2020.

[32]   R. Lo Gullo, S. Eskreis-Winkler, E. A. Morris, and K. Pinker, "Machine learning with multiparametric magnetic resonance imaging of the breast for early prediction of response to neoadjuvant chemotherapy," *Breast*, vol. 49, pp. 115–122, 2020.

[33]   J. Witowski, L. Heacock, B. Reig, *et al.*, "Improving breast cancer diagnostics with deep learning for MRI," *Sci. Transl. Med.*, vol. 14, no. 664, p. 4802, 2022.

[34] A. Ashtaiwi, "Optimal histopathological magnification factors for deep learning-based breast cancer prediction," *Appl. Syst. Innov.* 2022, vol. 5, no. 5, p. 87, 2022.

[35] S. Zahoor, U. Shoaib, and I. U. Lali, "Breast cancer mammograms classification using deep neural network and entropy-controlled Whale Optimization Algorithm," *Diagnostics*, vol. 12, no. 2, p. 557, 2022.

[36] F. Gao, T. Wu, J. Li, *et al.*, "SD-CNN: a shallow-deep CNN for improved breast cancer diagnosis," *Comput. Med. Imaging Graph.*, vol. 70, pp. 53–62, 2018.

[37] J. Arevalo, F. A. González, R. Ramos-Pollán, J. L. Oliveira, and M. A. Guevara Lopez, "Representation learning for mammography mass lesion classification with convolutional neural networks," *Comput. Methods Programs Biomed.*, vol. 127, pp. 248–257, 2016.

[38] I. H. Sarker, "Machine learning: algorithms, real-world applications and research directions," *SN Comput. Sci.*, vol. 2, no. 3, pp. 1–21, 2021.

[39] T. M. Mitchell, *Machine Learning.* McGraw-Hill Science, 1997.

[40] J. Patel and R. Goyal, "Applications of artificial neural networks in medical science," *Curr. Clin. Pharmacol.*, vol. 2, no. 3, pp. 217–226, 2008.

[41] J. Zurada, *Introduction to Artificial Neural System.* West Publishing Company, 1992.

[42] S. Agarwal, *Data Mining: Data Mining Concepts and Techniques.* ACS, 2014.

[43] R. Pise, K. Patil, and N. Pise, "Automatic classification of mosquito genera using transfer learning," *J. Theor. Appl. Inf. Technol.*, vol. 100, no. 7, pp. 1929–1940, 2022.

[44] P. Pawar, B. Ainapure, M. Rashid, N. Ahmad, A. Alotaibi, and S. S. Alshamrani, "Deep learning approach for the detection of noise type in ancient images," *Sustain*, vol. 14, no. 18, pp. 1–20, 2022.

[45] L. Balkenende, J. Teuwen, and R. M. Mann, "Application of deep learning in breast cancer imaging," *Seminars in Nuclear Medicine*, vol. 52, no. 5, pp. 584–596, 2022.

[46] L. Shen, L. R. Margolies, J. H. Rothstein, E. Fluder, R. McBride, and W. Sieh, "Deep learning to improve breast cancer detection on screening mammography," *Sci. Rep.*, vol. 9, no. 1, 2019.

[47] "Breast_Cancer | Kaggle." https://www.kaggle.com/code/abeerabdelnasser/breast-cancer/data. [Accessed: 20-Dec-2022].

[48] N. Khan, R. Adam, P. Huang, T. Maldjian, and T. Q. Duong, "Deep learning prediction of pathologic complete response in breast cancer using MRI and other clinical data: a systematic review," *Tomography*, vol. 8, no. 6, pp. 2784–2795, 2022.

[49] T. Sujithra, M. I. Mahaboob, C. Iwendi, *et al.*, "IoMT with deep CNN: AI-based intelligent support system for pandemic diseases," *Electronics*, vol. 12, no. 2, pp. 424, 2023.

[50] K. A. Ayub, A. A. Shaikh, O. Cheikhrouhou, *et al.*, "IMG-forensics: multi-media-enabled information hiding investigation using convolutional neural network," *IET Image Process.*, vol. 16, no. 11, pp. 2854–2862, 2022.

[51] P. Napoletano, F. Piccoli, and R. Schettini, "Anomaly detection in nanofibrous materials by CNN-based self-similarity," *Sensors (Switzerland)*, vol. 18, no. 1, 2018.

[52] M. A. Aslam and D. Cui, "Breast cancer classification using deep convolutional neural network," In *Journal of Physics: Conference Series*, 2020, vol. 1584, no. 1.

[53] M. H. Yap, M. Goyal, F. Osman, *et al.*, "Breast ultrasound region of interest detection and lesion localisation," *Artif. Intell. Med.*, vol. 107, p. 101880, 2020.

[54] T. Zhao and H. Dai, "Breast tumor ultrasound image segmentation method based on improved residual U-Net *network,*" *Comput. Intell. Neurosci.*, vol. 2022, p. 3905998, 2022.

[55] G. Piantadosi, M. Sansone, and C. Sansone, "Breast segmentation in MRI via U-Net deep convolutional neural networks," In *Proceedings of the International Conference on Pattern Recognition*, vol. 2018, pp. 3917–3922, 2018.

[56] Y. Yan, Y. Liu, Y. Wu, H. Zhang, Y. Zhang, and L. Meng, "Accurate segmentation of breast tumors using AE U-net with HDC model in ultrasound images," *Biomed. Signal Process. Control*, vol. 72, p. 103299, 2022.

[57] S. I. Khan, A. Shahrior, R. Karim, M. Hasan, and A. Rahman, "MultiNet: a deep neural network approach for detecting breast cancer through multi-scale feature fusion," *J. King Saud Univ. – Comput. Inf. Sci.*, vol. 34, no. 8, pp. 6217–6228, 2022.

[58] M. Wu, X. Shen, C. Lai, *et al.*, "Detecting neonatal acute bilirubin encephalopathy based on T1-weighted MRI images and learning-based approaches," *BMC Med. Imaging*, vol. 21, no. 1, pp. 1–12, 2021.

[59] K. He and J. Sun, "Deep residual learning for image recognition," In *IEEE Conference on Computer Vision and Pattern Recognition (CVPR)*, 2016, pp. 770–778.

[60] G. Hemant, M. Awais, A. K. Bashir, *et al.*, "AI-enabled radiologist in the loop: novel AI-based framework to augment radiologist performance for COVID-19 chest CT medical image annotation and classification from pneumonia," *Neural Comput. Appl.*, pp. 1–19, 2022.

[61] R. A. Welikala, P. Remagnino, J. H. Lim, *et al.*, "Automated detection and classification of oral lesions using deep learning for early detection of oral cancer," *IEEE Access*, vol. 8, pp. 132677–132693, 2020.

[62] S. Misra, S. Jeon, S. Lee, R. Managuli, I. S. Jang, and C. Kim, "Multi-channel transfer learning of chest x-ray images for screening of covid-19," *Electronics*, vol. 9, no. 9, pp. 1–12, 2020.

[63] E. Kim, G. S. Dahiya, S. Løset, and R. Skjetne, "Can a computer see what an ice expert sees? Multilabel ice objects classification with convolutional neural networks," *Results Eng.*, vol. 4, no. 2019.

[64]   D. Sarwinda, R. H. Paradisa, A. Bustamam, and P. Anggia, "Deep learning in image classification using residual network (ResNet) variants for detection of colorectal cancer," *Procedia Comput. Sci.*, vol. 179, no. 2019, pp. 423–431, 2021.

[65]   N. Behar and M. Shrivastava, "ResNet50-based effective model for breast cancer classification using histopathology images," *C. – Comput. Model. Eng. Sci.*, vol. 130, no. 2, pp. 823–839, 2022.

[66]   Google Colab, "Welcome to Colaboratory – Colaboratory," *Getting Started – Introduction*, 2020. https://colab.research.google.com/notebook. [Accessed: 02-Jan-2023].

[67]   E. H. Dulf, M. Bledea, T. Mocan, and L. Mocan, "Automatic detection of colorectal polyps using transfer learning," *Sensors*, vol. 21, no. 17, 2021.

Chapter 3

Detection of autism spectrum disorder using artificial intelligence

Kaushal Oza[1], Shree Udavant[1] and Mamoon Rashid[1]

Artificial intelligence (AI) has the potential to help diagnose autism, a neurodevelopmental condition that affects communication, social interaction, and behaviour, which is often diagnosed through clinical observation and standardised assessments. This chapter explores different methods and methodologies that are commonly used to identify and treat autism. Addressing autism requires substantial effort over an extended period of time. The chapter discusses techniques such as eye-tracking and identifying patterns in behaviour, movement, and speech using various machine and deep learning methods. Additionally, the chapter proposes developing a comprehensive AI-based system to aid medical professionals in detecting autism by recognising patterns in behaviour through screening tools.

3.1 Introduction

Autism, commonly known as an autism spectrum disorder (ASD), is a disorder brought on by a glitch in neurodevelopment that has an impact on behaviour, social interaction, and communication. According to the World Health Organization, ASD affects one in 160 children worldwide [1]. Autism symptoms can appear in many different ways, and they can range in severity. In general, autistic symptoms can be recognised in kids before the age of three. Some of these symptoms include issues with social communication, such as being unable to start or maintain conversations, difficulty comprehending non-verbal cues, and problems making friends. Repetitive actions like hand flapping, swaying, or spinning things are also common in people with autism [2]. Also, they might have sensory issues, like a sensitivity to touch, light, or noise, and they might have a hard time adjusting to schedule changes [3].

Preventing autism is a huge challenge. While the medical community is uncertain of the exact cause of autism, they hypothesise that genetics plays the most crucial role in determining whether a child will be born with the condition [4]. For

[1]Reseach Center of Excellence for Health Informatics, Vishwakarma University, Pune, India

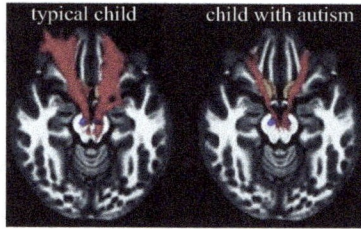

Figure 3.1   Nerve-fibre tracts in children

people with autism, there are many different therapies and interventions available, such as behavioural therapies, speech and language therapy, and medication. A typical form of therapy is applied behaviour analysis (ABA) therapy, which emphasises using positive reinforcement to increase positive behaviour and decrease negative behaviour. Autism sufferers who receive speech and language therapy are better able to communicate and form social relationships [5]. To treat symptoms like aggression, anxiety, or depression, doctors may give medications like antipsychotics or antidepressants. Children with autism have deficiencies in a brain region that often makes social engagement feel rewarding, according to MRI scans. In contrast to typically developing children, children with autism have less dense nerve-fibre tracts along the pathway (shown in red in Figure 3.1).

3.2   Early detection using artificial intelligence

Finding autism is a challenging undertaking that takes time and effort to improve cases. Many behavioural and physiological approaches have been utilised to successfully and accurately diagnose autism in young children. In addition to notifying scientific research centres about the proper remedies and treatments, predictive indicators are also required to alert parents to their children's behaviour, physiological status, and course extremely early [6–8]. Globally, autism prevalence rates vary widely depending on the country and the methods used to diagnose and assess the disorder. Some studies have reported rates as high as 1 in 38 children, while others have reported rates as low as 1 in 1,000 children. Despite the rising frequency of autism, the specific causes of the illness remain unknown. Further study is required to completely understand the origins and risk factors for the illness; however, it is thought that a mix of genetic and environmental factors may contribute to the emergence of autism [9–11].

3.2.1   ASD detection using eye tracking

Since it can be used on individuals of all ages and is quick, simple, and inexpensive to analyse, eye-tracking technology is one of the most significant and promising markers of ASD. Figure 3.2 shows a method of study known as "eye movement tracking" which creates, monitors, and records points while also computing eye movement via these locations. Several studies have demonstrated that eye

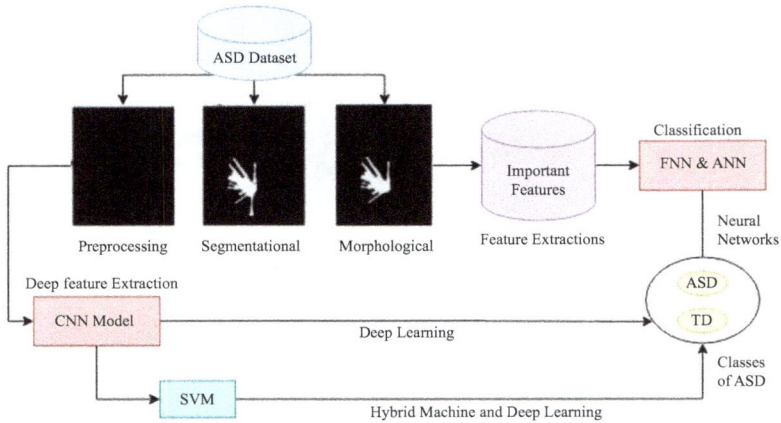

Figure 3.2   Techniques for applying AI to diagnose datasets with ASD

movements act as biomarkers of ASD by significantly influencing how people react to verbal and visual stimuli [12].

Also, some research have revealed a connection between eye movement tracking and clinical testing for ASD early diagnosis. Genetic factors are responsible for some of these connections. As a biomarker for evaluating autistic youngsters, eye-tracking technology has many benefits. First off, it makes eye tracking for young toddlers simple, allowing for early identification of autism concerns. Second, irregular visual focus is indicated by a variety of information from eye-tracking data, which is employed as a biomarker. Third, eye-tracking technology is a simple test connected to the diagnostic screening devices for ASD. ASD and eye-tracking models that measure social and non-social orienting performance have a significant association. These models make use of social attention deficits to detect ASD at an early age. The idea that effective eye-tracking results are a reliable indicator of long-term outcomes in children with ASD, however, is not well-supported by the available research [13].

3.2.2   Autism detection using machine learning and deep learning models

According to a study that attempted to use various machine learning and deep learning techniques to detect ASD. The performance of the models was evaluated using different metrics on non-clinical datasets from three age groups: children, adolescents, and adults. Figure 3.3 shows the methodology of how machine learning is used to perform autism detection. When all of the feature attributes listed in Table 3.1 were included after accounting for missing values, the study indicated that the CNN classifier outperformed the SVM classifier. After accounting for missing values, the accuracy of the SVM and CNN models for identifying ASD in the child dataset reached approximately 98.30%. The classification algorithm outperformed every other model-building method for the other two datasets, nevertheless. Table 3.2 shows that a CNN model could be used for detecting ASD instead of traditional machine learning classifiers used in previous research [14,15].

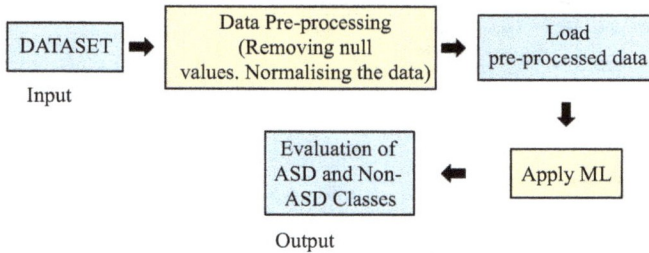

Figure 3.3   Methodology for autism detection using ML models

Table 3.1   Common attributes from the dataset used for detecting autism using AI

No.	Attribute description
1	Nationality of the patient
2	Age of the patient
3	Determining whether the user has ever used a screening application
4	Screening score
5	Answers to 10 questions based on the screening procedure
6	Members of the family that have severe developmental disorder
7	If the patient was suffered by jaundice from birth
8	Gender

Table 3.2   Results overall for adults screening for ASD using data from the UCI machine learning repository

Methodology	Accuracy	Sensitivity	Specificity
Logistic regression (LR)	96.69	0.9696	0.9575
SVM	98.11	0.8888	0.9574
Naive Bayes	96.22	96.96	0.9361
KNN	95.75	0.9696	0.9148
ANN	97.64	0.9757	0.9787
CNN	99.53	0.9939	01.00

3.2.3   ASD detection using behavioural analysis

Video and speech analysis: AI can examine video footage of behaviour to spot repetitive or unusual patterns, like hand-flapping or rocking, to detect early signs of autism or other behavioural disorders. A study provided a sizable dataset of videos of children engaging in social interactions that had been manually classified with behaviours crucial to the diagnosis of ASD [16]. This dataset will be analysed using a machine learning framework that has two stages: behaviours identification and ASD prediction based on statistical aspects of behaviours. They suggested two fundamental deep learning methods for behaviour detection, one based on end-to-end training on raw video frames and a second based on the child subject's facial characteristics. To predict ASD, feature selection was investigated, as class reba-lancing and neural network classifiers were to link the statistics of behaviours to ASD diagnosis. Artificial intelligence (AI) also can analyse speech patterns and detect vocal characteristics such as tone, pitch, and other factors that may indicate emotional states like anxiety [17].

In social interactions, people with ASD tend to avoid eye contact and their eye gazes display patterns of visual field scanning that are very dissimilar from those of neurotypical people. To automatically categorise autism symptoms from photographs and videos, a system that makes use of deep learning and computer vision was employed. To find behaviours connected to ASD, two pipelines were used. The video dataset included 1,707 movies of 365 newborns playing with either a parent or an examiner in a variety of activities. Each video was a 3-min clip of the interactive play session. The experiments were designed to observe children's social behaviours, such as eye contact, play behaviours, and interaction with others, as these could be signs of ASD. Researchers watched from behind a private glass window and oversaw the recording process while the interactive experiments were being done in a room equipped with cameras to record the movements of the testers and kids. A tester skilled in assessing autistic behaviour. The examiner was standing in front of the youngster and the child's parents might have been seated together. To get the child's attention and measure their reactions to various stimuli, the tester employed toys like dolls or miniature cell phones. All of the children's performances had been captured on tape, and each one had a camera to record the adult as well as the young person. Up to three play sessions might have been included in each visit, and the intention was to record a variety of social interactions to allow for efficient data analysis. With each film in this study, careful consideration was given to four different actions:

- Observing the partner's face to establish eye contact.
- Observing objects that the subject found interesting.
- Determining whether the subject was smiling.
- Detecting any vocalisations or speaking.

To provide baseline information for the supervised learning tasks, these behaviours were labelled or tagged by skilled coders. All movies were coded using the Noldus Observer 5.0 behavioural observation programme, and coders were instructed to achieve at least 90% agreement on all codes. To increase reliability, master coders double-coded 15% of the data, yielding strong intraclass correlation coefficients (ICCs) for all codes (0.95 for gaze to face, 0.98 for gaze to object, 0.96 for smile, and 0.93 for vocalisation).

Deep learning-based detection: Although the video collection is insufficient to effectively predict the diagnosis of ASD using deep neural networks, the challenge was addressed by treating it as an image-based classification task. They base their architecture on ResNet-18 and use binary cross-entropy as their loss function, SGD optimiser, and backend. The input image is horizontally flipped during training, and the learning rate is reduced by 10 times every 10 epochs.

Binary entropy: Loss= abs(Y_pred – Y_actual)

The final loss:

$$\alpha \, \Sigma Y + \log P(y = 1|X, W) + \beta \, \Sigma Y\_\log P(y = 0|X, W)$$

where |Y+| and |Y| stand for both the amount of samples for positive and negative samples, respectively. The input picture and network weight are denoted by X and W. Due to such a loss, the network is forced to pay less attention to larger negative samples, which leads to lower penalties.

3.2.4   *Behaviour detection based on facial key points as features*

On the look-face challenge, the model performed admirably based just on the child's characteristics, with a sensitivity of 0.59 and a specificity of 0.73. It had been logical to suppose that adding details about the interacting adult's head posture and facial features would have resulted in even more advancements in the look-face job. A sensitivity of 0.45 had room for improvement, but a specificity of 0.92 had proven fairly good for smile recognition. A review of the literature on emotion recognition indicated that facial landmarks and facial action units (FAUs) are very helpful features, particularly for detecting smiles when the face has been in a frontal or near-frontal posture [18]. The fact that the child's face was frequently out of its frontal position because of the camera position has hampered the performance of this dataset. Moreover, head movements or facial occlusions by toys have frequently happened and prevented successful face detections. Since a frame-based approach could not have taken full advantage of the movements of lips, the low sensitivity for vocal tasks suggested that this model might not have been well-suited for the detection of the vocalisation tasks. To enhance the detection of mouth movement, a temporal processing strategy would have been helpful [19].

The performance of the model utilising only a few characteristics was comparable to using all features. However, when synthetic minority over-sampling method (SMOTE) was used on the training set, it increased sensitivity but lowered specificity, showing that synthetic features produced by SMOTE can mostly enhance ASD class detection. Although the removal of the negative class links slightly improved the network's efficiency, the issue of the class imbalance was not completely resolved. The study presented a substantial video dataset of kids interacting socially for ASD diagnosis and suggested a machine learning architecture composed of behaviour detection and ASD prediction. For behaviour detection, feature selection, class rebalancing, and ASD prediction, two fundamental deep learning algorithms have been suggested. Neural net classifiers have also been given some attention. The strategy called for using auditory data, a temporal dimension, and self-supervised techniques to enhance behaviour detection.

3.2.5   ASD detection using wearable devices

The article suggested a novel deep learning application utilising multi-axis IMUs to enable automatic SMM detection, which is connected to ASD. In the interest of enhancing the detection rate on longitudinal data, parameter transfer learning was used for the CNN, and the temporal patterns in a series of multi-axis signals were modelled using LSTM. The study came to the conclusion that using an ensemble of LSTMs produced more accurate and reliable detectors [20] and that feature learning outperformed manually created features. The study's findings were a substantial advancement in the field of precise real-time SMM detection.

Children with ASD were shown to exhibit a large collection of unusual repetitive behaviours known as stereotypical motor movements (SMMs). SMMs were discovered to have detrimental effects on ASD children's quality of life, including their social interactions and learning capacities. Direct behavioural observation, paper-and-pencil assessment, and video-based procedures are examples of traditional ways of evaluating SMMs. These techniques are time-consuming and unusable as therapeutic tools, and they have a number of other drawbacks including subjectivity, difficulties reliably detecting the intensity, amount, and duration of SMMs [21].

It is crucial to create a system that can quickly and accurately identify stereotyped motor movements (SMMs) in kids with ASD. Researchers studying ASD, carers, families, and therapists might benefit from using such a system to assess how patients with ASD are adjusting and to lessen abnormal behaviours. Although there are still some issues to be resolved, the use of inertial measurement units (IMUs) for automatic real-time SMM detection is a promising development in the field of human activity recognition [22].

Figure 3.4 shows a system that can detect social motor movements (SMMs) in real-time that can be created by using inertial measurement units (IMUs) to collect

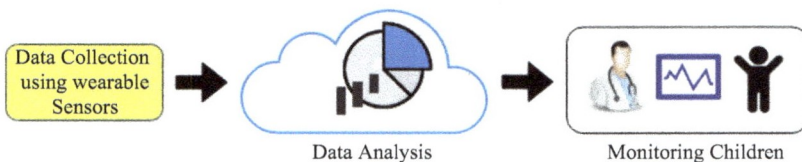

Data Collection using wearable Sensors

Data Analysis

Monitoring Children

Figure 3.4   Automatic stereotypical motor movement (SMM) detection system

data. To find any odd motions, the acquired data can subsequently be locally or remotely analysed. An alarm will always be issued to the parents, therapist, or carer if such movements are discovered.

To accurately detect stereotypical and repetitive movements in autistic children, the chapter discusses the shortcomings of current methods for measuring SMMs and suggests a deep learning architecture that combines a convolutional neural network (CNN) and long short-term memory (LSTM) to learn temporal patterns in IMU signal sequences. The chapter also explores the benefits of parameter transfer learning and ensemble learning for improving detection rates, and the potential for real-time SMM detection systems. Experimental results show that the proposed architecture outperforms handcrafted features and improves classification performance, particularly for unbalanced training sets. The article concludes with a discussion of future directions and limitations.

To predict the affective states of enjoyment, excitement, anxiety, and relaxation, a recent study developed a model based on CNN. Using signals from blood volume pulses and skin conductance, their suggested model was evaluated. The benefits of using CNN to analyse accelerometer signals to identify human activity were also demonstrated.

In three benchmarked datasets, the study assessed the effectiveness of several feature spaces and learning methodologies for SMM identification. The outcomes show that feature learning works better than unprocessed and manually created feature spaces. Moreover, parameter transfer learning enhances the CNN classifier's performance. The effectiveness of feature learning and transfer learning, however, suffers from uneven training sets. This problem is partially resolved by using an LSTM network to extract dynamic information from the signal. Moreover, compared to utilising a single LSTM classifier, the ensemble of LSTMs offers a more consistent performance. It was found that compared to each individual LSTM classifier, an ensemble of LSTMs offers a more trustworthy SMM detector. The LSTM's architectural layout is depicted in Figure 3.5. Although being a big step forward for a real-time, accurate automatic SMM detection system, the deep architecture that this study suggests has a serious drawback. For its online adaptability, the fully supervised training method for the SMM detection model is

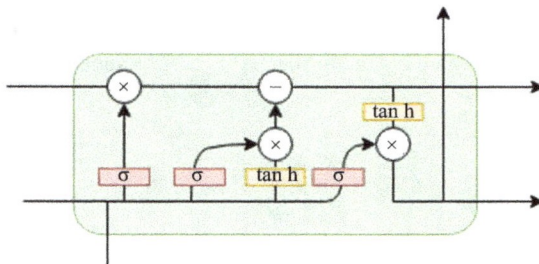

Figure 3.5   LSTM architecture

challenging. This problem occurs because, in actual applications, a new user cannot read the labels of incoming samples while using the system. As a result, only the input unlabelled data should be used to perform adaptation to fresh unseen data. This restriction calls for more investigation into the system's unsupervised online adaptation. Transductive transfer learning, which assumes the absence of labelled data in the target domain, is one option in this direction. One potential avenue for the future of this study is the adoption of a transductive transfer learning technique during the adaption phase.

In this study, the issue of automatic SMM detection was tackled inside the deep learning framework. To extract a robust feature space from multi-sensor/modal IMU inputs, a three-layer CNN architecture was used. It was shown how the suggested architecture may have been used for parameter transfer learning to improve the SMM detection system's capacity to adapt to fresh data. Additionally, it was demonstrated that by combining the CNN architecture with an LSTM unit, the temporal dynamics of the signal were included in the feature learning process and enhanced the SMM detection rate in real-world scenarios, particularly in the case of unbalanced data. The benefit of ensemble learning for producing more dependable and stable SMM detectors was also demonstrated. The outcomes illustrated the deep learning paradigm's tremendous potential for overcoming significant obstacles to real-time SMM detection systems employing wearable devices. With the examination of behavioural and other data patterns, AI can identify possible issues and help in developing specialised treatment plans for patients with behavioural disorders, resulting in more effective therapies and better outcomes [23].

3.3 Datasets available for ASD diagnosis

- **Autism Brain Imaging Data Exchange (aBIDE)**: This is a sizable, multi-site dataset that contains structural MRI and fMRI resting-state data from people with ASD and normally developing people. Data from more than a thousand people at 17 different sites are included in the dataset.
- **Autism Centers of Excellence (ACE) network:** This dataset includes fMRI data from individuals with ASD and typically developing individuals, as well as genetic and behavioural data. The dataset includes data from over 500 individuals from four different sites.
- **Longitudinal studies of brain function in autism (LongSCAN):** This dataset includes fMRI data from individuals with ASD and typically developing individuals, as well as genetic and behavioural data. The dataset includes data from over 200 individuals from two different sites.
- **Simons Foundation Autism Research Initiative (SFARI) Autism BrainNet:** This collection contains fMRI data from post-mortem brain tissue from people with ASD and people who are typically developing. More than 50 people's data are included in the dataset.
- **National Database for Autism Research (NDAR):** This is a large database that includes a variety of data types, including fMRI data, from individuals

with ASD and typically developing individuals. The dataset includes data from over 25 different studies.

- **Autism Genetics Resource Exchange (AGRE):** This dataset includes fMRI data from individuals with autism and their family members, as well as genetic and behavioural data. The dataset includes data from over 200 individuals from two different sites.
- **Autism Phenome Project (APP):** This dataset includes fMRI data from individuals with autism and typically developing individuals, as well as genetic and behavioural data. The dataset includes data from over 100 individuals from three different sites.
- **Developmental Connectomics Study of Autism (DCSA):** This dataset includes fMRI data from infants and toddlers with autism and typically developing infants and toddlers, as well as behavioural and clinical data. The dataset includes data from over 200 individuals from two different sites.
- **Human Connectome Project (HCP):** This dataset includes fMRI data from individuals with autism and typically developing individuals, as well as structural MRI data and other measures of brain function. The dataset includes data from over 1000 individuals from two different sites.
- **EU-AIMS Longitudinal European Autism Project (LEAP):** This dataset includes fMRI data from individuals with autism and typically developing individuals, as well as genetic and behavioural data. The dataset includes data from over 200 individuals from four different sites.
- **Autism Research Centre (ARC):** This dataset includes fMRI data from individuals with autism and typically developing individuals, as well as behavioural and genetic data. The dataset includes data from over 100 individuals from two different sites.
- **Autism-MAPS:** The Multi-Site Autism Study on the Pharmacogenomics of Social Communication and Behavioural Domains (Autism-MAPS) is a large-scale dataset that includes fMRI data from individuals with autism and typically developing individuals, as well as genetic and behavioural data. The dataset includes data from over 400 individuals from six different sites.
- **Philadelphia Neurodevelopmental Cohort (PNC):** This dataset includes fMRI data from individuals with autism and typically developing individuals, as well as genetic and behavioural data. The dataset includes data from over 900 individuals from the Philadelphia area.

3.4   Algorithms used to detect autism using AI

Support vector machine (SVM)

SVM is a supervised machine learning method that is used for regression and classification, as seen in Figure 3.6. It solves problems involving pattern recognition. The overfitting issue is not a result of it. A decision boundary is set by SVM to distinguish the classes. For classification and regression analysis, the SVM

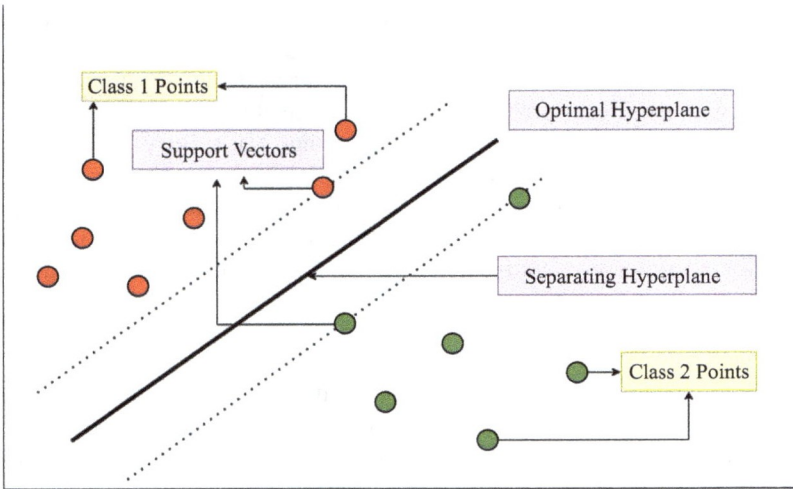

Figure 3.6   An SVM diagram in which two different categories are classified using a decision boundary or hyperplane

machine learning technique is helpful. Both linear and nonlinear datasets can be used with this approach to perform regression and classification. The SVM method finds a hyperplane that divides the data into discrete groups effectively, maximising the distance between the two nearest points from each class. The position and orientation of the hyperplane are determined by the nearest data points from each class, known as the support vectors. SVMs employ the kernel method to map datasets that cannot be separated linearly into a higher dimensional space where a hyperplane can be found to divide the data. The kernel function, which can be linear, polynomial, radial basis function (RBF), or sigmoid depending on the data and problem being studied, is crucial in establishing the geometry of the hyperplane in the transformed feature space. SVMs have a number of benefits, including the capacity to handle datasets with small sample sizes, high dimensionality, and the ability to prevent overfitting. However, they can be computationally expensive, especially for large datasets, and the choice of kernel function and other hyper-parameters can affect how well they perform [24].

Naive Bayes (NB)
Machine learning algorithms like naive Bayes are commonly employed for cate-gorisation tasks like detecting whether a person has autism. By using Bayes' the-orem and prior knowledge of the relevant conditions, it determines the likelihood that an event will occur. In the context of autism, naive Bayes can evaluate various factors linked to the disorder, such as environmental factors, genetic predisposition, and behavioural symptoms. Although it assumes that each factor is independent of the others, which is not always the case, it can still offer accurate results in many

cases. To use naive Bayes for autism classification, it is necessary to train it on a dataset containing both autism and non-autism cases. Subsequently, the probability that a new case belongs to each group is computed based on the factors considered. The group with the higher probability is then assigned to the new case, indicating whether the individual is likely to have autism or not. Naive Bayes is considered to be an effective tool for autism classification, with high accuracy rates reported in several studies. However, the accuracy of the algorithm depends on the quality of the training data and the relevance of the factors analysed. Naive Bayes is not suitable for all types of classification tasks, and other algorithms may be more appropriate for specific problems [25].

CNN

For image and video recognition tasks, the CNN deep learning method is frequently utilised. To find patterns or anomalies that may be connected to the illness, CNN can be used to analyse brain imaging data from MRI scans in the context of autism research. CNN extracts features from the input data through convolutional layers, pooling layers, and activation functions, and the final classification is made by fully connected layers. CNN can be trained on brain imaging data from individuals with and without autism to identify patterns that are more common in one group than the other. CNN has been shown to effectively identify brain imaging biomarkers associated with autism, such as alterations in brain connectivity and grey matter volume. These biomarkers can help in the early detection and diagnosis of autism and can inform treatment strategies. However, CNN is a complex algorithm that requires large amounts of data for training and may be computationally expensive. The accuracy of the algorithm depends on the quality of the training data and the relevance of the features extracted (Figure 3.7). Despite these challenges, CNN has the potential as a tool for autism research and diagnosis [26].

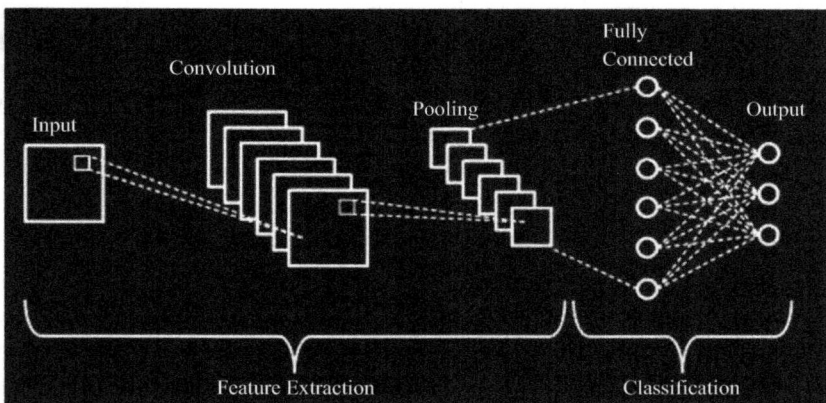

Figure 3.7   CNN architecture

LR

LR is a type of statistical analysis that is often used in medical research, including studies related to autism. The method involves analysing data to determine the relationship between one or more predictor variables and a binary outcome, such as whether a person has autism or not. In this context, logistic regression (LR) can be used to identify potential risk factors for autism and to develop models that can accurately predict whether a person is likely to have the disorder. To use LR for autism research, researchers typically start by collecting data on a set of potential predictor variables, such as age, gender, genetic factors, and environmental exposures. They then use statistical software to analyse the data and identify which variables are most strongly associated with autism. The results of this analysis can be used to develop a model that can predict the likelihood of autism based on the values of the predictor variables. While LR is a widely used statistical method in medical research, it has some limitations. For example, the accuracy of the model depends on the quality and completeness of the data used for analysis, and it may not be able to capture all of the complex interactions between different risk factors for autism. Nevertheless, LR can be a useful tool for identifying potential risk factors and developing predictive models in autism research [27].

K-Nearest neighbour (KNN)

KNN, or K-nearest neighbours, is a machine learning algorithm that can be used in autism research to classify individuals based on their similarity to other known cases. The algorithm works by identifying the KNNs to the input data point in a training dataset and using their classifications to determine the classification of the input data. In the context of autism, KNN can be used to analyse various factors that may be associated with the disorder, such as genetic predisposition, environmental factors, and behavioural symptoms. The algorithm requires a training dataset that includes both known cases of autism and non-autism cases to accurately classify new cases. KNN has been shown to be a useful tool in autism research, with several studies reporting high accuracy rates in classification tasks. However, the algorithm's performance depends on the quality of the training data and the relevance of the factors analysed. Additionally, KNN may not be suitable for all types of classification tasks, and other algorithms may be more appropriate depending on the specific problem being addressed [28].

3.5   Conclusion

The chapter discussed various AI methods used for detecting autism. It was highlighted that while there are many techniques available, none of them have sufficient accuracy or reliability on their own. One method that shows promise is eye tracking, which is fast, inexpensive, and easy to analyse. However, there is not enough evidence to support its long-term reliability. Another method is analysing video and audio for behavioural patterns, such as repetitive movements or unusual speech. Advanced deep learning and computer vision techniques can also be applied to detect autism. While eye tracking is a real-time detection method, it is not reliable on its own but can be used as part of a broader test for autism detection. Wearable devices are a more dependable option, as they contain sensors that collect and analyse patterns together, making them more accurate than detecting facial key points, speech, or eye-tracking separately, despite their limitations. Further study is required for more techniques that can be used for detecting autism.

We propose to create an AI-based system that can assist medical professionals in detecting autism more efficiently by identifying patterns in patient behaviour. The system can be developed with the help of AI, step-by-step, with an appealing interactive user interface that uses tools like modified checklist for autism in toddlers (M-Chat), ages and stages questionnaires (ASQ), and social communication questionnaire (SCQ) for screening. This can be the initial step in identifying children who require further evaluation and intervention for autism. Additionally, the system can be integrated with eye-tracking and machine and deep learning techniques to identify patterns in behaviour, and it can also be incorporated into wearable technology such as the Apple Watch to reduce costs. An application or software can also be created to help people with autism handle daily tasks through speech and by creating a visual schedule for the day. Games designed to help individuals with ASD develop communication skills can be included in the system. It is important to note that assistive technology should not be the sole solution, and individuals with autism should also seek medical care such as psychotherapy and appropriate treatment. It is best to use assistive technology in conjunction with other treatments to support individuals with ASD in their daily lives.

References

[1]   Rad, N. M., Kia, S. M., Zarbo, C., *et al.* (2018). Deep learning for automatic stereotypical motor movement detection using wearable sensors in autism spectrum disorders. *Signal Processing*, 144, 180–191. https://doi.org/10.1016/j.sigpro.2017.10.011.

[2]   Ahmed, I. A., Senan, E. M., Rassem, T. H., *et al.* (2022). Eye tracking-based diagnosis and early detection of autism spectrum disorder using machine learning and deep learning techniques. *Electronics*, 11(4), 530. https://doi.org/10.3390/electronics11040530.

[3]   Nah, Y. H., Young, R. L., and Brewer, N. (2014). Using the autism detection in early childhood (ADEC) and childhood autism rating scales (CARS) to predict long term outcomes in children with autism spectrum disorders. *Journal of Autism and Developmental Disorder,* 44, 2301–2310. https://doi.org/10.1007/s10803-014-2102-1.

[4]   Dawson, G. (2008). Early behavioural intervention, brain plasticity, and the prevention of autism spectrum disorder. *Development and Psychopathology,* 20(3), 775–803.

[5]   Foxx, R. M. (2008). Applied behaviour analysis treatment of autism: the state of the art. *Child and Adolescent Psychiatric Clinics of North America,* 17(4), 821–834.

[6] Sethuraman, S. K., Malaiyappan, N., Ramalingam, R., Basheer, S., Rashid, M., and Ahmad, N. (2023). Predicting Alzheimer's disease using deep neuro-functional networks with resting-state fMRI. *Electronics*, 12(4), 1031.

[7] Saxena, P., Goyal, A., Bivi, M. A., Singh, S. K., and Rashid, M. (2023). Segmentation of nucleus and cytoplasm from H&E-stained follicular lymphoma. *Electronics*, 12(3), 651.

[8] Rana, A., Dumka, A., Singh, R., Rashid, M., Ahmad, N., and Panda, M. K. (2022). An efficient machine learning approach for diagnosing Parkinson's disease by utilizing voice features. *Electronics*, 11(22), 3782.

[9] Madan, P., Singh, V., Chaudhari, V., *et al.* (2022). An optimization-based diabetes prediction model using CNN and bi-directional LSTM in real-time environment. *Applied Sciences*, 12(8), 3989.

[10] Ghayvat, H., Awais, M., Bashir, A. K., *et al.* (2022). AI-enabled radiologist in the loop: novel AI-based framework to augment radiologist performance for COVID-19 chest CT medical image annotation and classification from pneumonia. *Neural Computing and Applications*, 35, 1–19.

[11] Kumar, A., Rawat, J., Kumar, I., *et al.* (2022). Computer-aided deep learning model for identification of lymphoblast cell using microscopic leukocyte images. *Expert Systems*, 39(4), e12894.

[12] Frye, R. E., Vassall, S., Kaur, G., Lewis, C., Karim, M., and Rossignol, D. (2019). Emerging biomarkers in autism spectrum disorder: a systematic review. *Annals of Translational Medicine*, 7(23).

[13] Balachandar, V., Mahalaxmi, I., Neethu, R., Arul, N., and Abhilash, V. G. (2022). New insights into epigenetics as an influencer: an associative study between maternal prenatal factors in autism spectrum disorder (ASD). *Neurology Perspectives*, 2, 78–86.

[14] Jha, N., Prashar, D., Rashid, M., *et al.* (2021). Deep learning approach for discovery of in silico drugs for combating COVID-19. *Journal of Healthcare Engineering*, 2021, 1–13.

[15] Raj, S. & Masood, S. (2020). Analysis and detection of autism spectrum disorder using machine learning techniques. *Procedia Computer Science*, 167, 994–1004.

[16] Siddiqui, U. A., Ullah, F., Iqbal, A., *et al.* (2021). Wearable-sensors-based platform for gesture recognition of autism spectrum disorder children using machine learning algorithms. *Sensors*, 21(10), 3319. https://doi.org/10.3390/s21103319.

[17] Rad, N. M. and Furlanello, C. (2016). Applying deep learning to stereotypical motor movement detection in autism spectrum disorders. In *2016 IEEE 16th International Conference on Data Mining Workshops (ICDMW)*, Barcelona, Spain, 2016, pp. 1235–1242, doi:10.1109/ICDMW.2016.0178.

[18] Wilson, K. P., Carter, M. W., Wiener, H. L., *et al.* (2017). Object play in infants with autism spectrum disorder: a longitudinal retrospective video analysis. *Autism & Developmental Language Impairments*, 2. https://doi.org/10.1177/2396941517713186.

[19]   Wu, C., Liaqat, S., Helvaci, H., *et al.* (2021). Machine learning based autism spectrum disorder detection from videos. In *Healthcom. International Conference on e-Health Networking, Applications and Services*, 2020. https://doi.org/10.1109/healthcom49281.2021.9398924.

[20]   Raj, S. and Masood, S (2020). Analysis and detection of autism spectrum disorder using machine learning techniques. *Procedia Computer Science*, *167*, 994–1004. https://doi.org/10.1016/j.procs.2020.03.399.

[21]   Kosmicki, J. A., Sochat, V., Duda, M., and Wall, D. P. (2015). Searching for a minimal set of behaviours for autism detection through feature selection-based machine learning. *Translational Psychiatry*, 5(2), e514. https://doi.org/10.1038/tp.2015.7

[22]   Anagnostopoulou, P., Alexandropoulou, V., Lorentzou, G., Lykothanasi, A., Ntaountaki, P., and Drigas, A. (2020). Artificial intelligence in autism assessment. *International Journal of Emerging Technologies in Learning (iJET)*, 15(6), 95–107. https://www.learntechlib.org/p/217192/.

[23]   Moridian, P., Ghassemi, N., Jafari, M., *et al.* (2022). Automatic autism spectrum disorder detection using artificial intelligence methods with MRI neuroimaging: a review. *Frontiers in Molecular Neuroscience*, 15. https://doi.org/10.3389/fnmol.2022.999605.

[24]   Eman, D. and Emanuel, A. W. (2019, November). Machine learning classifiers for autism spectrum disorder: a review. In *2019 4th International Conference on Information Technology, Information Systems and Electrical Engineering (ICITISEE)* (pp. 255–260). IEEE.

[25]   Reeta, R., Pavithra, G., Priyanka, V., and Raghul, J. S. (2018, April). Predicting autism using naive Bayesian classification approach. In *2018 International Conference on Communication and Signal Processing (ICCSP)* (pp. 0109–0113). IEEE.

[26]   Haweel, R., Shalaby, A., Mahmoud, A., *et al.* (2021). A robust DWT–CNN-based CAD system for early diagnosis of autism using task-based fMRI. *Medical Physics*, 48(5), 2315–2326.

[27]   Thabtah, F., Abdelhamid, N., and Peebles, D. (2019). A machine learning autism classification based on logistic regression analysis. *Health Information Science and Systems*, 7, 1–11.

[28]   Haque, M. M., Rabbani, M., Dipal, D. D., *et al.* (2021). Informing developmental milestone achievement for children with autism: machine learning approach. *JMIR Medical Informatics*, 9(6), e29242.

Chapter 4

Lossless medical image compression and noise removal using deep learning models

N. Karthikeyan[1], N. Pooranam[2], D. Surendran[3] and M. Sivakumar[4]

With the rapid expansion of the medical industry and advancements in medical sensors, mobile computing, and connectivity, data storage is increased by collecting, processing, and uploading medical data from remote sites for remote medical collaboration and diagnosis. In medical imaging, image reduction is essential for reducing data storage. To balance a good compression ratio (CR), greater image quality after decoding, and minimum processing time is the main problem of the compression technique in medical imaging. Due to increasing the CR, the loss of information in the decoded image impacts major issues in processing medical images. This research chapter presents a new lossless image compression and noise removal scheme using deep learning (DL) models. It focuses on compressing the data without loss of information using deep neural networks and an entropy coding scheme and takes minimum computation time to process the noise removal using different types of DL models. This scheme's performance is measured using the standard performance metrics of CR%, mean square error (MSE), and peak signal-to-noise ratio (PSNR), and its results are compared with JPEG and JPEG-2000.

4.1 Introduction

In the digital field, the data is growing every data to so many applications that deal with digital data. Digital data is more important for analyzing to predict the decision and extracting its features for further process. Image processing is one of the dominant fields that is used in different areas like healthcare, retail, government sector, security, academic, gaming, museums, galleries, etc. Some of the major

[1]School of Computer Science and Engineering, Vellore Institute of Technology, Chennai, India
[2]Department Computer Science and Engineering, Sri Krishna College of Engineering and Technology, Coimbatore, India
[3]Department of Information Technology, Karpagam College of Engineering, Coimbatore, India
[4]Department of Computer Science and Engineering, Saveetha School of Engineering, SIMATS Deemed University, Chennai, India

areas of image compression are feature extraction, clustering, classification, segmentation, image retrieval, security, compression, etc. To process the digital image, the storage is the major concern, that is, increasing the computation time while in analysis. Image compression plays a major role in representing the original image with the lowest number of bits. After minimizing the number of bits needed to represent the image, the network can transmit data very quickly, which also reduces the processing time. Lossless compression [1,2] and lossy compression [3,4] are two forms of image compression that are classed based on the produced image. No data is lost during lossless image compression, leaving the reconstructed image equivalent to the original. The various techniques of lossless image compression are shown in Table 4.1.

The number of bits needed to represent an image with information loss is reduced through lossy compression. In lossless image compression, the resultant image with acceptable information loss is based on the level of quantization such that it is not equivalent to the original image. The techniques of lossy image compression are shown in Table 4.2.

Some features of lossless coding are (i) no damage in the reconstructed image, (ii) ease to implement in hardware and software, and (iii) ease of use and no need for parameters. It is applied to deal with some sensitive data in the area of the medical field like lung cancer detection, tumor cell detection, and some feature

Table 4.1   Lossless image compression techniques

Techniques	Description
Huffman encoding	Based on the frequencies of corresponding characters, minimum-redundancy codes are constructed
Arithmetic coding	Most common lossless encoding technique with wavelet transformation
Run-length (RL) encoding	A single data value and its counts are retained for consecutive items of the same data
Area image compression	Encoding is performed based on identifying large areas of contiguous 1s and 0s
Difference pulse code modulation (DPCM) and predictive coding	The predicted value is found and quantized after which encoding is applied

Table 4.2   Lossy image compression techniques

Techniques	Description
Chroma subsampling technique	It stores color information at a lower resolution than intensity information
Transform coding	It converts the spatial image into frequency domain coefficients. So that, correlation is removed between the pixels of an image
Fractal compression	It reassembles the encoded image by converting data portions into mathematical data termed "fractal codes"

extraction in the specific region of an input image whereas lossy compression is applied to data processing in some fields where the data lost does not impact the result. Spatial and frequency domain-based image compressions are the two important categories of image compression. The data of the original image are directly applied to the computation process in the spatial domain [5], where there is no information loss throughout the inverse compression scheme process. In frequency domain compression, the original pixels are transmitted into transform coefficients value using some popular transformations such as discrete cosine transformation (DCT) [6] and discrete wavelet transformation (DWT) [7]. The most popular transform coding of DCT is used in JPEG compression [8] and DWT is used in the JPEG-2000 compression scheme [7]. When compared to spatial domain compression, frequency domain compression yielded a higher compression ratio. The major steps of JPEP and JPEG-2000 image compression are transformation, quantization, and encoding and decoding. After analysis of spatial and frequency-based image compression schemes, both techniques are treated for medical imaging for the lossless compression scheme. The medical field is one of the major and dominant field where a huge volume of medical data in the form of images are treated to analyze and predict patient diseases.

Recently, convolutional neural network (CNN)-based models [9] are applied to image compression to deal with large quantities of data, and to produce an efficient processing system. These algorithms train the new compression models of more than 1,000 layers. DL-based image coding in the medical field is the most challenging task to analyze it. It saves human life by predicting the disease and identifying issues like brain tumor, cancer cells, etc. The study of artificial intelligence neural networks gives way to deep learning (DL). One of the best examples of deep structure models is pre-fed neural networks with multiple hidden layers, or deep neural networks (DNNs).

Machine learning (ML) and DL [10–12] lead to new models to use in various applications. Image compression is improved through ML–DL in different ways such as remove artifact, determine the quantization coefficients, retrieval the features from the compressed image, color compression, etc. A brief classification of improved JPEG standard and comparative analysis is shown in Figure 4.1.

Over the recent years, DL technology has made tremendous progress in a number of fields, including image processing and computer vision. However, DL for video compression is currently in its development. The democratic work on DL for image and video codecs that have been actively progressing for a few years is

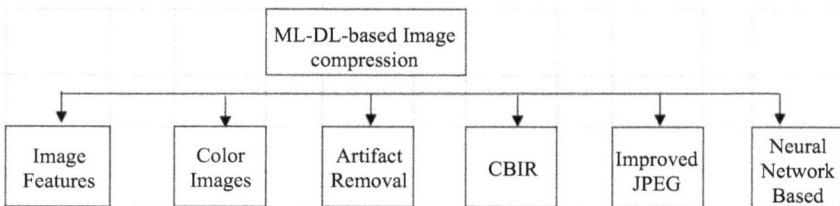

Figure 4.1   ML–DL-based image compression model

examined. The research investigates intelligent image compression techniques developed over the previous 4 years using DL. The structure of the chapter is as follows. JPEG-based compression techniques and their performance are presented in Section 4.2. Section 4.3 briefly describes the DL-based compression models [13] such as convolutional neural network, recurrent neural network, FMM method, autoencoder, and different schemes of image denoising methods and results comparison of JPEG-based coders and DL-based coders, respectively. Finally, the conclusion is reported in Section 4.4.

4.2   JPEG compression schemes

The major steps of JPEG compression scheme are transformation, quantization, and encoding and decoding. The main objective of transform coding is to minimize pixel correlation in the input image. So that, it compresses the image by assigning the minimum number of bits. The popular transform coding used in the JPEG image compression scheme is reported in this section.

4.2.1   DCT

After color conversion, the original grayscale image is split into a number of blocks with a size of (8×8). The original pixel value ranges from 0 to 255 for each block. To translate the original pixel value into transform coefficients, DCT [14] is performed on each block. It reduces the correlation between the pixels in the transformed domain and provides better efficiency of compression. Each DCT block is applied to the inverse DCT technique to produce the original image. Both forward and inverse DCT formula is reported in (4.1) and (4.2).

$$F(u,v) = \frac{2}{N} C(u)C(v)$$
$$\sum_{x=0}^{N-1}\sum_{y=0}^{N-1} f(x,y)\cos\left[\frac{\pi(2x+1)u}{2N}\right]\cos\left[\frac{\pi(2y+1)v}{2N}\right] \tag{4.1}$$

For $u = 0 \ldots N-1$ and $v = 0 \ldots N-1$

Here, $N = 8$ & $C(k) = \left\{ \begin{array}{l} \dfrac{1}{\sqrt{2}} \;\; \text{for} k = 0 \\ 1 \;\;\;\; \text{otherwise} \end{array} \right\}$

$$f(x,y) = \frac{2}{N} \sum_{u=0}^{N-1}\sum_{v=0}^{N-1} C(u)C(v)F(u,v)\cos\left[\frac{\pi(2x+1)u}{2N}\right]\cos\left[\frac{\pi(2y+1)v}{2N}\right] \tag{4.2}$$

For $x = 0 \ldots N-1$ and $y = 0 \ldots N-1$, where $N = 8$.

4.2.2   DWT

In DWT, image pixels are transformed into coefficients that are real values in which the image is split into four sub-bands using low-pass and high-pass filtering techniques

[15]: Low Level (LL), High Level (HL), Low High (LH), and High High (HH) bands are four parts of DWT. The upper left of this region, called LL, is the low-resolution sub-band that concentrates the energy of the image. Then, it is combined with the other sub-bands to obtain the original reconstructed image, which is shown in Figure 4.2. HL and LH carry high-frequency values, not contain much information to reconstruct the image. LL carries only high-frequency values. To recreate the decoded image with maintaining the better quality of PSNR, these three regions are considered in the reverse process [16]. The wavelets transform disintegrates a signal into a collection of basic functions. These functions are known as wavelets as follows:

$$\Psi_{x,y}(z) = \frac{1}{\sqrt{x}} \Psi\left(\frac{z-b}{x}\right) \tag{4.3}$$

To achieve a high compression ratio, three bands, LH, HL, and HH, are ignored in the reverse process [17], which lies in lossy compression. Merits of DWT are to produce a high compression ratio, to remove blocking artifact that is obtained during DCT compression process by dividing the image into non-overlapping 8 × 8 block, to allow both spatial and spectral resolution. An image band contains S1 rows and S2 columns. 2DWT four sub-band images namely A, H, V, and D, each containing S1/2 rows and S2/2 columns is obtained. The forward 2DWT of the function $h(x, y)$ with size coordinates S1 and S2 is given in terms of coefficients as:

$$W_\varphi(s_1, s_2) = \frac{1}{\sqrt{S_1 S_2}} \sum_{y=0}^{S_2-1} \sum_{x=0}^{S_1-1} h(x,y)\varphi_{s_1,s_2}(x,y) \tag{4.4}$$

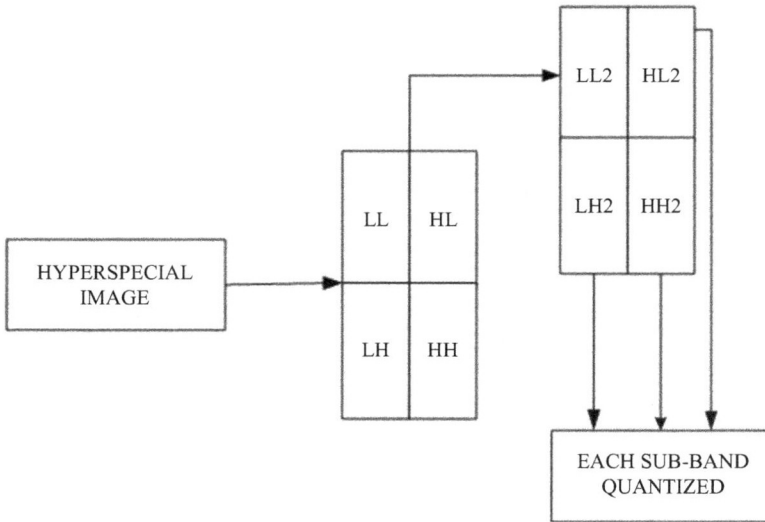

Figure 4.2 Decomposition of HSIs images using filters

$$W_\Psi^m(q,s_1,s_2) = \frac{1}{\sqrt{S_1 S_2}} \sum_{y=0}^{S_2-1} \sum_{x=0}^{S_1-1} h(x,y) \Psi_{q,s_1,s_2}^m(x,y) \tag{4.5}$$

where $m = \{H, V, D\}$,

Here, $m = \{H, V, D\}, \varphi$ denotes the scaling function, and Ψ represents the wavelet function. The coefficients $W_\varphi(s_1,s_2)$ give an approximation of $h(x,y)$. The coefficients $W_\psi^m(q,s_1,s_2)$ provide the horizontal, vertical, and diagonal information.

Conventionally, $s_1 = s_2 = 2^q$ is chosen, so that $q = 0, 1 \ldots Q - 1$. The functions $\varphi_{s_1,s_2}(x,y)$ and $\psi_{q,s_1,s_2}^m(x,y)$ are expressed in terms of wavelet filter coefficients c_φ and c_Ψ, respectively. The wavelet filtering is performed by a biorthogonal wavelet. The inverse 2DWT is calculated as:

$$\begin{aligned} h(x,y) &= \frac{1}{\sqrt{S_1 S_2}} \sum_{s_2} s_1 W_\varphi(s_1,s_2) \varphi_{s_1,s_2}(x,y) \\ &+ \frac{1}{\sqrt{S_1 S_2}} \sum_{m=\{H,v,D\}} \sum_{q=0}^{Q-1} W_\psi^m(s_1,s_2) \psi_{q,s_1,s_2}^m(x,y) \end{aligned} \tag{4.6}$$

4.2.3 Quantization techniques

The obtained transform coefficients after DCT/DWT are then quantized to achieve a higher compression ratio. The technique of quantization involves minimizing the number of possible values for a quantity. It reduces the number of bits required to represent the input image using a quantization matrix, which is provided below:

$$Q_{(i,j)} = round * \frac{DCT_{(i,j)}}{Quantum_{(i,j)}} \tag{4.7}$$

Here $Q_{(i,j)}$ is the corresponding coefficient DCT's quantized value $_{(i,j)}$.

The formula, which is provided below, is used to generate the quantum $_{(i,j)}$ values:

$$Quantum_{(i,j)} = 1 + ((1 + i + j) * qf) \tag{4.8}$$

where qf is a user-inputted quality factor that is usually in the range of 0–255. By decreasing the precision or number of transform coefficients, $Q_{(i,j)}$ is granted the fewest possible bits. Vector quantization (VQ) [18] is another popular quantization technique used in image compression. VQ evaluates the entire data vector before using a look-up table to approximate the coded vector. After transformation and quantization, quantized transform coefficients (QTC) are arranged as 1D array components using zigzag to remove the continuous zero coefficients, which are presented in each (8 × 8) block in 2D. By avoiding these zeroes, it can store the last nonzero quantized transform coefficient and attain a larger CR. Finally, the encoder is performed on each QTC (8 × 8) block and turns the coefficients into a compressed image bitstream. The inverse encoder method is applied to encoded bits to obtain the original image, which is referred to as a decoded image.

4.2.4   Encoding techniques

The encoder plays an essential role in image compression and is subjected to transform coefficients to store the image in terms of 0s and 1s as bit-stream. Some of the encoding techniques are listed below.

4.2.4.1   Huffman coding

The Huffman encoding technique is a well-known entropy encoding and it achieves a good lossless compression due to no information loss in the reverse process of encoding. This algorithm assigns the minimum number of bits to the variable length pair value. It reduces the coding redundancy due to assigning code words that were generated from the Huffman table to the input source symbol [19]. In this process, the most frequently occurring values are assigned with a lower number of bits, and low-frequency occurring values are assigned with higher bits.

4.2.4.2   Arithmetic coding

To increase the compression ratio and storage, arithmetic coding is used to apply in compression technique. It is a well-known lossless compression algorithm, such as JPEG2000. It reads the entire file as a sequence of source symbols as a single unit. This input source symbol is applied to multiple iterations by dividing the initial interval into subintervals to encode it [20]. Each source symbol is encoded differently depending on the probability assigned to it, with a starting range of 0–1. Maximum bits are assigned to lower-frequency source symbols and lower bits are assigned to higher-frequency source symbols. On the observation of experimental results, arithmetic coding achieves higher compression than Huffman coding, and implementation of Huffman coding is easier than arithmetic coding.

4.2.4.3   Golomb_Rice coding

Golomb_Rice (GR) coder [21] is an optimal encoding technique with infinite prefix codes. Each code for the probability of the source symbol is classified into a nonnegative integer value as k. To encode the nonnegative integer "i" by using GR coder of k, it constructs the prefix codeword $[i/2k]$ using unary code then construct suffix code word $[i \bmod 2k]$ using binary codes for the corresponding values. To generate the codebook, the above process is considered as two sections: quotient (Q) and remainder (R). The computation formula of Q is: $Q = \text{int } [n/m]$, where m denotes the parameter value of the GR code. The formula to find R is: $R = n$ modulo m. The output bits for Q are made up of Q number of "1" followed by a "0" and for R is the binary or offset value of R. The code words are defined individually based on their input value and make reference to the codebook.

4.2.4.4   Modified Huffman coding

To increase the transmission efficiency and increase the storage capacity, Modify Huffman encoding techniques [22] are reported by the researchers in the compression area. This modified Huffman coding algorithm consists of two phases to compress the quantized transform coefficients with a minimum number of bits. In the first phase, a unique source symbol and its occurrence were found then it is applied to generate binary codes. Finally, the compressed binary codes of the first level are applied to Huffman coding to generate bitstream to compress the bits further. This modified algorithm increases the compression ratio, and higher compression ratio slightly than Huffman coding.

4.2.4.5 LLEC coding

It refers GR_Fundamental Sequence (GR_FS) code and Zero Tree Coding (ZTC). The GR_FS code [23] yields a code word for a value of n, which consists of two parts. One finds the length of the bits of n, denoted as L, and the binary value of n. The output bits of L are made up of an L number of "0" followed by a "1." The LLEC output for the quantized transformed coefficient value n=42 is split into L and the binary value of n. L bits are 0000001 and the binary value of m is 101010. Hence, the output bits are 0000001101010. ZTS bit is presented either as 0 or 1, after the GR_FS code word. If the last bit of the code word is 0, the first level coefficient value has a child with a non-zero coefficient value in three child-parent relationships else the child has all zeros. The codeword is generated from the first level (parent) to child levels with a non-zero coefficient and starts with 0 bit after the GR_FS bit. However, the code words used in this work are individually specified by their input value; therefore, a codebook is not necessary. So, compressing the image requires less computational effort.

4.2.4.6 FELE coding

JPEG-based image encoding technique [24] is used to compress the image with low processing time and low memory, that is called "Fast and Efficient Lossless Encoder." The transform coefficients are applied to differential pulse code modulation (DPCM), then directly applied to FELE coding to produce bitstream. The binary bitstream is converted for each transform coefficient. The length of b is calculated and is denoted by L, and it is used to split even or odd series of b. The formula in the equation is used to calculate the lesser number of bits in an even series "p" if L is an even series of length b (4.9):

$$p = \frac{n}{2} \tag{4.9}$$

Here "p" number of "0" bits is included in the encoding section, followed by "1" bits, to reduce the correlation period between the pixels that contain fewer reference bits. The binary bit representing n is then added following the reference bits.

Eq. (4.10) can be used to calculate the lesser number of bits in an even series "q" if L is an odd series with length b:

$$q = \frac{n-1}{2} + 1 \tag{4.10}$$

In the encoding section, "q" number of "1" bits is included, followed by "0" bits used as reference bits. After the reference bits, the binary bit of n is added. Let *n* be 19. *L* is 5, where "b" of *n* is 10011. *L* is used to solve the odd series equation and get the value of *q*, which is 3. As a result, the reference bit for n is 1110, while the *b*-bit for *n* is 10011. Using the FELE coder, the bitstream for 19 is 100111110. If *n* is negative, such as −16, then b is 01111 (1'se complement of 10000), and b's *L* is 5. *L* is used to solve for *q*, which equals 3, in the odd series equation. As a result, the reference bit of *n* is 1000 and the *b* of *n* is 01111. Finally, using the suggested coder, the bitstream for −16 is 100001111.

4.2.4.7   ZTC coding

The transform coefficients are subjected to ZTC processing to take advantage of the zero-tree structure and improve the CR% by using fewer bits to encode the zero trees. To find the bitstream using the ZTC technique, some parameters are computed that are transform coefficients (*n*), bitstream (b), length of bitstream (L), odd series of bitstream (4.10), and even series bitstream (4.9). From the DCT $f^{\wedge}(x,y)$ block series as 74,8,−4,2, −2,0,0,0,0,0,0, 0,0,0,0,0,0,0,0,0,0,0,0,0 ,0,0,0,0,0,0,0, 0,0, 0,0,0,0,0,0,0,0,0,0,0,0,0,0,0,0, 0,0,0,0,0,0,0,0,0,0,0,0,0,0,0,0, Let *n* is 74. The reference bit for *n* is 11110, and 1001010 is used as bit "b" of *n*. The *L* of bit "b" is 7, and bit "b" of *n* is 1001010. Using the recommended FELE coder, the bitstream for 74 is 111101001010. Once generated the bits for "n" are then applied to ZTC. All the "s" values of 74 are not zero coefficients. So that, add "1" bit in 1 bit and pass 8, 2, and −4 "s" to FELE. The bitstream of 8, 2, and −4 using the proposed FELE coder are 0011001, 0110, and 110011, respectively. All the "ss" values of 8 are not zero. So that, add "1" bit in 1 bit by ZTC, and −2, 0, 0, and 0 "s" are passed to FELE. The bitstream of −2, 0, 0, and 0 using the proposed FELE coder are 0011001, 0110, and 110011, respectively. All the "ss" values of −2 are zero then add '0' bit. All the 'ss' values of 2 are zero. So that, add '0' bit in 1 bit by ZTC. All the 'ss' values of −4 are zero. So that, add '0' bit in 1 bit by ZTC. Once all the 'ss' values are zero, the process is immediately stopped after adding the '0' bit for every 's' value. Finally, the bitstream of ZTC-FELE proposed coder is 111101001010 1 001100101101 1 001110011001 0 0 0 0 0. Zero coding (add '0' bit when all 'ss' are zero for 'n' and add '1' bit when all 'ss' are non-zero for 'n') bit is mentioned with box symbol.

4.2.5   *JPEG encoding process*

The following is a detailed explanation of the encoding algorithm's steps:
   Input: An image in monochrome that is the size of (ROW × COL)
   Output: Bitstream encoded with the suggested JPEG coder
   Begin

1. Create 8 × 8 non-overlapping subblocks from the input image.
2. As described in Section 4.1, apply DCT to each block of *I(i,j)*.
3. Perform scalar quantization (SQ) on transform coefficients with various qf as mentioned in Section 4.2.
4. As stated in Section 4.2, apply scalar quantization (SQ) to the transform coefficients.

5. To find the last non-zero coefficient in the zigzag quantization block.
6. Apply DPCM for each block's DC coefficient (i,j)
7. Apply the JPEG coder, as described in Section 4.4, to transform the quantization block into the bitstream.

    End

The JPEG-based coder's reverse approach is used to retrieve the lossless reconstructed image. The described system is tested using more than 200 example images with a (256×256) resolution and evaluated with various encoding methods. Various encoder schemes are used to examine the obtained results.

4.2.6   JPEG decoding process

The following is a detailed explanation of the decoding algorithm's steps:
   Input: Bitstream encoded with the suggested JPEG coder
   Output: Reconstructed image
   Begin

1. Start a disc and load the image's bitstream
2. Use the JPEG coder's reverse method to convert the bitstream into QTC.
3. Divide the coefficient values into (8×8) blocks to create the image's decoded blocks.
4. Apply the differential DC inverse procedure to each block.
5. Perform the de-quantization.
6. Execute the inverse transformation on each block before merging the partition to get the reconstructed image.

    End

4.2.7   JPEG compression: experimental results

The experiments and an analysis of various parameters have been described in this section for the JPEG and JPEG-2000 approaches. The performance of the presented techniques has been tested with other JPEGs' techniques such as modified Huffman, LLEC, and Golomb-Rice coding techniques. To conduct the experiments, the different sets of sample images are tested using JPEG, JPEG-2000, and compared with other standard schemes. Figure 4.3(a–c) displays sample images of brain tumors that are (256×256) in size. These sample images are subjected to JPEG transformation like DCT and DWT, then the results are subjected to quantization with various quality scales. The JPEG scheme gives an average value of 84 CR% with 34.56 dB PSNR for different sets of brain tumor images, as shown in Figure 4.4(a–c). The JPEG-2000 scheme achieves an average value of 86 CR% with 37.25 dB PSNR for different sets of brain tumor images, are shown in Figure 4.5(a–c). For performance analysis, the results of JPEG and JPEG-2000 are compared to LLEC, GR, and FELE coder. LLEC-based JPEG gives an average value of 83 CR% and 32.56 dB PSNR, whereas GR gives 79 CR% and 31.5 dB

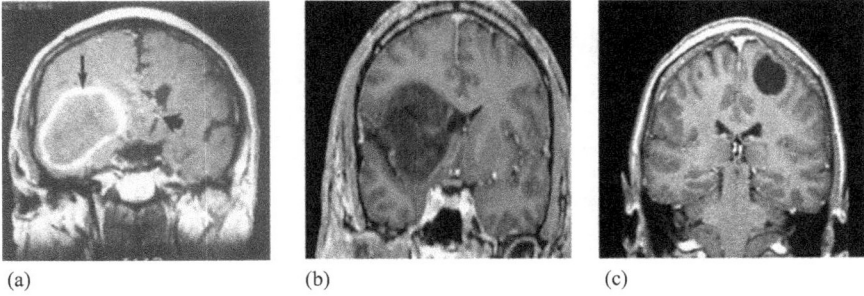

(a)   (b)   (c)

Figure 4.3   Brain tumors – test images (256 × 256)

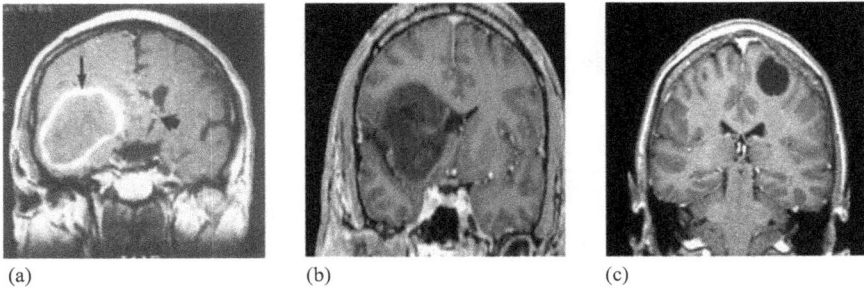

(a)   (b)   (c)

Figure 4.4   Resultant images of JPEG-based Huffman for test images

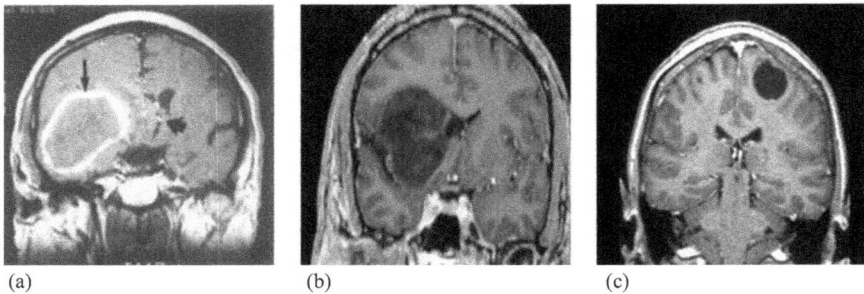

(a)   (b)   (c)

Figure 4.5   Resultant images of JPEG-2000-based arithmetic for test images

PSNR, are shown in Figure 4.6(a–c). LLEC-based JPEG gives an average value of 83 CR% and 32.56 dB PSNR, are shown in Figure 4.6(a–c). whereas GR gives 79 CR% and 31.5 dB PSNR, are shown in Figure 4.7(a–c). The FELE-based JPEG achieves 83 CR% and 32.56 dB PSNR for the same sets of brain tumor images, are shown in Figure 4.8(a–c).

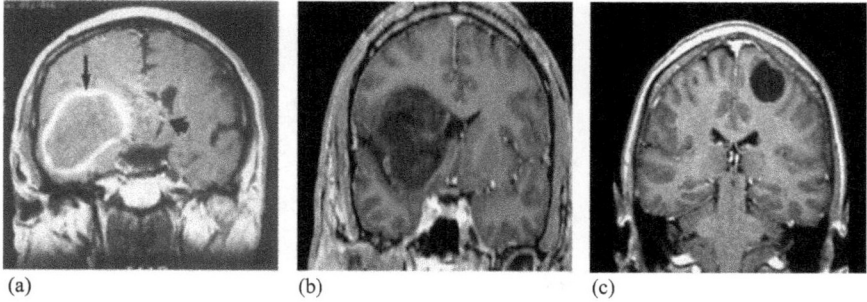

Figure 4.6   Resultant images of JPEG-based LLEC for test images

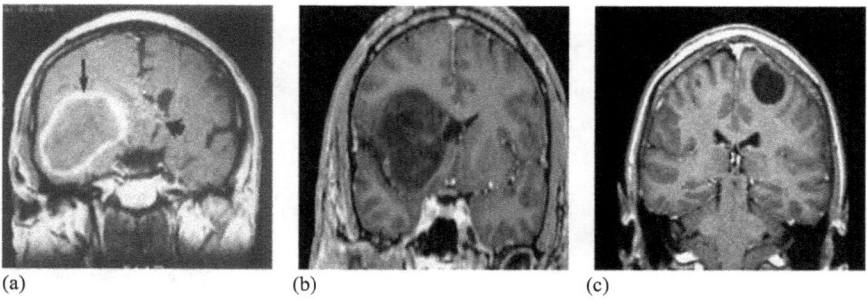

Figure 4.7   Resultant images of JPEG-based GR for test images

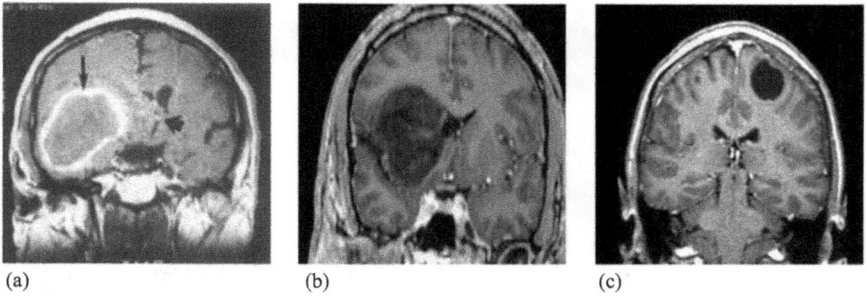

Figure 4.8   Resultant images of JPEG-based FELE for test images

4.3   Types of compression schemes and noise removal techniques using DL

The popular JPEG/JPEG-2000 compression techniques produce a lossless image while in the inverse process of encoding techniques. In the medical industry, it is really utilized to analyze essential characteristics of images to locate disease-causing cells or predicting problems that could save lives. In recent years, new schemes are required to find important properties and analyzing the features of complex problems. Due to the large data set and their processing time, the researchers used DL and machine learning-based models [25,26] like different types of neural networks, auto-encoder scheme, and end-to-end compression scheme. These schemes perform well along with traditional compression schemes. It is useful for the researchers to be aware of the present trends and future developments. For image compression, deep neural networks, artificial neural networks, recurrent neural networks, and convolutional neural networks are some of the various neural networks required. To achieve superior image compression with high accuracy, minimize loss, and enhance the quality of the reconstructed image, this chapter explored how to apply the DL rule to various neural networks. Therefore, to achieve these things, DL is required, along with its justified application to various image types and distinct analyses. Some of the DL techniques are discussed in the section, as follows.

4.3.1   Five modulus method (FMM) for image compression

A new type of image compression [11,13] was built to compress the image with more reliable and error free, which is called FMM. It treats the spatial value of an input image in which the whole image is treated into a number of equal size blocks with a size of 8×8. In each block, the pixel values are multiplied by 5 to construct the 6-bit length value. It has less storage than compared to the original length size of 8-bit pixel value.

The FMM algorithm [13] checks the following constraints to design the newly processed pixel values with a length of 6-bit.

If $I(i, j)$ mod 5 is EQUALS to 4,
   SET $I(i, j)$ +1 to $I(i, j)$
ELSE IF $I(i, j)$ mod 5 EQUALS to 3,
   SET $I(i, j)$ +2 to $I(i, j)$
ELSE IF $I(i, j)$ mod 5 EQUALS to 2,
   SET $I(i, j)$ −2 to $I(i, j)$
ELSE IF $I(i, j)$ mod 5 EQUALS to 1,
   SET $I(i, j)$ −1 to $I(i, j)$

Figure 4.9 shows that original pixel values of 8×8 block and its transformed pixel value using FMM.

Again, the resultant FMM values are divided by 5 to find the remainder between 0 and 51. Even it performs well when compared to the traditional JPEG compression scheme, it is observed that it is not the optimal compression method, considered as an existing technique.

4.3.2   Recurrent neural network

Recurrent neural networks (RNN) are artificial neural networks [11,27] that employ sequential data or time series data (RNN). These DL techniques are frequently used for speech recognition, natural language processing (NLP), picture captioning, and

Old	New		Old	New
0	0		90	90
1	1		91	90
2	0		92	95
3	5	. . .	93	95
4	5		94	95
5	5		95	95
6	5		96	95
7	5		97	95
8	10		98	100
9	10		99	100
10	10		100	100

Figure 4.9   Sample RGB values and their transformed FMM values

RNNs like feedforward and convolutional neural networks (CNNs). Based on the data that is retained in their memory, these approaches can be distinguished from one another. It makes use of information from earlier inputs to enable the present input and output. As opposed to standard deep neural networks, which assume that inputs and outputs are independent of one another, recurrent neural networks' outputs are dependent on the previous components in the sequence. These stand out due to their "memory," which allows them to affect the current input and output by using data from previous inputs. Recurrent neural networks' outputs are dependent on the previous parts in the sequence, unlike typical deep neural networks, which presume that inputs and outputs are independent of one another. Uni-directional RNNs are useful for forecasting the result of specific sequences, but they are unable to account for future occurrences in their predictions.

Other than mentioned the above applications, image compression is one of the major parts where the bitstream of the image is reduced and gives good results in terms of MSE and PSNR. The RNN structure includes both fully and partially linked networks, and several layer feedforward networks have specific input and output layers. The entirely (fully) connected networks, as shown in Figure 4.9(a) and (b), do not have distinct input layers of nodes; rather, each node serves as the input for every other node. It is feasible for the node to provide feedback.

The simple partial recurrent neural network is used to learn character strings, as shown in Figure 4.10(a). The sequential context of other nodes will be presented since certain nodes are a feedforward framework, and feedback from other nodes is obtained. Backpropagation [27,28] will be used to process the context unit weights (C1 and C2) in the same manner as the input unit weights. In the case of a simple RNN, the context units get a time-delayed response from the layer units. Training

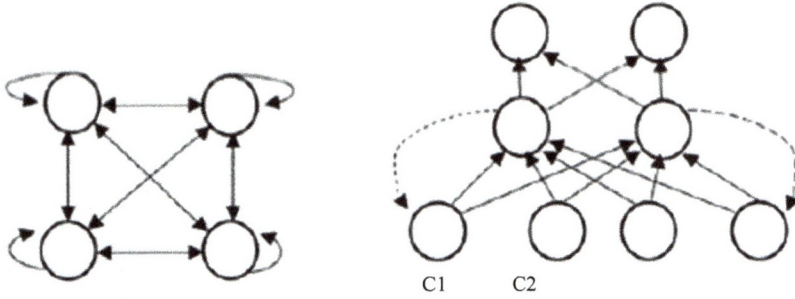

Figure 4.10   (a) RNN fully connected. (b) Simple RNN.

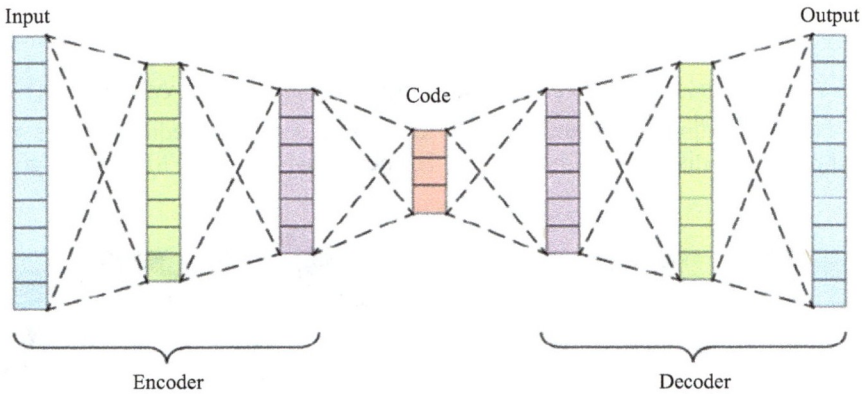

Figure 4.11   SAE architecture with encoder and decoder

data consists of inputs and the outputs that are intended to replace them. A character string's next letter can be predicted by the net, which can also be trained to evaluate a character string.

4.3.3   Autoencoder

DL is mostly used in the current field to analyze the image by learning different patterns from the input image, then It transforms it into a different pattern with fewer parts. By varying the weight of connections among the layers, the neural network learns the model. Supervised and unsupervised learning are two important learning mechanisms. One of the unsupervised learning models preferred in the research domain is auto-encoder. The major aim of auto-encoder is to represent or encoding the dataset, which is achieved by learning the network to ignore the noise reduction. It creates an encoding in the inverse process. In generative data models, the auto-encoder concept is widely employed. The input layer is used by the Autoencoder to compress data and create a short code. The code is then converted into a form that is similar to the original data and decompressed [9]. Figure 4.11

shows the encoder and decoder layers of the simple autoencoder (SAE) architecture.

The major applications of autoencoder are image compression and image denoising. In image compression. In this approach, the size of the hidden layer in the autoencoder is exactly smaller than the size of the output layer. The auto-encoder is forced to learn the low-dimensional representation of the input data when trained using the same input values as the target values through back-propagation. The data is compressed by the active hidden layer. Image de-noising: a non-linear feature architecture of autoencoder is used in denoising the image. It removes the noise which occurred in the processed image, using some random noise methods like Gaussian noise, linear and non-linear filter, and threshold method. This approach trains the network to build the reconstructed image without any noise. A sample image with de-noising process and compression scheme is shown in Figures 4.12–4.14.

4.3.4   DL-based compression scheme: experimental results

DL-based encoding techniques are applied to various sets of medical images and their results are discussed in this section. The performance of the FMM model gives

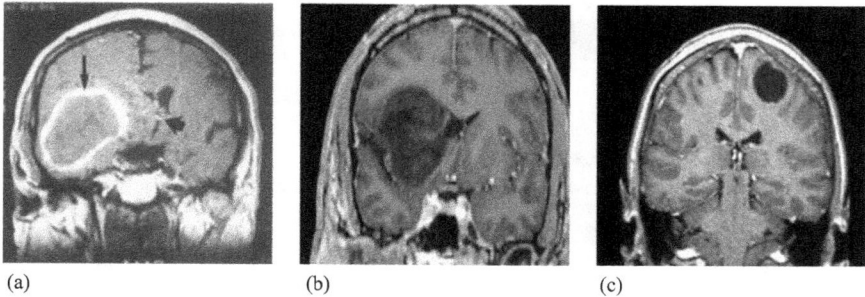

(a)   (b)   (c)

Figure 4.12   Resultant images of the FMM method for test images

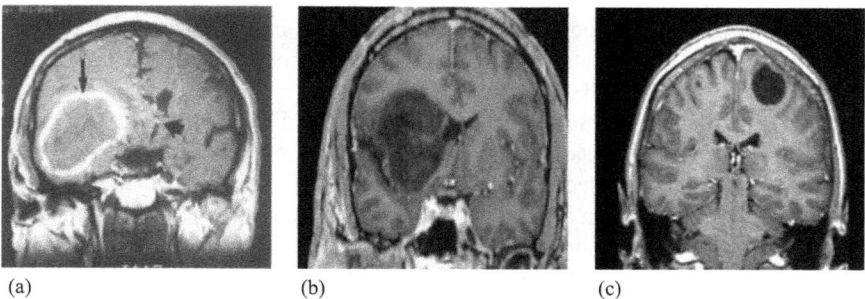

(a)   (b)   (c)

Figure 4.13   Resultant images of the RNN method for test images

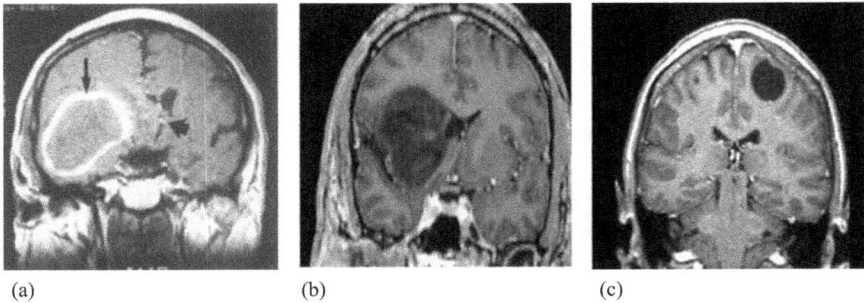

(a)   (b)   (c)

Figure 4.14   Resultant images of the auto-encoder method for test images

Table 4.3   CR % values obtained by JPEG-based coders and DL-based coders for different images

Test images (256 × 256)	JPEG	JPEG-2000	LLEC	GR	FELE	FMM method	RNN	Autoencoder
Set 1	95.52	95.53	92.03	74.92	91.43	92.48	96.06	96.10
Set 2	95.39	95.40	91.91	74.03	90.79	91.82	95.48	95.64
Set 3	93.51	93.81	89.33	42.52	94.09	94.08	96.82	96.90
Set 4	96.23	96.30	91.89	56.74	93.95	93.99	96.77	96.79
Set 5	95.66	95.72	92.21	72.67	95.36	95.72	97.28	97.31

achieves an average value of 89.52 CR% with 35.87 dB PSNR for different sets of brain tumor images, are shown in Figure 4.12(a)–(c). RNN-based compression scheme gives an average value of 91.12 CR% with 38.87dB PSNR for different sets of brain tumor images, are shown in Figure 4.13(a)–(c). Autoencoder-based compression scheme achieves an average value of 92.31 CR% with 38.85 dB PSNR for different sets of brain tumor images, are shown in Figure 4.14(a)–(c).

For performance analysis, the results of JPEG and JPEG-2000 are compared to DL-based methods such as FMM, RNN, and autoencoder. The results of CR%, BPP, and PSNR of JPEG-based coders and DL-based coders are tabulated in Tables 4.3, 4.4, and 4.5, respectively. The average results of CR%, BPP, and PSNR are shown in Figures 4.15, 4.16, and 4.17, respectively.

4.3.5   DL-based noise removal models

A process that involves an image to remove the noise from it. It can occur in different ways like low-resolution images captured in low light intensity, sensor illumination of camera and bit error due to faulty memory location, etc. The various noise types [29,30] are impulse noise (IN) and additive white Gaussian noise. The original pixels are completely different from the surrounding pixels whereas

Table 4.4   BPP values obtained by JPEG-based coders and DL-based coders for different images

Test images (256 × 256)	JPEG	JPEG-2000	LLEC	GR	FELE	FMM method	RNN	Autoen-coder
Set 1	0.36	0.36	0.64	2.01	0.69	0.60	0.32	0.31
Set 2	0.37	0.37	0.65	2.08	0.74	0.65	0.36	0.35
Set 3	0.52	0.50	0.85	4.60	0.47	0.47	0.25	0.25
Set 4	0.30	0.30	0.65	3.46	0.48	0.48	0.26	0.26
Set 5	0.35	0.34	0.62	2.19	0.37	0.34	0.22	0.22

Table 4.5   PSNR values obtained by JPEG-based coders and DL-based coders for different images

Test images (256 × 256)	JPEG	JPEG-2000	LLEC	GR	FELE	FMM method	RNN	Autoen-coder
Set 1	36.65	36.65	36.65	36.65	36.65	28.25	38.12	39.68
Set 2	36.03	36.03	34.57	36.03	34.57	27.32	38.61	40.21
Set 3	36.03	36.03	29.70	36.03	29.70	28.94	38.28	39.47
Set 4	30.21	30.21	31.09	30.21	31.09	32.47	37.56	38.85
Set 5	31.76	31.76	36.76	31.76	36.76	33.56	38.40	39.45

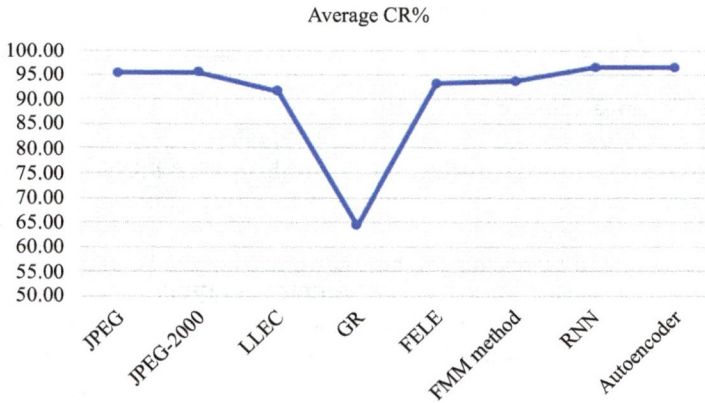

Figure 4.15   Comparison of CR% of JPEG-based encoders and DL-based encoders

AWGN has pixels that will be changed from its original pixels. Salt-and-pepper impulse noise (SPIN) and random valued impulse noise are the two varieties of IN (RVIN). The common challenge to the researchers or medical industry is to remove the noise or unwanted signal which occurred in the image and recover the original

Average BPP

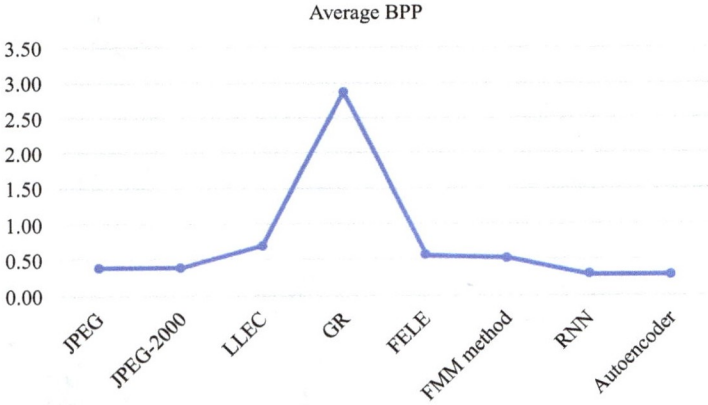

Figure 4.16   Comparison of BPP of JPEG-based encoders and DL-based encoders

Average PSNR

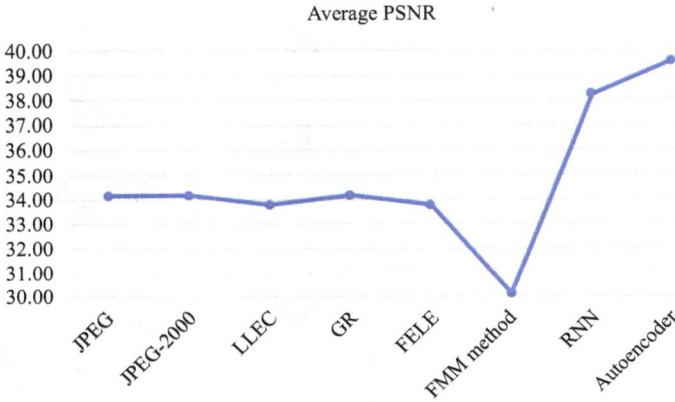

Figure 4.17   Comparison of PSNR of JPEG-based encoders and DL-based encoders

image from its degradation. The performance measurement is also important that are computation and performance level of quality. To deal with these issues, neural network-based models are developed and applied to the processed image to get good results. In the beginning, the first cut technique builds input pipelines that accept input data patches and add some random noise to it. The common convolutional autoencoder model is designed with TensorFlow keras using these noisy patches. Some of the DL model architectures are deep neural networks, CNN models, deep CNN, etc. The Sample dataset images, and its corresponding noise images denoising images using autoencoder and median filter images are shown in Figure 4.18(a)–(c), respectively.

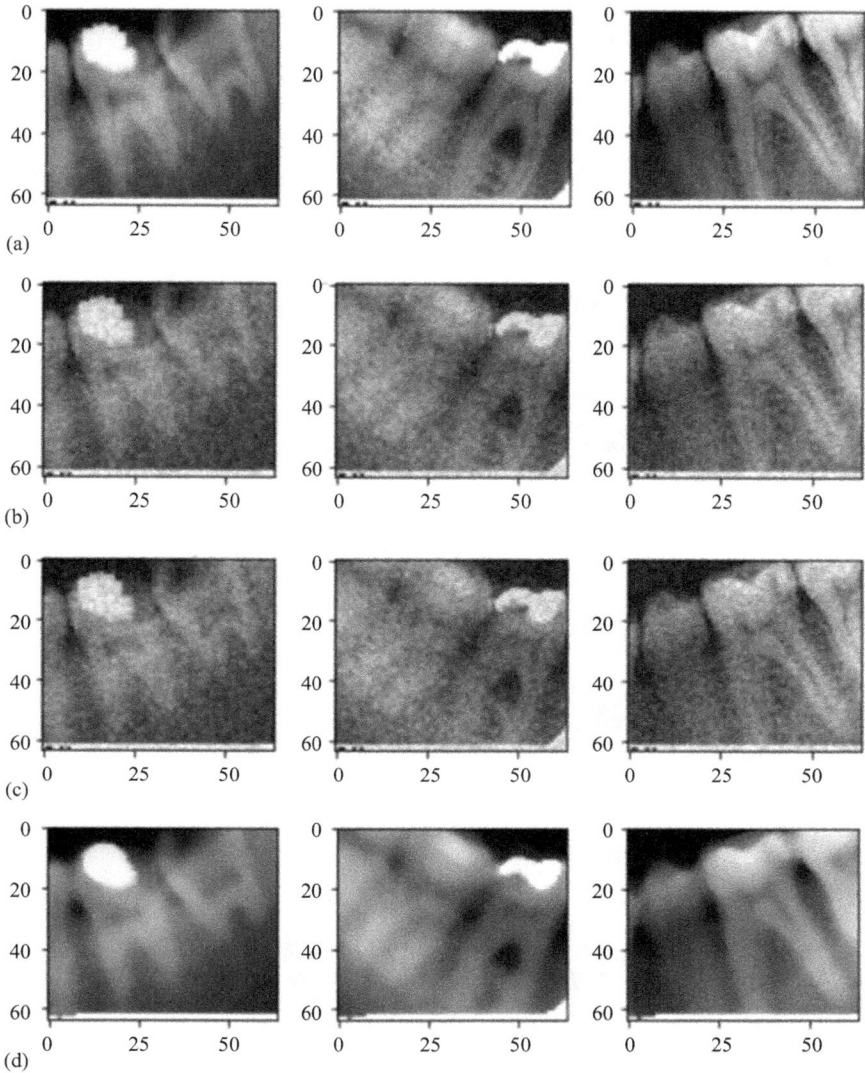

Figure 4.18   (a) Sample dataset images with corresponding noise images, (b) denoising images using autoencoder and (c) median filter images

4.4   Conclusion

This survey investigates the problem of image compression using JPEG, JPEG-2000, and DL-based schemes to provide efficient CR% and better quality of PSNR in the decoded images. Initially, the different types of compression schemes in both spatial and frequency domains are discussed in the literature review. It helps to identify the issues in image compression and indicates that deeper research is required for image compression. This research focuses on different types of image compression schemes using DL to achieve higher CR% and maintain good PSNR with low computation time. The algorithms of image compression in both JPEG and DL are analyzed for different sets of medical images with size of (256 × 256). The performance of DL-based schemes is better than JPEG coders in terms of CR% and PSNR. From the analysis, JPEG-based arithmetic coder achieves a CR of 95.35%, BPP of 0.37, and PSNR of 34.14. DL-based coders achieve higher CR of 96.55%, BPP of 0.28, and PSNR of 39.53 compared to JPEG coders.

References

[1]   A. Tariq Bhatti and J. Kim, 'Implementation of lossless Huffman coding: image compression using K-means algorithm and comparison vs. random numbers and message source', *International Research Journal of Engineering and Technology*, 2015, vol. 2, no. 5, pp. 497–505.

[2]   H. Wu, X. Sun, J. Yang, W. Zeng, and F. Wu, 'Lossless compression of JPEG coded photo collections', *IEEE Transactions on Image Processing*, 2016, vol. 25, no. 6, pp. 2684–2696.

[3]   N. Karthikeyan, N.M. Saravana Kumar, and S.R. Mugunthan, 'Comparative study of lossy and lossless image compression techniques', *International Journal of Engineering & Technology*, 2018, vol. 3, no. 34, pp. 950–953.

[4]   A.A. Shah, S. A. Parah, M. Rashid, and M. Elhoseny. 'Efficient image encryption scheme based on generalized logistic map for real time image processing', *Journal of Real-Time Image Processing*, 2020, vol. 17, no. 6, pp. 2139–2151.

[5]   M. George, M. Thomas, and C.K. Jayadas, 'A methodology for spatial domain image compression based on hops encoding', *Procedia Technology*, 2016, vol. 25, pp. 52–59.

[6]   T. Prabakar Joshua, M. Arrivu Kannamma, and J.G.R. Sathia Seelan, 'Comparison of DCT and DWT image compression', *International Journal of Computer Science and Mobile Computing*, 2016, vol. 5, no. 1, pp. 62–67.

[7]   R. Starosolski, 'Application of reversible denoising and lifting steps to DWT in lossless JPEG 2000 for improved bitrates', *Signal Processing: Image Communication*, 2015, vol. 39, pp. 249–263.

[8]   G. Lakhani, 'Modifying JPEG binary arithmetic codec for exploiting inter/ intra-block and DCT coefficient sign redundancies', *IEEE Transactions on Image Processing*, 2012, vol. 22, no. 4, pp. 1326–1339.

[9]   H.M. Yasin and A.M. Abdulazeez, 'Image compression based on deep learning: a review', *Asian Journal of Research in Computer Science*, 2021, vol. 8, no. 1, pp. 62–76.

[10] Sethuraman, S. Kumar, N. Malaiyappan, *et al.* 'Predicting Alzheimer's disease using deep neuro-functional networks with resting-state fMRI', *Electronics*, 2023, vol. 12, no. 4, p. 1031.

[11] https://heartbeat.comet.ml/image-compression-using-different-machine-learn-ing-techniques-5787c88515f8

[12] L. Theis, W. Shi, A. Cunningham, and F. Huszar, 'Lossy image compression with compressive autoencoders', *CoRR, abs/1703*.00395, 2017.

[13] https://heartbeat.comet.ml/a-2019-guide-to-deep-learning-based-image-com-pression-2f5253b4d811

[14] M. Rashid, H. Singh, and V. Goyal, 'FFTPSOGA: Fast Fourier Transform with particle swarm optimization and genetic algorithm approach for pattern identification of brain responses in multi subject fMRI data', in: *Multimedia Tools and Applications*, 2023, Springer, New York, NY, pp. 1–20.

[15] L. Yang, X. He, G. Zhang, L. Qing, and T. Che, 'A low complexity block-based adaptive lossless image compression', *Optik*, 2013, vol. 124, no. 24, pp. 6545–6552.

[16] J.C. Goswami and A.K. Chan, *Fundamentals of Wavelets – Theory, Algorithms and Applications*, Wiley-Interscience, 2010.

[17] R. Starosolski, 'Application of reversible denoising and lifting steps to DWT in lossless JPEG 2000 for improved bitrates', *Signal Processing: Image Communication*, 2015, vol. 39, pp. 249–263.

[18] M.A. Brifcani and J.N. Al-Bamerny, 'Image compression analysis using multistage vector quantization based on discrete wavelet transform', in: *Proceedings of the 2010 International Conference on Methods and Models in Computer Science (ICM2CS)*, 2010, pp. 46–53.

[19] R. Patel, V. Kumar, V. Tyagi, and V. Asthana, 'A fast and improved image compression technique using Huffman coding', in: *International Conference on Wireless Communications, Signal Processing and Networking*, 2016, IEEE, pp. 2283–2286.

[20] G. Langdon and J. Rissanen, 'Compression of black-white images with arithmetic coding', *IEEE Transactions on Communications*, 1981, vol. 29, no. 6, pp. 858–867.

[21] R. Sugiura and N. Harada, 'Optimal golomb-rice code extension for lossless coding of low-entropy exponentially distributed sources', *IEEE Transactions on Information Theory*, 2018, vol. 64, no. 4, pp. 3153–3161.

[22] N.D. Salih, A. Abid, and C. Eswaran, 'Efficient retinal image compression based on modified Huffman algorithm', *International Journal of Engineering Research and Technology*, 2019, vol. 12, no. 7, pp. 942–948.

[23] D. Zhao, W. Gao, S. Shan, and Y.K. Chan, 'LLEC: an image coder with low-complexity and low-memory requirement', in: *Advances in Multimedia Information Processing*, 2001, Springer, New York, NY, pp. 957–962.

[24] N. Karthikeyan, N.M. Saravanakumar, and M. Sivakumar, 'Fast and effi-cient lossless encoder in image compression with low computation and low memory', *IET Image Processing*, 2021, vol. 15(6), pp. 2494 –2507.

[25] D. Erdogmus and J.C. Principe, 'Entropy minimization algorithm for mul-tilayer perceptrons neural networks', in *2001 International Joint Conference on Proceedings of IJCNN'01*, 2001, vol. 4.

[26]   G. Toderici, 'Full resolution image compression with recurrent neural networks', 2016, arXiv preprint arXiv:1608.05148.

[27]   M.I. Patel, S. Suthar, and J. Thakar, 'Survey on image compression using machine learning and deep learning', in: *IEEE – International Conference on Intelligent Computing and Control Systems*, 2019, pp. 1103–1105.

[28]   A.S. Abd-Alzhra and M.S.H. Al-Tamimi, 'Image compression using deep learning: methods and techniques', *Iraqi Journal of Science*, 2022, vol. 63, pp. 1299–1312.

[29]   https://medium.com/analytics-vidhya/noise-removal-in-images-using-deep-learning-models-3972544372d2#:~:text=Noise%20removal%20in%20images%20using%20deep%20learning%20models,...%208%208.%20Model%20Analysis%20...%20More%20items

[30]   C. Tian, L. Fei, W. Zheng, Y. Xu, W. Zuo, and C.-W. Lin, 'Deep learning on image denoising: an overview', *Neural Networks*, 2020, vol. 131, pp. 251–275.

Chapter 5

Prediction of diabetes using voting classification algorithms

Sunil Gupta[1], Neha Sharma[1], Gagandeep Kaur[1] and Anita Sardana[2]

Data mining is a process that sifts through enormous amounts of data to find valuable information. Using our statistical and artificial intelligence capabilities, we could examine and analyze large patterns found in massive databases. Data mining can be used to make predictions about the future or discover previously unknown patterns. Classification, clustering, association rules, and regression are some of the techniques used in data mining. The healthcare industry makes extensive use of data mining. Many bioinformatics researchers employ "data mining" techniques. Bioinformatics is the study of how biological sequences and molecules can be saved, retrieved, organized, interpreted, and used. Foretelling the future based on current conditions is called forecasting. Using machine learning techniques, scientists hope to improve their ability to forecast the onset of diabetes-related problems. Type 2 diabetes has a multistage prognosis. Based on how people vote, a new strategy for predicting diabetes was established in this study. The performance of the proposed algorithm in predicting whether or not someone has diabetes has increased by 2%, and the vote classifier approach is being used instead. (1) Because of this, the new method is 98.05 percent accurate. (2) The rate of accuracy is 97.12%. (3) 98% of the values, which is better than other methods.

5.1 Introduction

In the last 20 years, the amount of information kept in databases has grown a lot. Businesses and tech companies are also using databases more and more. The main reasons for the growth of electronic data storage are the success of the interactive data storage paradigm and the development and growth of techniques for extracting and handling information. Companies have realized, however, that there may be useful information hidden in these huge amounts of data that were once thrown away.

[1]Chitkara University Institute of Engineering and Technology, Chitkara University, India
[2]Chandigarh University, Mohali, India

5.1.1   Data mining

Data from many different organizations will be gathered and used to help the company make decisions more quickly. The goal of data mining is to get useful information from large amounts of data. From these patterns, you can figure out a set of rules. So that different goals can be met, the patterns found in the research must be useful. There is a chance that the relevant patterns could be useful in more than one way. This system can help with many things, like making decisions, researching in the bazaar, and the growth of the economy. To find these kinds of patterns, you need a lot of data [1]. Under this umbrella are a number of different fields, such as risk control, healthcare management, customer relationship management (CRM), financial analysis, and the operational activities of an organization. Data mining (DM) is a big part of the knowledge discovery in databases (KDD) method. Mathematicians, people who work with databases, and businesses all use the term "data mining." KDD is a broad term for the process of getting useful information from data stored in data repositories. Data mining is a very important part of KDD. It is a more advanced version of traditional data analysis, which is based on numbers. Some of the ways this technology works are through artificial intelligence (AI), machine learning (ML), and online analytical processing (OAP).

Data mining architecture

It has many parts. These parts compose DM's framework. These components are needed for data management [2]. Figure 5.1 shows data mining's high-level architecture. The actual data sources are the database, data warehouse, World Wide Web (WWW), text files, and other documents. Massive volumes of historical data are necessary for efficient data mining. Databases and data warehouses are common places for organizations to store their information. Databases, text files, spreadsheets, and other information repositories make up data warehouses. Plain text files and spreadsheets may occasionally contain data. The Internet and the WWW are the other sources of information [3].

Graphical user interface (GUI)

Interface (GUI): The GUI is how the user and the management system talk to each other (DM). The user does not need to know anything about how complicated the system is to use it successfully. DM talks to the GUI when the user enters a question or task, and the result is shown to the user in a way that is easy to understand.

Knowledge base: The DM process is aided by this component. The database of information from which the search is guided or the probability of finding a pattern is calculated. DM practitioners may find it useful to consult this document because it contains information gleaned from user feedback and observations. The DM engine may use this component to achieve a more accurate and trustworthy output. Obtaining and updating input from the pattern assessment module is done on a regular basis through communication between the two components.

5.1.2   Data mining and classification

Data mining extracts useable information from huge, heterogeneous datasets to make economic decisions or locate comparable samples. To find new examples,

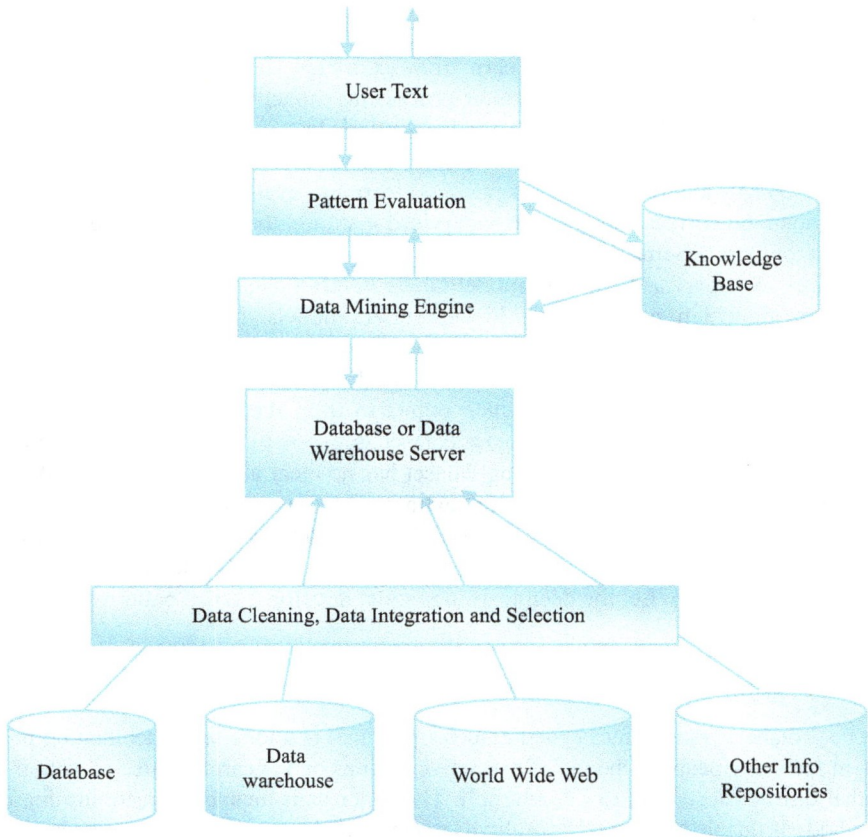

Figure 5.1   General data mining structure

similar connections between information, and co-relationships, it can be used to find answers, create rules from old data, decide on the best ad-hoc business arrangements, uncover hidden information design from datasets, and predict future yield, i.e., practices and patterns [4]. The key tasks of data-driven model are sorting the dataset and marking the informational index. A system scans the informative index to apply a gathering mark or predict class names. Categorization aims to create new, highly predictive models. Well-formed models can reliably recognize dataset properties and class names. The order shows which class gives the dataset to another class. First is the training index, then the test dataset (step 2). First, gather data and create a list of class names. The grouping model breaks a dataset into groups and names to build a new model. Prepare a new grouping model using the set. Stage 2's informative index includes non-classified events. This demonstration is linked to the exam index so students can predict their grades. The model's performance is measured using several metrics. Correct predictions vs. total projections.

5.1.3 ML

ML studies how computers can learn from examples, data, and past experience. Greater data availability and computer processing capacity have boosted ML systems' analytical skills [5]. Algorithmic innovations have helped ML in supervised, semi-supervised and unsupervised learning. Unsupervised, supervised, and semi-supervised ML algorithms. In unsupervised learning, examples do not have labels (other than the correct ones), but in supervised learning, they do (the corresponding correct outputs). Semi-supervised learning [6] combines unlabeled and labeled instances. A supervised learning model labels training data with an answer key to measure algorithm performance. In supervised models, the algorithm is given labeled data to extract features and patterns.

Supervised learning helps classification and regression in two ways: it works best when there are enough reference points to train the algorithm. Not always available. In unsupervised learning, a dataset is given to a deep learning model without instructions [7]. The training dataset has no clear answers or results. When a neural network examines data and extracts features, it tries to automatically uncover structure. Without a "ground truth," it is hard to evaluate an unsupervised-learning algorithm's accuracy. In many scientific domains, labeled data is hard to collect or expensive. Let the deep learning model develop its own patterns for high-quality results.

5.1.4 *Data mining and diabetes prediction*

Type 2 diabetes (sometimes called diabetes mellitus) is a long-term, debilitating problem for many people. One out of every five persons on the earth is infected with this lethal disease, according to a recent poll. The pancreas is unable to create insulin, or the body is unable to utilize the insulin that is produced to meet the body's needs. This causes a spike in blood sugar levels [8]. A person's body can be damaged and many tissues and organs can fail if their blood sugar levels are constantly raised.

T1DM, a type of diabetes that originates in the pancreas, is one of the three main types of diabetes. The other two common types are T2DM and gestational diabetes mellitus (GDM), which typically develops during the later stages of life. T1DM can affect persons of any age; however, it is most typically seen in children and adolescents. The human body produces little or no insulin in this state. This disease can only be managed by administering insulin injections on a regular basis to those who have it. Age is a risk factor for type 2 diabetes. The most common type of diabetes [9] is diabetes mellitus. The key to preventing this illness is to live a healthy lifestyle. To keep their blood sugar levels in check, diabetics use oral medications. The third sort of diabetes, known as gestational diabetes mellitus (GDM), affects predominantly pregnant women and normally goes away after the baby is born. The medical business generates a tremendous amount of data on a daily basis. Extracting valuable information from large amounts of data is a common practice in medicine. Predicting diseases and analyzing clinical data have been the subject of numerous data mining techniques throughout the years. Several diabetes-related indicators can be combined to diagnose the disease early. Diabetes mellitus study uses a vast

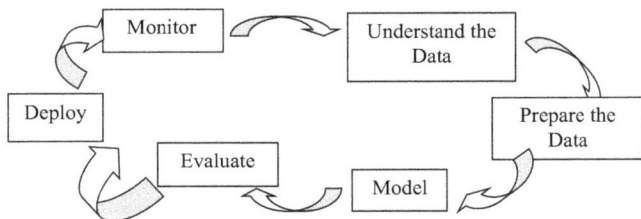

Figure 5.2   Cycle of predictive analytics

amount of preexisting diabetes information for knowledge discovery via ML and data mining approaches [10]. A great amount of data is generated as a result of the disease's social and economic impact, making it a high priority in medical research. ML and data mining are unquestionably important in the diagnosis, treatment, and other aspects of medical administration for diabetes mellitus.

5.1.5   Prediction analysis in data mining

All data saved in large databases is useless unless and until significant information is extracted from them. Predictive analytics [11] is used to provide sophisticated analytics for anticipating future events. Data gathering, modeling, statistics, and deployment are all bundled together with predictive analytics. Unstructured data refers to information found on social media that is extracted via a model-building method. The steps of the predictive analysis are illustrated in Figure 5.2.

5.1.5.1   Introduction to prediction using data mining

Your body is made up of cells that are all linked to each other. In a healthy organism, cells divide, grow, and die all the time. Cancer happens when the cells of a body part take over the area around them. Normal cell growth is different from the growth of cancer cells. These cancer cells do not die, so they keep making more of themselves in the same place. Over time, many different kinds of cancer have been found. They can move to any part of the body and make new tissues there. Some of the most common types of cancer are breast cancer, lung cancer, and skin cancer.

5.1.5.2   Architecture of data mining-based diabetes prediction system

Today, it is hard for doctors and nurses to tell if a patient has diabetes. Patients with diabetes have not yet found a full treatment that will get rid of the disease from their bodies completely. Several tests can tell if someone will get diabetes [12]. But, even though diabetes can be cured if caught early, it is hard to tell when it is in its early stages. Data mining can help predict how likely it is that this disease will spread quickly. Because of this, there are ways to predict the risk of this disease early on through data mining. When using the diabetes prediction tool to figure out the different types of diabetes, both genetic and non-genetic information given by the user is taken into account. So, as soon as this system finds a risk, the user is told to take the steps that are needed based on the risk level [13]. This shows how

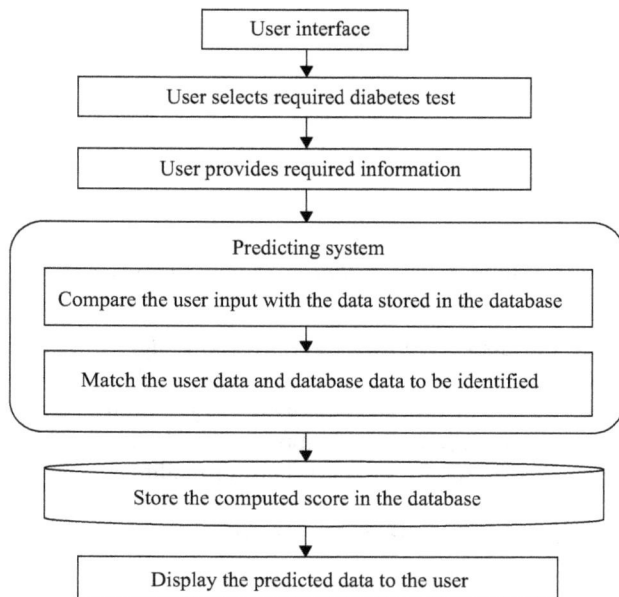

Figure 5.3   Architecture of data mining-based diabetes prediction system

decision trees can be used as the architectural framework for a data mining strategy. A decision tree can help you figure out what data mining is all about [14]. Before making a decision tree, the rules from the training dataset are taken out. Diabetes information will be shown when you log in to the cancer prediction system. Diabetes can be predicted by a system that looks at the following information [15]. There is also a list of the things that make a person more likely to get diabetes. If you have any of these symptoms, see a doctor immediately [16]. If a patient's symptoms indicate diabetes, they will be evaluated and treated immediately. Users must answer all first-level diabetes prediction test questions to advance. Each question is monetary. The questions' values were only determined after consulting doctors and previous research [17]. The cancer prediction system scores each user response. Allocating cancer risks requires comparing the result to the specified risk. Low, medium, high, and extremely high are prediction levels. Once a risk is assigned, user information is saved [18]. User results will be delivered via database. The architecture of data mining-based diabetes prediction system is shown in Figure 5.3.

5.2   Literature review

According to Deeraj Shetty *et al.* [19], data mining is a subfield of software engineering. A methodical search of massive databases turned up the images. It was the primary objective of this data mining technique to draw conclusions from the data.

For future reference, this content was arranged in a logical manner. As a result, this medical conclusion was a focus of the study, which used diabetic data to inform its design. It was a great therapeutic decision for doctors to form an expressive support network. The primary objective of this research was to develop a system that could accurately predict the onset of diabetes. This method made use of a database of people with diabetes to assess the condition. Based on data from diabetic patients, K-nearest neighbor (KNN) and Bayesian algorithms were recommended for use in this system. These approaches were tested on a variety of diabetic characteristics.

Santosh Rani *et al.* (2018): The healthcare system's massive amounts of patient records have been analyzed. Because of its huge size, this data was difficult to evaluate and extract for study. However, a wide range of ML-based algorithms were used to analyze the data. Using a machine-learning approach, we were able to gather the most accurate and useful data. This method may one day be applied to the prediction of a patient's prognosis for an illness. Rukhsar Syed *et al.* (2018): A tree-based partitioning method was given in [20]. The adaptive support vector machine (SVM) technique was also used in our system for categorization in our system. Sampling SMORT was used to prepare the data for trimming in this method. Weka was used for the experiment on the diabetes dataset. The round trip time (RTT) method, J48, and tree-based algorithms were all put to the test. Data processing and data categorization for diabetes improved using the proposed method, according to the findings of the studies.

Bhargavi Chatragadda *et al.* (2018): It was possible to foretell the onset of diabetes using data mining [21]. It was primarily the goal of this data mining technique to extract useful information from the dataset. It was also used to look for patterns in data. There are a wide range of illnesses among the people, some of which went unnoticed by those who were infected. The most important health problem was diabetes mellitus. Diabetic patients affected a vast number of individuals. This disease has had an effect on people of various ages. Predictive analysis was used by HUE to determine which diseases would arise. When putting the data together, the Pima Indian Database was used. An effective method for predicting the number of diabetes in the United States was developed using this framework with SVM classification.

The stacked ensemble methodology [22] was created by the researchers as a meta-learning process. We predicted that LOS would be variable among diabetes patients. Results show that stacked ensemble methods can be used well in this field. Stacking multiple classification learning algorithms outperformed other fundamental approaches in terms of prediction accuracy.

Geetha Guttikonda *et al.* (2019): Prediction of diabetes via data mining [23]. Using data mining, we were able to glean useful information and discover patterns in a large dataset. For a long time, many medical problems have gone unnoticed. One of these conditions was diabetes mellitus. Children were also affected by this disease. These illnesses were predicted using the HUE. They had no hope of recovery. Using the Pima Indian database, the dataset was built out. SVM classification and the given framework were used to calculate the prevalence of diabetes in the community.

Wenqian Chen *et al.* (2017): Type-2 diabetes can be detected using a hybrid predictive technique, as proposed by [24]. K-means and a J48 decision tree were used to categorize the data. An experiment was conducted using the Pima Indians Diabetes Dataset. When compared to earlier studies, the results demonstrated that the proposed model achieved superior precision. Type-2 diabetes can be accurately diagnosed using the previously mentioned method, as research has shown.

Zhongxian Xu *et al.* (2019) suggested a risk prediction model for type-2 diabetes. This model was created using the ensemble learning method [25]. The best characteristics were selected using the RF-WFS approach. Test results and several performance measures were used to verify the technique's effectiveness. When it came to predicting accuracy, this method outperformed the competition. The data from the Pima Indian diabetes study at the University of California was used to verify the findings. The proposed model's accuracy and classification performance were superior to those of other studies reported in the literature. Early diabetes detection was made possible because of this model.

Baiju *et al.* (2019) inquired about the results of a thorough survey that was designed to forecast ill health. Data mining algorithms based on diabetic datasets were used in this study. The illness could be detected with the use of a variety of symptoms [26]. As a result, varying levels of precision were achieved in this poll. Differences in prediction outcomes were found when compared to earlier methods. The diabetic prediction based on the DIM was explained during the diabetes prediction. After the data was pre-processed, the noisy records were deleted [27]. Data point attributes were used to calculate a DIM in the second stage. Value-based prediction of diabetes has been completed. The results of a study on disease prediction methods were presented.

Bakshi Rohit Prasad *et al.* (2014): It was shown how to develop a model that predicts the risk of T2DM in a person [28]. The risk of developing diabetes had been predicted by the most accurate set of markers. These signals were identified using the GBRE algorithm. After training, a variety of classifiers were tested for their accuracy. The voting policy method was used to select the best classifier.

Beschi Raja *et al.* (2020): A new model for predicting T2DM was developed based on DM techniques [29]. The PSO-FCM was created by fusing the particle swarm optimization (PSO) and FCM together. A collection of medical data about a diabetes diagnosis challenge was compiled using this newly discovered technology. There were a number of tests conducted utilizing PIDD. The reliability of the offered system was estimated using the evaluation measures. The prototype's accuracy was more than 8.26% higher than that of other methods. The suggested technique outperformed other models, as evidenced by the results.

Krittika Kantawong *et al.* (2020): Prioritizing the development of diabetes complications forecasting models [30]. The main conceptual framework was the ID3 DT-based binary number vector modified prediction model. Using the 10-fold cross-validation method, the model's performance was evaluated. As a result of these findings, the model's accuracy was estimated at 92.35%. A smartphone app was developed to test the concept with patients of all ages and backgrounds. The projected outcomes were 100% accurate.

Dipak R. Nemade *et al.* (2020): T2DM was predicted by utilizing ML to carry out diagnostics by learning classification [31]. The BPSO was used to choose the features. Features that were selected were classified using the DT algorithm. A method for predicting diabetes was suggested based on the use of supervised ML algorithms. The DT classifier was run on the PIDD to obtain the diabetes prediction results. After that, the best learning classifier, DT, had its precision, sensitivity, and accuracy increased. Unlike previous algorithms, this one had a higher categorization rate: 96.1%. Ramya Akula *et al.* (2019) introduced the methods for ML According to the authors of [32], the evaluation parameters were used to calculate each model's performance. In this investigation, all approaches save the NB classifier were found to be inaccurate. A weighted average or soft voting ensemble model was created, in which each algorithm generated a majority vote to determine if the patient was diabetic or not. Practice fusion's ensemble model yielded an accuracy of 86%. Aside from helping to recover from inaccurate predictions and accurately anticipate T2DM, the weighted average ensemble model also performed well in terms of overall metrics. As a cautionary tale, the proposed model was utilized to encourage individuals to seek immediate medical attention.

Amelec Viloria *et al.* (2020): To predict diabetes diagnosis using criteria indicated by patients [33], the authors proposed SVM, which was employed [33]. Diabetic, non-diabetic, and diabetic propensity were the three categories of output variables. With Colombian patients, the accuracy of the recommended strategy was found to be 99.2%, while the accuracy of other ethnic groups was found to be 65.6%. The proposed classification algorithm's accuracy and predictability will be improved in the future by combining these algorithms with additional computational methodologies like genetic algorithm (GA) or PSO.

Srabani Patikar *et al.* (2020): The goal was to use a modified version of the Fuzzy-KNN classification algorithm. The proposed technique relies on two variables: the fuzzy coefficient and the nearest neighbor classes. To turn a crisp collection into a fuzzy one, we employed the Gaussian membership function. The performance of the algorithm was evaluated on a range of diabetes data sets. According to the results of the study, the planned modified fuzzy-K-nearest neighbor technique performed better than traditional algorithms.

Md. Tanvir Islam *et al.* (2020): If proper precautions are followed in the early stages of diabetes, it may be possible to successfully treat the disease. As a result, it was suggested that the Random Forest (RF) algorithm be used to forecast diabetes. There were 340 diabetics who provided examples for this study, and the examples included 26 different qualities. Typical and non-typical symptoms were found, and they were classified as such.

This study focused on identifying type 1 diabetes accurately. For this, an ensemble ML technique, the proposed algorithm, was constructed. Up to 98.24% of the proposed algorithm's accuracy was found.

Aeshah Saad Alanazi *et al.* (2020): Diabetes was viewed as a long-term condition. In the last few decades, the risk of developing diabetes has skyrocketed, creating a serious health hazard. Two ML classifiers, SVM, and RF were coupled in the framework to predict diabetes. Security Force Primary Health Care provided the dataset from which the provided system was built.

The suggested framework was found to be 98% accurate, while the ROC was found to be 99% accurate. In addition, RF's accuracy was superior to SVM's accuracy.

Maha S. Diab *et al.* (2020) established neural network models for predicting and classifying the likelihood of diabetes onset [34]. There are three neural network (NN)-based approaches to predict and classify diabetes. These ideas enabled the creation of a feed forward neural network (FFN), pattern network, and a cascade forward architecture. Algorithms were evaluated on a variety of metrics, including accuracy, sensitivity, and specificity. MATLAB® was used to implement and test the new approach. The accuracy percentage for this technique was 91.1%.

Md. Tanvir Islam *et al.* (2020): To predict diabetes, researchers employed algorithms like AdaBoost, Bagging, and RF [35]. It was hoped that the real-time data would be used to train and evaluate the proposed models. There were 464 occurrences in this dataset, each with its own unique set of 22 risk factors. AdaBoost's accuracy in predicting diabetes disease was 97.84%, Bagging's accuracy was 98.28%, and RF's accuracy was 99.35%.

Md Shafiqul Islam *et al.* (2020): Diabetes prevention or postponing its start was found to be crucial [36]. We used ML to identify the characteristics most closely associated with diabetes's likely future growth. Diabetes prediction algorithms were then developed as a result of this. Data from a long-term clinical trial was used to quantify the proposed model. An 81.01% accuracy in prediction, 81.2% specificity, 79.50% sensitivity, and an AUC score of 87.1% were the outcomes of the suggested technique.

Biswajit Giri *et al.* (2020): Diabetic information can be extracted from a medical information source using a hybrid technique, according to [37]. The medical diagnostic was accomplished swiftly thanks to the use of this technique, which provided a clear and comprehensible diagnosis. The PIDD dataset was utilized to assess the hybrid approach. An increase in accuracy of 86% was observed when the suggested technique, which included pre-processing, was implemented. To determine if the patient was diabetic, a variety of procedures were employed.

Gulam Gaus Warsi *et al.* (2019): Ensemble learning can forecast diabetes onset [38]. This technique predicts future diabetes risk and risk likelihood. The dataset is a collection of surveys used to train the model using classifiers or experts. Scikit-Learn, Pandas, and Numpy are libraries. Based on a lifestyle questionnaire, the model can predict early diabetes onset [39].

5.3 Diabetes prediction

Data mining and trend/behavior pattern prediction are components of predictive analytics. Unnamed refers to future significant events. PA can be utilized to learn about the past, present, and future. This model's effectiveness depends on how well the explanatory factors correlate with the predicted variables, which are drawn from past events. Data analysis and assumptions often determine results. Predictive analytics can offer more detailed forecasts, allowing certain organizational components to be given projected ratings. PA defies the forecast. PA uses two models to describe prediction systems:

Predictive models: When predicting the value of one attribute, these models take into account the values of other characteristics. The projected attribute can be found by looking at the target or dependent variable. Explanatory or independent variables are the characteristics that are used to construct forecasts. Classification, prediction analysis (PA), and estimation are some of the tasks that the prediction DM algorithm seeks to do. This DM algorithm [40] predicts future outcomes based on previously obtained data and previously provided responses.

Descriptive models: The primary goal of these DM models is to find patterns to examine the data's existing relationships. The exploratory behavior of descriptive DM tasks is frequently required in post-processing procedures to authenticate and explain the results. The fundamental goal of these models is to identify patterns and linkages in massive data sets to better understand the examined system.

Descriptive analytics is widely acknowledged as a major substitute for predictive analysis. The focus of descriptive analytics is on identifying patterns in data. When descriptive analytics and predictive analytics are combined, the term KDD is used; nevertheless, this word is also appropriate for descriptive analytics. When studying patterns, it is frequently seen to be more appealing and useful. However, achieving a direct advantage from descriptive analytics is more difficult than with predictive analytics.

5.3.1   Diabetes mellitus

DM, or diabetes mellitus, is the medical term for a condition affecting the body's glucose metabolism. This disorder causes the blood sugar level to rise. Glucose is transported into human cells via insulin, a hormone.

Endocrine cells store and utilize insulin for energy production [41]. As a result, either the body does not create enough insulin or it does not utilize it well. Several organ systems can be damaged if this condition is not addressed quickly enough. Nerves, eyes, kidneys, and other organs may be affected.

There are numerous subtypes of this disease:

Type 1 diabetes or (T1DM): To put it simply, T1DM is an autoimmune condition. If you have type 1 diabetes, your immune system attacks and damages your pancreas cells. No one knows what set off the strike. One in ten people are affected by this form of diabetes. There are several common symptoms of this illness, including hunger, thirst, weight loss that is unintentional, frequent urination, hazy eyesight, and fatigue.

Type 2 diabetes or (T2DM): In this form of diabetes, the human body is unable to make use of insulin, which results in glucose being produced in the plasma of the individual affected. The general symptoms may include acute famine, excessive thirst, an increased need to urinate, frequent urination, blurred vision, weariness, and other symptoms [42].

Prediabetes: This type of diabetes is characterized by abnormally high blood sugar levels. Although the elevated sugar level is insufficient for doctors to identify the condition, it is still a good indicator. More than a third of Americans are afflicted by this condition, which is mostly undetected by the general public. Prediabetes raises a person's risk of acquiring T2DM, as well as coronary artery disease. These disorders can be prevented to a great extent with regular physical activity and a reduced body mass index (BMI).

Gestational diabetes: Pregnant women are most likely to suffer from this illness. Because of the hormonal changes that occur during pregnancy, pregnant women's insulin sensitivity decreases. Pregnancy-related gestational diabetes does not affect all of the women who are carrying children. The diabetes went away on its own after the delivery. A standard blood glucose test is commonly used to detect this particular type of disease. If this condition is present in the pregnant woman, she may have frequent urges to urinate or drink excessive amounts of water.

5.3.2 Diabetes prediction using data mining

Data mining is a common practice in healthcare databases. A growing number of clinical forecasts are being generated using data mining algorithms [43]. In recent years, many scholars have claimed that vital data collected from patients might be used to develop medically useful support and prediction patterns. Studies in the field of DM illness PA are mostly focused on increasing the accuracy rate. A data mining-based approach for predicting the likelihood of diabetes in a person includes a number of steps as shown in Figure 5.4.

In this order, these are the steps you need to take:

(a) Data selection
(b) Data preprocessing
(c) Data analysis
(d) Result database
(e) Knowledge evaluation and prediction

Following is a rundown of everything that needs to be done to accurately predict diabetes:

Data selection: To begin, the data must first be selected. Various sources were used to acquire the information. The data gathered included critical risk factors

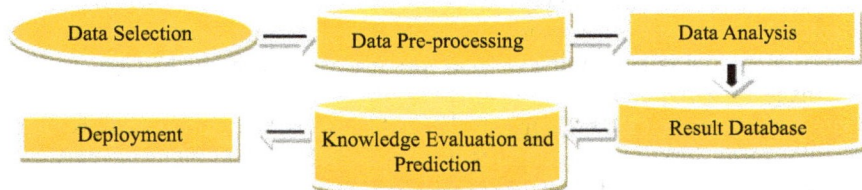

Figure 5.4   General process of diabetes prediction

such as observable symptoms, analyses, and demographics. All of these risk factors must be taken into account when attempting to predict a person's likelihood of developing diabetes. These diagnostic criteria can be used to identify if someone has diabetes. This is the fundamental reason for making use of the data. Health and clinical test results are included in this data set [44]. There is information on the number of births, blood pressure, BMI, and age of the participants in this dataset.

Data pre-processing: Most databases are vulnerable to data that is unreliable, missing, or otherwise incoherent. To account for their enormous size and the fact that they may have originated from any number of places, this is the reason. When it comes to using data mining to find and predict disorders, the features of the data matter a lot. Data of poor quality can lead to inaccurate or less predictive outcomes. Many different pre-processing techniques are employed to enhance the data's utility and applicability for diabetes prediction as a result. Data preprocessing is carried out using all of the KDD processes. The data must be enhanced in terms of time, cost, and quality before it can be used for data mining and analysis. Data pre-processing is divided into three stages:

> ***Data cleaning:*** This process comprises the replacement of any missing values as well as the elimination of any unnecessary data. In noisy data, outliers can be detected. These outliers must be eliminated to resolve anomalies. In a diabetic dataset, all of the variables sugar, blood pressure, weight, insulin, and BMI have zero values. As a result, the median value of the feature was used to replace all zeros.

> ***Data reduction***: Data reduction is used to lower the dataset size once it has been gathered. There is no difference in the conclusions that can be drawn from this smaller dataset. Dataset properties can be reduced using the dimensional reduction technique [45]. A variety of methods can be used to extract the most important properties from a large dataset. Sugar, BMI, hypertension, and age are among the dataset's most important characteristics.

> ***Data transformation***: This task refers to the process of transforming data from one format into another one, which can be thought of as an interchange. There are three stages involved in the process of transforming data: smoothing the data, normalizing the data, and aggregating the data. The technique of binning is utilized pretty frequently these days for smoothing out the data.

The step of preprocessing the data is an essential part of the data analysis process.

Data analysis: In this stage of the research process, the data are analyzed to achieve the objectives that have been set for the study. In this procedure, making the right choice in terms of the target values to shoot at is of the utmost importance. A data mining platform will often incorporate a collection of algorithmic methods as part of its data mining strategies. KNN, SVM, naive Bayesian, artificial neural network, and other similar programs are examples of well-known predictive algorithms for diabetes.

Result database: During this stage of the process, the preferred algorithmic technique and associated metrics are chosen. During this stage of the process, we will employ a specialized piece of software to process the raw data and create the finished database.

Knowledge evaluation and pattern prediction: At this stage, the resultant database is mined for new information or templates to use as a starting point. This step is responsible for the generation of an informative knowledge database that will facilitate the pattern prediction based on the possibilities, as well as therapy [46].

Deployment: Here, a model that has been selected in advance will be applied to new data to generate predictions.

5.4   Research significance

The key goals are to undertake a predictive analysis of diabetes condition. Various diabetic detection methods are broken down into phases. The diabetes dataset was gathered from the UCI database. A number of pre-processing procedures are also used to increase the quality of this dataset. It was then that the dataset's most relevant features were eliminated. In the last stage, the acquired attributes are used to predict diabetes using k-mean and logistic regression approaches. In this study, a new classification algorithm for diabetic prediction must be provided, which boosts prediction accuracy.

Here are the study's objectives:

1. To review and examine different diabetic prediction algorithms of data mining.
2. To design a voting classification method for predicting diabetic disease.
3. To apply a new method and perform its comparison against the earlier methods in regard to certain metrics.

Research methodology: The practice of using data-mining methods to forecast levels of blood sugar is becoming increasingly common. Data-mining technologies do not necessitate significant model assumptions to create models for predicting blood sugar levels. Data mining is used to uncover the underlying patterns and relationships in the data that people have collected through their experiences. Because of this, data mining can reliably forecast blood sugar levels. There have been a number of studies that have used data-mining techniques to predict blood sugar levels, whether they were fasted or not. A different approach has used data-mining algorithms to predict or classify postprandial blood sugar as regular or irregular. A continuous glucose monitoring device is also used in current investigations of diabetes blood sugar levels. Prediction of diabetes is broken down into the following stages:

1. *Data set input*: The dataset used for diabetic risk assessment was taken from the UCI database. The dataset includes a variety of characteristics that will go towards the final forecast.
2. *Attribute selection*: In this stage, the principal components analysis (PCA) method is used, which sorts through a huge number of attributes to determine which ones are most important. The selection of pertinent features may result in a reduction in the amount of time needed for execution.

3. *Clustering*: The process of deciding which features should be included will take place during this phase. k-clustering, a technique for improving classification, will be used in this stage to group similar and dissimilar attributes together.

4. *Classification*: During this stage of the process, a voting classifier will be utilized to make a diabetic disorder prediction. This voting classifier will be a mixture of several other voting classifiers, and the results of each voting classifier will be merged to make a forecast of the ultimate result. to apply voting classification to the entire collection of data, it will first be partitioned into training and testing sets. Some eminent data mining algorithms for diabetes prediction have been elaborated below.

5.4.1 Support vector machine

Classification and regression rules are learned from data using a support vector machine (SVM), a machine learning technique. The SVM employs statistical learning principles. In a way, this algorithm solves the basic problem, but not the more difficult one. The bias-variance trade-off problem can be solved comprehensively using SVM. This algorithm can be implemented in two ways. Using mathematical programming is the first approach while using kernel functions is the second. In this method, the data is divided into two categories: P and N.

There are two classes: one for situations where $yi=+1$ and the other for situations where it is equal to or less than 1. It seeks out a hyperplane that is equally distant from each class on the shortest separation surface it can find [47]. Hyperplane features a variety of statistically significant properties. The term "kernel functions" refers to decision surfaces that are non-linear. In the event that the training data are linearly separable, a pair (w,b) will exist, as stated in (5.1) and (5.2) below:

$$W^T X_i + b \geq 1 \text{ for all } X_I \in P \tag{5.1}$$

$$W^T X_i + b \leq -1 \text{ for all } X_I \in P \tag{5.2}$$

Here, x_i & b represents a weight vector and denotes a bias. The predictive rule is specified by (5.3):

$$f = sign(W.X) + b \tag{5.3}$$

5.4.2 Artificial neural network

A connection can be seen between the ANN technique and artificial intelligence. The process of data mining makes use of this technology. The most basic form of an artificial neural network (ANN) has only one hidden layer; yet, due to the extensive connections that exist between the neurons in each successive layer, it is quite analogous to the neuronal network that can be found in the human brain.

The input layer is transformed into the output layer by these units. The output of the previous layer of neurons serves as the input for the next layer. Complex patterns can be discovered using artificial neural networks. Its ability to learn is based on these patterns. There are billions of neurons in the human brain, which is why we are so clever. Axons and a single neuron connect these cells to other cells in a system known as a perceptron [48]. Dendrites receive the info and process it as a stimulus for the brain. There are a lot of nodes in the artificial neural network. There is a connectivity between every node. To explain the relationship between different units, we will utilize a weight scale. This strategy's primary goal is to turn raw data into something that can be processed. Input is the term used to describe the set of weight vector input values. It can be either positive or negative in terms of weight. The weights are added with the help of a function, and the final result is displayed as a map. The weight of a unit affects its ability to be commanded. neurons communicate through the synapses that link them. This study was conducted using the supervised learning method, and the results are reflected in the model shown below. A predetermined value is used to control both the input and the output of this method. The actual result is compared to the desired outputs after the processing is complete. The weaknesses in a system can be fixed by using backward propagation. Many times throughout the training cycle, a network is used in weight-balancing and refinement to analyze data.

5.4.3   Random forest (RF)

The RF method is a simple machine-learning strategy that is quick to implement and flexible to change. The tree predictors are integrated into this technique [49]. With this approach, you can nearly always expect success. Increasing its efficiency is difficult. Numerical, binary, and nominal data can all be processed with this method. In RF, there are many trees. These trees offer accurate and appropriate outcomes when put together. Use the RF algorithm to classify and regression data. Classification is the most essential task in machine learning. Hyperparameters such as decision trees and bagging classifiers fall within this category. It is easy to figure out RF, or random forest, because of the way the trees in this scenario overlap each other randomly. For example, seven randomly selected trees can be used to discover a variable. There are four trees that agree with each other, whereas there are three that do not. To build a machine learning model, the majority of votes are used. The RF randomly selects a subset of dataset attributes to produce more precise results. Rather than trying to identify the exact threshold, a random threshold provides more random trees for all qualities. Overfitting can be avoided by combining the RF algorithm with other approaches.

5.4.4   K-means clustering

Clustering is the act of forming groups out of things that share some characteristic. The characteristics of these goods determine their classification. It is possible to learn without supervision by using a technique known as clustering. Data that is not labeled is grouped in the same way as data with labels. Clusters like this one share many similarities. Things in one cluster are distinguished from those in other clusters by this distinction. Inter-cluster similarity is low during clustering, whereas intra-cluster similarity is high. Clustering can take a variety of shapes. Examples include partitioned clustering and hierarchical clustering, among many others. K-means clustering was used in this investigation, though. It is a lot simpler and less time consuming to implement this clustering method. The cluster center is indicated by K in the numerical data. Each data point is assigned to a cluster based on its distance from the center of the graph. Using a cluster, you may find the average value of all of the points in your data. A new location for the cluster's core will be chosen, and the process will be repeated as many times as the cluster's core moves.

5.4.5 K-nearest neighbor (KNN)

K-nearest neighbors (KNN): Supervised machine learning algorithms fall within the category of algorithms. Classification and regression problems can be solved with this approach. Lacking a training stage, this approach is considered a lazy algorithm. Classification for training has made use of all of the data. KNN is a non-parametric learning technique since it cannot make any assumptions about the core data. The KNN method uses feature similarity to forecast the values of new data points. We are going to assign a numerical value to this new data point. Because of its closeness to the points in the training set, this was selected as the value to be used [50].

5.4.6 Decision tree

Groups of instances are separated by a recursive classifier A root tree can be constructed using the nodes in this paradigm. As a result, the Decision Tree's root node is a distributed tree with no outbound edges. Each additional node necessitates the use of a corresponding incoming edge. If a node is labeled as "internal" or "test node," it has no outbound connections. Leaves refer to the remaining nodes. Using a discrete function of the input values, this approach separates the instance space into two or more sub-spaces. Single attributes may be used to partition the instance space for each test [4]. There must be a range of numbers for the condition to apply. Assigning a single class to each leaf yields the final goal value. In each leaf, a probability vector indicates how likely it is that a particular feature will be present. To classify the instances based on the test results along the route, the features are transported down the leaf from the tree's root. The DT model is an easy-to-follow manner. Branch nodes with the property are given labels, and the labels are complemented by values indicating what they represent. As a result of using this classifier, an analyst can predict a potential customer's response and learn about the complete population of possible customers. A collection of orthogonal hyperplanes, each one orthogonal to an axis, can be constructed geometrically from DTs with numerical features. These classifiers are deemed to be more thorough by decision-makers.

5.4.7 Linear regression

A key objective of the linear regression (LR) is the identification of relationships and connections among different variables. One or more explanatory variables (*X*) and a continuous scalar-dependent variable (D) are said to have a modeling relationship (*y*). To anticipate a continuous variable, regression analysis can be utilized; classification is used to predict a label from a finite set [43]. Modeling a linear combination of input variables in a multiple regression has the form of (5.4):

$$y = \beta_0 + \beta_1 x_1 + \beta_2 x_2 + .. + e \qquad (5.4)$$

LR also belongs to the group of supervised learning algorithms. This implies the model is trained on a set of labeled data. After that, these labels are predicted on unlabeled data using this model.

5.4.8   Naive Bayes

Bayesian classification combines supervised learning and statistical techniques to produce classifications. Consider the underlying probability model. To explain the model's uncertainty in an ethical manner, the probability of results is established. Prediction is at the heart of the Bayesian approach to classifying data in statistical models. Classification based on the monitoring system's data gives a realistic method of learning. This classification. Understanding and calculating learning algorithms becomes easier when using Bayesian classification. Probabilities for hypotheses are also examined [5,6]. Assume the distribution of probabilities has two values. To keep the equation as generic as possible, the Bayes rule is used to represent it in the form of (5.5):

$$P(x_1, x_2) = P(x_1 | x_2) P(x_2) \qquad (5.5)$$

Similarly, if there is another class variable *c*, as depicted in (5.6) is:

$$P(x_1, x_2 | c) = P(x_1 | x_2, c) P(x_2 | c) \qquad (5.6)$$

If the generalization of the situation is done using two variables to a conditional independence assumption for a set of variables x_1 . . . . .x_N conditional on another variable *c* in (5.7):

$$\boldsymbol{P(x|c)} = \prod_{i=1}^{N} P(x_i | c) \qquad (5.7)$$

5.5   Results and discussion

The focus of this study is on diabetes prediction. The information comes from the University of California at Irvine's database. The dataset for PA comprises 20 attributes and is a multivariate data set (predictive analysis). The two approaches are implemented and compared based on a set of metrics. Figure 5.5 represents the dataset used for the testing of the proposed model.

```
 1 Pregnancies,Glucose,BloodPressure,SkinThickness,Insulin,BMI,DiabetesPedigreeFunction,Age,Outcome
 2 6,148,72,35,0,33.6,0.627,50,1
 3 1,85,66,29,0,26.6,0.351,31,0
 4 8,183,64,0,0,23.3,0.672,32,1
 5 1,89,66,23,94,28.1,0.167,21,0
 6 0,137,40,35,168,43.1,2.288,33,1
 7 5,116,74,0,0,25.6,0.201,30,0
 8 3,78,50,32,88,31,0.248,26,1
 9 10,115,0,0,0,35.3,0.134,29,0
10 2,197,70,45,543,30.5,0.158,53,1
11 8,125,96,0,0,0.232,54,1
12 4,110,92,0,0,37.6,0.191,30,0
13 10,168,74,0,0,38,0.537,34,1
14 10,139,80,0,0,27.1,1.441,57,0
15 1,189,60,23,846,30.1,0.398,59,1
16 5,166,72,19,175,25.8,0.587,51,1
17 7,100,0,0,0,30,0.484,32,1
18 0,118,84,47,230,45.8,0.551,31,1
19 7,107,74,0,0,29.6,0.254,31,1
20 1,103,30,38,83,43.3,0.183,33,0
21 1,115,70,30,96,34.6,0.529,32,1
22 3,126,88,41,235,39.3,0.704,27,0
23 8,99,84,0,0,35.4,0.388,50,0
24 7,196,90,0,0,39.8,0.451,41,1
25 9,119,80,35,0,29,0.263,29,1
26 11,143,94,33,146,36.6,0.254,51,1
27 10,125,70,26,115,31.1,0.205,41,1
28 7,147,76,0,0,39.4,0.257,43,1
29 1,97,66,15,140,23.2,0.487,22,0
30 13,145,82,19,110,22.2,0.245,57,0
31 5,117,92,0,0,34.1,0.337,38,0
```

Figure 5.5   Dataset of diabetes

```
17 import time
18 data.head()
19 data.shape
20 print(data.describe())
21
22
23 pca=PCA(n_components=2)
24
25 X_train=pca.fit_transform(x)
26
27 model = KMeans(n_clusters=2, random_state=0).fit(X_train)
28
29 abc=model.predict(X_train)
30
31 from sklearn.model_selection import train_test_split
32
33 X_train, X_test, y_train, y_test = train_test_split(x, abc, test_size = 0.10, random_state=100)
34 from sklearn.metrics import accuracy_score
35 from sklearn.metrics import classification_report
36
37 classifier1 = LogisticRegression(random_state=0)
38
39 clf_1 = classifier1.fit(X_train, y_train)
40 y_pred1 = clf_1.predict(X_test)
41 print('Accuracy of PCA + Kmean + Logistic Regression is {}'.format(accuracy_score(y_test,y_pred1 )*100))
42 start_time = time.time()
43 print(classification_report(y_test,y_pred1))
44 print("The execution time is %s seconds ---" % (time.time() - start_time))
45
46
Accuracy of PCA + Kmean + Logistic Regression is 97.40259740259741
          precision    recall  f1-score   support

       0       0.97      1.00      0.98        59
       1       1.00      0.89      0.94        18
```

Figure 5.6   PCA+KMEAN+LR

Figure 5.6 represents the results obtained from the first method that uses a PCA, *K*-means, and logistic regression combination. For diabetic forecasting, the second method uses PCA, K-means, and voting classification algorithms. Figure 5.7 represents a combination of logistic regression, RF, and SVM to

```
Editor - C:\Users\hp\Desktop\ANU\prpsd.py
 fin.py    untitled0.py - thesis1    untitled0.py - ANU    prpsd.py
32
33 abc=model.predict(X_train)
34
35 from sklearn.model_selection import train_test_split
36
37 X_train, X_test, y_train, y_test = train_test_split(x, abc, test_size = 0.20, random_state=100)
38 from sklearn.metrics import accuracy_score
39 from sklearn.metrics import classification_report
40
41 classifier1 = LogisticRegression(random_state=0)
42
43 clf_1 = classifier1.fit(X_train, y_train)
44 y_pred1 = clf_1.predict(X_test)
45 print('Accuracy of PCA + Kmean + Logistic Regression is {}'.format(accuracy_score(y_test,y_pred1 )*100))
46 start_time = time.time()
47 print(classification_report(y_test,y_pred1))
48 print("The execution time is %s seconds ---" % (time.time() - start_time))
49
50
51 clf1= MLPClassifier(solver='lbfgs', alpha=1e-5,hidden_layer_sizes=(5, 2), random_state=1)
52 clf2 = RandomForestClassifier(n_estimators=100, random_state=123)
53 clf3 = GaussianNB()
54 model = VotingClassifier(estimators=[('lr', clf1), ('rf', clf2), ('gnb', clf3)],
55                          voting='soft',
56                          weights=[3, 2, 1])
57
58 clf_1 = model.fit(X_train, y_train)
59 y_pred1 = clf_1.predict(X_test)
60 print('Accuracy of proposed is {}'.format(accuracy_score(y_test,y_pred1 )*100))
61 start_time = time.time()
62 print(classification_report(y_test,y_pred1))

Accuracy of proposed is 98.05194805194806
              precision    recall  f1-score   support
         0       0.98      0.99      0.99       116
         1       0.97      0.95      0.96        38
```

Figure 5.7   Voting classifie

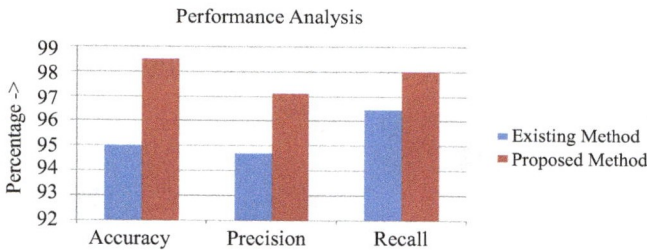

Figure 5.8   Performance analysis

classify votes. Figure 5.8 illustrates the performance analysis of the existing algorithms and proposed model. It is quite evident from the results obtained that the proposed model is better.

The following is a list of significant metrics to take into consideration while assessing the effectiveness of these algorithms:

1. Precision: The degree to which identical results are produced by repeated measurements carried out under constant conditions is referred to as precision and is expressed as (5.8):

$$Precision = (True\ Positive) / (True\ Positive + False\ Positive) \qquad (5.8)$$

Table 5.1 Comparative analysis

Parameters	Existing method	Proposed method
Accuracy	97.4	98.05
Precision	97	97.12
Recall	97	98

2. Recall: It is the proportion of correctly anticipated positive observations to the total number of observations in the initial class, as in (5.9), below:

$$\text{Recall} = (\text{True Positive})/(\text{True Positive} + \text{False Negative}) \qquad (5.9)$$

3. Accuracy: It is the proportion of subjects that have been correctly labeled relative to the total number of subjects (refer (5.10)):

$$\text{Accuracy} = (\text{Number of points correctly classified})/(\text{Total Number of Points}) * 100 \qquad (5.10)$$

Figure 5.5 shows the diabetes dataset obtained from the UCI database [51]. Figure 5.6 shows the use of the diabetes dataset for PA. PCA, K-mean, and logistic regression were utilized to carry out the task of diabetes prediction. To conduct an analysis of the prediction outcomes, the entire dataset is partitioned into two subsets: the training set and the testing set. The use of the diabetes dataset is illustrated in Figure 5.7 for PA. To make a prediction on diabetes, a voting classifier combination that included multi-layer perceptron (MLP), RF, and NB was used. To conduct an analysis of the prediction outcomes, the entire dataset is partitioned into two subsets: the training set and the testing set. As shown in Figure 5.8, a comparison is made between the effectiveness of an existing algorithm and that of a new algorithm with regard to specific metrics. It has been determined through research that the new algorithmic approach has a larger percentage of each of the three factors. Table 5.1 illustrates the comparison of the existing techniques with the proposed model using three different parameters such as accuracy, precision, and recall.

5.6 Conclusion and future work

In the process of forecasting blood sugar levels, data-mining algorithms have been applied quite frequently. The creation of accurate models for forecasting blood sugar levels does not require the use of large model assumptions when data mining technologies are utilized. Data mining is the process of searching for hidden patterns and connections among large amounts of data that have been compiled by individuals as a result of their experiences. Data mining allows for an accurate prediction of blood sugar levels as a result of this. There have been a number of studies that have used data-mining techniques to predict blood sugar levels, whether they were fasted or not. A different approach has used data-mining algorithms to predict or classify postprandial blood sugar as regular or irregular. A continuous glucose monitoring device is also used in current investigations of diabetes blood sugar levels. In this chapter, diabetics are predicted in different stages. To reduce the number of features, the PCA technique is applied. The k-means approach is used to group data into clusters based on similarities and differences. Finally, a vote classifier strategy is employed to predict diabetes and non-diabetic status. The proposed approach is having a beneficial impact by obtaining (a) better accuracy 98.05%, (b) precision 97.12%, and (c) recall 98% values as compared to existing methods. The future work can include further improving the capabilities of the proposed algorithm by using transfer learning for diabetes prediction and comparative analysis of recently developed algorithms with those developed in the past is able to be carried out for diabetes prevention.

References

[1]   R. Tamilselvi and S. Kalaiselvi, "An overview of data mining techniques and applications", *International Journal of Science and Research (IJSR)*, 2013, 2(2).

[2]   F. Ståhl, R. Johansson, Eric Renard, "Post-prandial plasma glucose prediction in type I diabetes based on impulse response models", in: *Annual International Conference of the IEEE Engineering in Medicine and Biology*, Buenos Aires, Argentina, 2010, pp. 1324–1327.

[3]   S. Chemlal, S. Colberg, M. Satin-Smith, *et al.*, "Blood glucose individualized prediction for type 2 diabetes using iPhone application", in: *IEEE 37th Annual Northeast Bioengineering Conference (NEBEC)*, Troy, NY, USA, 2011, pp. 1–2.

[4]   N. Barakat, A.P. Bradley, and M.N.H. Barakat, "Intelligible support vector machines for diagnosis of diabetes mellitus", *Transactions on Information Technology in Biomedicine,* 2011, 14, 1114–1120.

[5]   A. Rana, A. Dumka, R. Singh, M. Rashid, N. Ahmad, and M.K. Panda, "An efficient machine learning approach for diagnosing Parkinson's disease by utilizing voice features", *Electronics*, 2022, 11(22), 3782.

[6]   A. Kumar, J. Rawat, I. Kumar, *et al.*, "Computer-aided deep learning model for identification of lymphoblast cell using microscopic leukocyte images," *Expert Systems*, 2022, 39(4), e12894.

[7]   M. Rashid, H. Singh, and V. Goyal, "The use of machine learning and deep learning algorithms in functional magnetic resonance imaging—A systematic review", *Expert Systems*, 2020, 37(6), e12644.

[8]   Mr. R. Sengamuthu, Mrs. R. Abirami, and Mr. D. Karthik, "Various data mining techniques analysis to predict diabetes mellitus", *International Research Journal of Engineering and Technology (IRJET)*, 2018, 05(05).

[9]   B. Suvarnamukhi and M. Seshashayee, "Big data processing system for diabetes prediction using machine learning technique", *International Journal of Innovative Technology and Exploring Engineering (IJITEE)*, 2019, 8(12).

[10] A. Azrar, M. Awais, Y. Ali, and K. Zaheer, "Data mining models comparison for diabetes prediction", *International Journal of Advanced Computer Science and Applications*, 2018, 9(8).

[11] M. Koklu and Yauz Unal, "Analysis of a D. population of diabetic patients databases with classifiers", *International Journal of Medical, Health, Pharmaceutical and Biomedical Engineering*, 2013, 7(8).

[12] S. Rao and V. Arun Kumar, "Applying data mining technique to predict the diabetes of our future generations", *ISRASEeXplore Digital Library, 2014.*

[13] V. Vijayan and A. Ravikumar, "Study of data mining algorithms for prediction and diagnosis of diabetes mellitus", *International Journal of Computer Applications (0975-8887)*, 2014, 95(17).

[14] P. Madan, V. Singh, V. Chaudhari, *et al.*, "An optimization-based diabetes prediction model using CNN and Bi-directional LSTM in real-time environment", *Applied Sciences*, 2022, 12(8), 3989.

[15] A. H. Abed and M. Nasr, "Diabetes disease detection through data mining techniques", *International Journal of Advanced Networking and Applications,* 2019, 11(01).

[16] S. Mondal, K. Agarwal, and M. Rashid, "Deep learning approach for automatic classification of x-ray images using convolutional neural network", in: *2019 Fifth International Conference on Image Information Processing (ICIIP)*, IEEE, 2019, pp. 326–331.

[17] G. Srivastav, M. Rashid, R. Singh, A. Gehlot, and N. Sharma, "Breast cancer detection in mammogram images using Machine Learning Methods and CLAHE Algorithm", in: *2022 5th International Conference on Contemporary Computing and Informatics (IC3I)*, IEEE, 2022, pp. 1187–1192.

[18] K. Priyadarshini and I. Lakshmi, "A survey on prediction of diabetes using data mining technique", *International Journal of Innovative Research in Science, Engineering and Technology*, 2017, 6(11)

[19] D. Shetty, K. Rit, S. Shaikh, and N. Patil, "Diabetes disease prediction using data mining", in: *International Conference on Innovations in Information, Embedded and Communication Systems* (ICIIECS), 2017.

[20] R. Syed, R. Kumar Gupta, and N. Pathik, "An advance tree adaptive data classification for the diabetes disease prediction", in: *International Conference on Recent Innovations in Electrical, Electronics & Communication Engineering (ICRIEECE)*, 2018.

[21] B. Chatragadda, S. Kattula, and G. Guthikonda, "Diabetes data prediction using spark and analysis in hue over big data", in: *3rd IEEE International Conference on Recent Trends in Electronics, Information & Communication Technology (RTEICT)*, 2018.

[22] A. Alahmar, E. Mohammed, and R. Benlamri, "Application of data mining techniques to predict the length of stay of hospitalized patients with diabetes", in: *4th International Conference on Big Data Innovations and Applications (Innovate-Data)*, 2018.

[23] Geetha Guttikonda, M. Katamaneni, and M. L. Pandala, "Diabetes data prediction using spark and analysis in hue over big data", in: *3rd International Conference on Computing Methodologies and Communication (ICCMC)*, 2019.

[24] W. Chen, S. Chen, H. Zhang, and W. Tianshu, "A hybrid prediction model for type 2 diabetes using K-means and decision tree", in: *8th IEEE International Conference on Software Engineering and Service Science (ICSESS)*, 2017.

[25] Z. Xu and Z. Wang, "A risk prediction model for type 2 diabetes based on weighted feature selection of random forest and XGBoost ensemble classifier", in: *Eleventh International Conference on Advanced Computational Intelligence (ICACI)*, 2019.

[26] B.V. Baiju and D. J. Aravindhar, "Disease influence measure based diabetic prediction with medical data set using data mining", in: *1st International Conference on Innovations in Information and Communication Technology (ICIICT)*, 2019.

[27] WenxiangXao, F. Shao, J. Ji, R. Sun, and C. Xing, "Fasting blood glucose change prediction model based on medical examination data and data mining techniques", in: *IEEE International Conference on Smart City/SocialCom/SustainCom (SmartCity)*, 2015.

[28] B. R. Prasad and S. Agarwal, "Modeling risk prediction of diabetes—a preventive measure", in: *9th International Conference on Industrial and Information Systems (ICIIS)*, 2014.

[29] J. Beschi Raja and S. Chenthur Pandian, "PSO-FCM based data mining model to predict diabetic disease", *Computer Methods and Programs in Biomedicine*, 2020, 196, 105659.

[30] K. Kantawong, S. Tongphet, P. Bhrommalee, N. Rachata, and S. Pravesjit, "The methodology for diabetes complications prediction model", in: *Joint International Conference on Digital Arts, Media and Technology with ECTI Northern Section Conference on Electrical, Electronics, Computer and Telecommunications Engineering (ECTIDAMT&NCON)*, 2020.

[31] D. R. Nemade and R. Kumar Gupta, "Diabetes prediction using BPSO and decision tree classifier", in: *2nd International Conference on Data, Engineering and Applications (IDEA)*, 2020.

[32] R. Akula, N. Nguyen, and I. Garibay, "Supervised machine learning based ensemble model for accurate prediction of type 2 diabetes", 2019, SoutheastCon.

[33] A. Viloria, Y. Herazo-Beltran, D. Cabrera, and O. B. Pineda, "Diabetes diagnostic prediction using vector support machines", *Procedia Computer Science*, 2020.

[34] Md. T. Islam, M. Raihan, N. Aktar, Md. S. Alam, R. Rahman Ema, and T. Islam, "Diabetes mellitus prediction using different ensemble machine learning approaches", in: *11th International Conference on Computing, Communication and Networking Technologies (ICCCNT)*, 2020.

[35] Md S. Islam, M. K. Qaraqe, H. T. Abbas, M. Erraguntla, and M. Abdul-Ghani, "The prediction of diabetes development: a machine learning framework", in: *IEEE 5th Middle East and Africa Conference on Biomedical Engineering (MECBME)*, 2020.

[36] B. Giri, N. S. Ghosh, R. Majumdar, and A. Ghosh, "Predicting diabetes implementing hybrid approach", in: *8th International Conference on Reliability, Infocom Technologies and Optimization (Trends and Future Directions) (ICRITO)*, 2020.

[37] O. Geman, I. Chiuchisan, and R. Toderean, "Application of adaptive neuro-fuzzy inference system for diabetes classification and prediction", in: *E-Health and Bioengineering Conference (EHB)*, 2017.

[38] G. G. Warsi, S. Saini, and K. Khatri, "Ensemble learning on diabetes data set and early diabetes prediction", in: *International Conference on Computing, Power and Communication Technologies (GUCON)*, 2019.

[39] M. B. Schulze, K. Hoffmann, H. Boeing, *et al.*, "An accurate risk score based on anthropometric, dietary, and lifestyle factors to predict the development of type 2 diabetes", *Diabetes Care*, 2007, 30(3), pp. 510–515.

[40] W. A. Sandham, E. D. Lehmann, D. J. Hamilton, and M. L. Sandilands, "Simulating and predicting blood glucose levels for improved diabetes healthcare", in: *4th IET International Conference on Advances in Medical, Signal and Information Processing - MEDSIP 2008*, 2008.

[41] C. Huang, G. Jiang, Z. Chen, and S. Chen, "The research on evaluation of diabetes metabolic function based on Support Vector Machine", in: *3rd International Conference on Biomedical Engineering and Informatics*, 2010.

[42] N. Barakat, A. P. Bradley, M. N. H. Barakat, "Intelligible support vector machines for diagnosis of diabetes mellitus", *IEEE Transactions on Information Technology in Biomedicine*, 2010, 14(4).

[43] F. Stahl and R. Johansson, "Short-term diabetes blood glucose prediction based on blood glucose measurements", in: *30th Annual International Conference of the IEEE Engineering in Medicine and Biology Society*, 2008.

[44] C. J. Steele, A. H. Marshall, A. Kouvonen, F. Kee, and R. Sund, "Modelling the time taken to experience a type 2 diabetes related complication using a survival tree in order to advise general practitioners", in: *IEEE 29th International Symposium on Computer-Based Medical Systems (CBMS)*, 2016.

[45] H.-C. Chan, J.-C. Chen, S.-W. Chien, Y.-F. Chen, and Cho-TsanBau, "Evaluation of intelligent system to the control of diabetes", in: *International Symposium on Computer, Consumer and Control*, 2012.

[46] D. A. Finan, C. C. Palerm, F. J. Doyle, *et al.*, "Identification of empirical dynamic models from type 1 diabetes subject data", in *American Control Conference, 2008*.

[47] C. Zecchin, A. Facchinetti, G. Sparacino, G. De Nicolao, and C. Cobelli, "A new neural network approach for short-term glucose prediction using continuous glucose monitoring time-series and meal information", in: *Annual*

International Conference of the IEEE Engineering in Medicine and Biology Society, 2011.

[48]   E. Georga, V. Protopappas, A. Guillen, *et al.*, "Data mining for blood glucose prediction and knowledge discovery in diabetic patients: the METABO diabetes modeling and management system", in: *Annual International Conference of the IEEE Engineering in Medicine and Biology Society*, 2009.

[49]   N. Khan, C.A. Ikejiaku, and S. Rahman, "Prediction of type II MODY3 diabetes using backpercolation", in: *18th IEEE Symposium on Computer-Based Medical Systems (CBMS'05)*, 2005.

[50]   K. Yadav and Sunil Gupta, "Hybridization of K-means clustering using different distance function to find the distance among dataset", in *International Conference on Information and Communication Technology for Intelligent Systems*, Springer Science, 2020.

[51]   J. Eggermont, J. N. Kok, and W. A. Kosters. *Genetic Programming for Data Classification: Partitioning the Search Space.* SAC, 2004.

Chapter 6

Use of deep learning approaches for the prediction of diseases from medical images

Amrita Thakur[1], Kushagra Nagori[2], Ayushman Rao[2] and Neeta Rai[1]

Medical imaging is indispensable in the study or prediction of various medical conditions, early identification, surveillance, diagnosis, and therapy assessment. Understanding medical images for disease analysis using computer vision requires two key concepts: deep learning (DL) and artificial neural networks (ANNs). This chapter explains the DL approach (DLA), which uses medical picture analysis to determine if a disease is present or not. The creation of ANNs and a thorough examination of DLA, which have intriguing applications for medical imaging, will also be covered in this chapter. The majority of DLA implementations concentrate on digital histology, computed tomography, mammography, and X-ray pictures. It offers a thorough analysis of the articles for DLA-based classification, detection, and segmentation of medical images. This book chapter concludes by providing researchers, medical professionals, scientists, advanced students, and academics with valuable information to comprehend medical images and the significant role of ANNs and DLA, in predicting diseases.

6.1 Introduction

Prior to the last ten years, it was extremely challenging to obtain healthcare data, and if it was accessible, it was of a minimal scale. However, that is no longer the case in today's environment. The amount of data available for image analysis has increased dramatically due to the remarkable progress made in image acquisition technologies. Radiologists, doctors, and other medical specialists worked long hours to significantly improve digital biomedical imaging and modalities. Digital image analysis, in particular, necessitates enormous variances in examination and diagnosis based on subject matter specialists. Machine learning (ML) may address these problems, although typical ML methods are unsuitable for complicated

[1]School of Pharmacy, Vishwakarma University, Pune, India
[2]Rungta College of Pharmaceutical Sciences & Research, Rungta Educational Campus, Bhilai, India

situations. When solving complex challenges, high-performing computing (HPC) and ML work together to provide promising outcomes [1]. Deep learning (DL) is the ultimate consequence of HPC and ML cooperation, and this will yield the best results on massive medical picture datasets. Accurate findings will be obtained with this method. Automated feature selection, as well as the capacity to quantify prognosis goals and produce convoluted estimate models, is provided by DL, which further enhances the diagnostic abilities of medical specialists. Among the many applications of ML, the most significant are decision-making, recommendation, image analysis, and online search engines. ML techniques such as neural networks, random forests (RFs), hidden Markov models, SVM support vector machines (SVMs), and Gaussian networks are all used in the processing of medical images.

Bioinformatics is a branch of medical study that deals with image processing. Data modalities used in bioinformatics include medical digital image processing. Moreover, it includes omics and biomedical signaling. Medical image processing has recently seen a significant uptick in applying sophisticated DL algorithms. Such systems have been shown by IBM's WATSONS and Google's DeepMind. Several bioinformatics issues were addressed with the application of DL algorithms in these initiatives. IBM's Watson uses Doctors' patient health records to determine the best possible remedies. To tackle health-related issues and terminology, Google's DeepMind designed a DeepMind health system. The raw data in medical imaging may not be compatible with conventional ML algorithms. This is because medical pictures have a sophisticated structural design (the number of features is very high). Medical image analysis does not benefit from handmade feature selection methods (ML). Among many classic techniques, feature vector extraction is the most important for image analysis. For input data, neural network design relies heavily on feature vectors. Data from photos in the medical area must be processed for feature vectors before being fed into neural networks. Moreover, raw data like this requires much more work to preprocess and takes a long time. By using DL, a deep neural network (DNN) can assist in resolving these issues. DL phenomena may be studied in a wide range of bioinformatics applications. Merriam-Webster describes the field of bioinformatics as "a collection of data, to undertake classification and prediction utilizing feature extraction by the study of biochemical properties and biological information using computers." Protein structure prediction, gene expression control, protein categorization, and anomaly classification are the subjects of study in bioinformatics [2]. Some of the data available in bioinformatics include omics (RNA, DNA, RNase, protein sequences, etc.), biomedical imaging (CT scan, MRI, PET, etc.), and biomedical signal processing (ECG, EEG, EMG, etc.). As a result, this chapter will teach readers how to use medical image processing and analysis to forecast the development of disease. Additionally, this chapter will give a thorough explanation of the DL and ML methods used in biomedical image research, which aid in the diagnosis and prognosis of diseases.

6.2   Overview of the medical imaging

Medial imagining was a part of biological imaging, developed after the 19th century. Let us first understand a radiological image of a whole human body. In a radiological image, some kind of energy must enter the body, interact with it, and then send a signal to a detector, usually outside the body. Visible light may be utilized in dermatology and other areas of medicine for observation; however, the fundamental objective of radiological imaging is to create pictures that reflect anatomy or physiological function much below the skin's surface electromagnetic spectrum is put to extensive use for medical imaging in diagnostic radiology. This includes the use of X-rays in mammography, radiography, fluoroscopy, and computed tomography (CT); radiofrequency (RF) waves are utilized in magnetic resonance imaging (MRI); and gamma rays are used in nuclear medicine. In ultrasonic imaging, the mechanical energy produced by a transducer undergoing fast vibration is converted into sound waves operating at excessively high frequencies [3].

In the same way, all fields of medical imaging, except for nuclear medicine, need the energy used to enter the body's tissues and interact with those tissues. If the energy went through the body without interacting in any way, like being absorbed or scattered, then the energy that was picked up would not contain any useful information about the body's internal structure. With the information that was found, it would not be possible to make an image of the body. Radioactive chemicals are either injected or swallowed as part of nuclear medicine imaging. The information in the pictures comes from how the radioactive material moves through the body, which is called the "physiologically mediated biodistribution of the agent."

The diagnostic value of a medical picture is directly proportional to the image's level of technical quality and the circumstances under which it was acquired. When using medical imaging devices, there is often a trade-off between the quality of the images and the amount of radiation. This can be explained as the more the rays a patient absorbs the higher the ultrasonic power level and the better the pictures will be. When capturing medical pictures, however, the patient's safety and comfort must be a top priority. As a result, administering an excessively high dose of radiation to the patient to achieve the ideal image is unacceptable. Because of this, the power and energy levels employed to produce medical pictures necessitate a trade-off between the patient's safety and the quality of the resulting image. The medical imaging and prediction of diseases are related to the study of ML. ML is a part of artificial intelligence and along with DL it does wonders in the presumption of severe diseases [4].

6.3 Overview of ML

Medical imaging can benefit from the pattern recognition method known as ML. The initial step in ML often involves computing the picture attributes that are thought to be crucial for producing the desired prediction or diagnosis. To classify the image or derive some metric for the selected part of the image, the system uses ML techniques to identify the optimal arrangement of those image properties. Moreover, there are numerous approaches that can help in calculating these images but all have their advantages and disadvantages. The majority of these ML techniques are available in open-source forms, making it simple to test them out and use them on pictures. There are many metrics available for evaluating an algorithm's effectiveness, but one must be aware of any potential flaws that could lead to inaccurate results. However, utilizing ML algorithms for computer-aided detection and diagnosis can speed up and assist physicians' interpretation of medical imaging results [5]. Also, these techniques could be used to do a variety of difficult things, such as segmenting brain tumors with magnetic resonance (MR) imaging, finding out how the brain works with functional MR imaging to diagnose neurological diseases (like dementia), and finding and diagnosing breast cancer with mammography [6–8]. Even though the readers of this chapter must be familiar with medical images, but many may not know about ML. That is the use of ML in medical image analysis and interpretation of data. One can easily understand the definition and use of ML by the following example: algorithms will be developed to predict any disease, here we will take the example of a brain tumor. The algorithms will be developed in such a way that we can classify brain tumors into benign and malignant. Then, the different medical images will be run which is commonly known as a data set. Based on the data set algorithms for benign and malignant, the tumors can be identified and categorized, respectively. The algorithm system is said to be learning if it increases its performance by optimizing its settings, i.e., by properly diagnosing more tests.

Let us now learn about various commonly used terms used in ML. These definitions will help to understand how ML works.

1. Classification: An algorithm is a way to give a cluster of images, like the pixels that make up that tumor, a class or label. In this case, the classifier might look for signs of benign or cancerous tissue in the segmented area that was labeled "abnormal brain" during image segmentation.
2. Model: Collection of consideration points in an ML system. After learning, the prototype can be used to figure out which class an unknown example relates to.
3. Algorithm: The procedure of creating a model that can be used to accurately forecast categories based on features observed in the simulation instances.
4. Labeled data: An arrangement of specimens (e.g., visual representations) that exhibit the appropriate "response." The response could potentially serve as a suitable indicator for specific occupations. For example, it can help to identify the presence of cancer or the type based on the lesion.
5. Training: The initial stage of the ML algorithm involves the provision of labeled example data, which includes answers in the form of labels. These labels may pertain to various aspects, such as tumor type or accurate lesion boundaries. The model's weights or decision points undergo iterative adjustments until a point is reached where there is no longer a statistically significant improvement in performance.
6. Validation set: It is also called the training set, they are basically a group of examples that are utilized for training.
7. Testing: A tertiary pair of samples is occasionally utilized for "actual world" testing, and the computer system may pick up on various elements of the training set as it replicates to increase its performance with the validation set. Gaining credibility for the algorithm's ability to reliably provide correct results in the

actual world requires it to perform well on an "unseen" test set. It is important to keep in mind that different communities equate validation with testing. This is indicative of the engineering background as opposed to the statistical one. This is why it is crucial to specify the meaning of these terms in context.

8. Node: A fundamental element of a neural network is a node, which comprises multiple inputs and an activation function. Mostly, an output is obtained when the initiation function adds up with the inputs

9. Layer: A layer is comprised of a set of nodes that perform computations on one or multiple input values to generate corresponding output values.

10. Weights: Weights are the values that result from multiplying every incoming feature by a certain amount. They are adjusted throughout training till the optimal configuration is determined.

6.4 Types of ML

There are three types of ML algorithms based on their aiming pattern. They are the following: supervised, unsupervised, and reinforcement learning [9]. These techniques are employed for the purpose of differentiating the regions on the brain showing either tumor (malignant or benign) region or normal tissue region. Let's discuss supervised learning. Images of benign and malignant brain tumors are used in supervised learning to gain experience and then apply the knowledge gained to predict the presence of benign and malignant neoplasia in new brain tumor images that have never been seen before (test data). A set of images of brain tumors, each labeled as benign or malignant, are fed to the algorithm system in this hypothetical example. Later, the system would be put to the test by having it attempt to classify findings on new images as either benign or malignant. SVMs, decision trees, linear regressions, logistic regressions, naive Bayes, k-nearest neighbors, RFs, AdaBoost, and neural network methods all fall under the umbrella of supervised learning techniques [10]. However, when using unsupervised learning, data, such as images of brain tumors, are treated with the intention of classifying the images into distinct categories; for instance, those depicting benign tumors are separated from those depicting malignant tumors. The most important distinction is that this is carried out in spite of the fact that the algorithmic system is not supplied with information concerning the identities of the groups. The algorithmic process decides how many groups there are and how to divide them up into distinct categories [11–13]. ML is an essential discipline for developing automated systems for tasks as diverse as decision-making, recommendations, image analysis, web searching, and more. Many different types of ML are employed in the field of biomedical image processing. These include artificial neural networks (ANNs), RFs, hidden Markov models, SVMs, gaussian networks, and others.

Supervised learning
It provides a computer system with a training set of cases with appropriate goals. Using this training set technique, it is feasible to accurately respond to a given set of inputs.

Supervised learning is divided into two categories: classification and regression.

- Actions must be taken by a trained system to assign concealed inputs to specific classes based on the classification algorithms used. Multi-labeling is one example of this. E-mails are identified as "spam" or "not spam" throughout the spam purification process.
- Rather than producing discrete results, regression is a supervised method. The root mean squared error (RMSE) is used as a performance measure for regression predictions, whereas accuracy is used for classification predictions.

Unsupervised learning
In this technique, instead of relying on a pre-existing dataset, the system will make a judgment on its own. The system that can be utilized to make predictions is given no labeling at all. It is possible to apply feature learning to uncover the hidden pattern using unsupervised learning.

To categorize the inputs, an unsupervised learning approach known as "clustering" was employed. These clusters are not discovered until later on. It creates groupings based on similarity.

Types of ML algorithms
Selecting optimal feature weights can be done using any number of available algorithms. These algorithms are dependent on various assumptions and methods for fine-tuning feature weights. Some of the most popular ones will be covered below; they consist of decision trees, the naive Bayes algorithm, SVMs, neural networks, k-nearest neighbors, and DL.

Neural networks
ML most frequently takes the form of neural network-based learning. The framework for learning in the aforementioned technique is composed of the three elements described below. First, the network weight modifies in response to the search function. These values are determined by the update function. The update function also helps to determine the direction and magnitude of change necessary to minimize the error function. Lastly, the error function will then evaluate the degree of correspondence between a given set of inputs and the output.

k-nearest neighbors
Classification using k-nearest neighbors works by placing an unlabeled example object into the category or categories to which it is most comparable. An input vector is another name for a set of features for this object. The variable k denotes the quantity of identified entities in close proximity to the exemplar entity, which collectively participate in a decision-making process to determine the potential classifications that may be attributed to the exemplar entity. According to this definition, an object's neighbors are those other known objects that are physically close by. If k is 1, the unknown item's class is simply taken to be that of the nearest known object. A method for quantifying the degree of similarity between two instances involves computing the Euclidean distance between the input

vector's values and those of the vector corresponding to the remaining cases. When compared to the vector values of the other cases, this distance provides useful information. It is crucial, however, that feature vector values be normalized properly.

SVMs
The SVM algorithm employs a transformation of the data to generate a support vector or plane with the maximum width. The data is subjected to a series of modifications to generate a support vector that distinguishes between the two classes. These machines exhibit high flexibility in terms of selecting a broad range of separation planes and the corresponding quantity of imprecise points that ensue from such planes. However, these systems attained prominence subsequent to the integration of fundamental functionalities that facilitate the mapping of points to alternate dimensions through nonlinear interactions [14]. They can also classify data that is not easily divided into discrete groups. As a result, the algorithms offer the most benefits among all ML techniques.

Decision tree
All the aforementioned ML methods have one major drawback in common. They are unable to retrieve the meaningful human-interpretable information from weights and activation function employed in a given model. The significant benefit that decision trees provide is the generation of rules that are comprehensible by humans for determining how a specific instance should be categorized [15]. The majority of people are familiar with decision trees, which often take the form of yes-or-no questions. One of these questions may ask if a specific numeric value is greater than another. In ML, the expedited exploration of potential decision point combinations to construct a concise decision tree yielding optimal accuracy is a crucial aspect of decision trees. This aspect of decision trees is known as the decision point combination search. When the algorithm is executed, one selects the maximum depth (i.e., the maximum number of decision points) and the maximum breadth (the maximum number of decision points) that are to be searched. One also determines the relative importance of having accurate findings and having more decision points. In certain circumstances, one's accuracy can be improved by employing an ensemble method, which involves the construction of more than one decision tree. Techniques known as bagging and RF are two ensemble methods that are frequently employed. Building numerous decision trees can be accomplished using boosting with aggregation, which is also known as bagging. The method entails iteratively resampling the training dataset with replacement, followed by aggregating the predictions of the decision trees through a voting mechanism to yield a consensus forecast [16]. The RF classifier employs multiple decision trees to enhance classification accuracy and typically exhibits superior performance, yet it does not engage in data resampling. The RF algorithm partitions each node in a decision tree by selecting the most influential attribute from a randomly selected subset of the entire feature set. In contrast, the bagging strategy chooses how to split a node based on all of its attributes.

Naive Bayes algorithm

The Bayes theorem, one of the earliest techniques of ML, argues that an event's probability depends on other events that are related to it [17]. $P(y|x) = [P(y) \, P(x|y)]/ P(x)$ is the formula for the Bayes theorem. In ML, given a matrix of input features, the probabilities of each feature must be chained together when there are many input features to determine the final probability of a class. Unlike other ML algorithms, the naive Bayes method uses only one computation to determine the relationship between the input feature set and output. The Bayes algorithms do not call for an iterative training process. Data from training and testing is still needed, therefore, the concerns raised above still apply. Due to the independent feature of one another, this technique is called a naive Bayes algorithm and not just Bayes algorithms. Because this is not always the case, taking this strategy can produce findings that are not accurate. To get useful estimates of performance despite the assumption being broken, this method can still be applied [18]. Additionally, compared to other methods that call for a high number of instances, employing this method can produce more trustworthy results when there are fewer examples available. The issue of pre-test probability and accuracy is also brought up: if a positive discovery was prevalent in 1% of cases, one could just label all cases as negative and get 99% accuracy. Frequently, 100% specificity and 99% accuracy would be considered acceptable, but this method would have no sensitivity. Prior probability is a crucial component that will affect how effectively a system works from this perspective, as accuracy alone is insufficient.

DL and its approaches

Using neural networks to learn and predict data makes this a sophisticated form of ML. In addition, it is a collection of several algorithms. Complex systems that can handle any type of problem and forecast the outcome are used in this method. As high-performance computing became more widely available, the popularity of DL algorithms such as neural networks increased. The ability to examine a large number of features has made DL more powerful and flexible than other ML methods when working with unstructured data. Using a DL method, the data is passed through multiple stages, each of which is capable of gradually extracting features and then passing them on to the next stage. The image's basic elements are gathered in the first layer, and the subsequent layers combine them into a more complete picture [19].

Convolutional neural networks

When analyzing photographs, convolutional neural networks, more commonly referred to simply as CNN, are frequently utilized. It accomplishes this by assigning different weights and biases to the various components of the image, which enables it to differentiate between the various components of the picture. When compared to other methods of classification, it has a lower threshold for the amounts of preprocessing that are considered appropriate. CNN accomplishes the goal of capturing the spatial and temporal correlations present in a picture by applying the necessary filters [20]. The different CNN designs include LeNet, AlexNet, VGGNet, GoogleNet, ResNet, and ZFNet. CNNs are most commonly utilized for a variety of applications, including Object Detection, Semantic Segmentation, and Captioning, among others [21].

Recurrent neural networks
When using recurrent neural networks, or RNNs, outputs from previous states are used as inputs for the present state. It is possible to store data in the RNN's hidden layers of memory. The previous state's output informs the updating of the concealed state. Time series prediction is possible because an RNN has "long-short term memory" that can recall previous inputs [22].

6.5 Use of artificial intelligence in medical imaging

6.5.1 Use of ML in medical imaging

Specific disorders can be easily studied by using ML algorithms in medical imaging. In medical image processing, different sorts of items, for example, lesions and organs, are too complicated to be represented by simple mathematical solutions. Medical image processing was the first field to use pixel analysis in ML, which uses particular values in pictures without first initially separating features from portions of input data [23]. It is a superior method as compared to basic feature-based classifiers for certain situations. It is difficult to study the image's qualities when it has low contrast. Pixel-based ML does not require the calculation and segmentation of features, unlike conventional classifiers that avoid errors caused by improper segmentation and feature calculation. Due to the high dimensionality of data (a large number of pixels in an image), pixel analysis requires extensive training time [24]. The expert systems utilize ML to produce premises based on patient information. To paradigmatized an expert system, input from specialists is mined for distinct rules. ML techniques may be used to develop a methodical description of clinical characteristics that specifically characterize the clinical situations. Knowledge of intelligent systems may be utilized to achieve the group of clinical problems that may be used as examples. As a result, information can be described as a decision tree or by grouping simple rules together. KARDIO, which was developed to translate ECGs, is a classic example of this type of approach [25]. A statistical analysis is regarded as the gold standard for examining image attributes in the field of medical image analysis.

The channelized Hoteling observer, often known as CHO, is a device that is frequently used for nuclear medicine imaging treatments. The notion that flexible topics are present in the human visual system activates the channels. This method is used to identify and rate picture quality, and it also has a justified and advantageous impact on medical imaging. An SVM, or channelized SVM, is the next algorithm (CSVM). Two medical physicists assessed the defect discernibility in a hundred distinct noisy images, and using a six-point scoring system, they estimated the score confidence of a lesion actuality contemporary. Following that, a training session will include an additional 60 images. For a total of six separate alternatives for the flattening filter and two distinct choices regarding the total number of repetitions in the OS-EM rebuilding phase, the human viewers were effective in completing this assignment [26].

6.5.2   Use of DL in medical imaging

DL principle depends upon the principle that computer programs can better understand how to classify certain types of data. Because of the gradual packing of high-level information into the models, the input photos are transformed into outputs regarding specific diseases by the models, which consist of several layers. Convolutional neural networks (CNNs) are a superior sort of model for image analysis. Convolution filters are used in multiple layers of CNNs to transform input data. DL approaches are commonly used in the medical profession to familiarize current architectures with unique input formats, such as 3D data. CNNs were formerly used to handle large amounts of data without having to deal with the enormous number of restrictions that come along with full 3D convolutions [27].

6.6   Computer-aided approaches for predicting diseases

There are different ways by which computer-aided approaches have proved to be very efficient in predicting medical images. They are described below:

- Image classification
  Identifying and analyzing clinically relevant issues are the primary goals of DL, which focuses on the classification of medical images. Multiple photos can be used as input for the categorization, and a single diagnostic can be modified as a result (disease yes or no). Rather than relying on large datasets like in computer vision, each diagnostic test is treated as a model in these circumstances instead. Studies showed that after using a DL method like CNN, there was a fine modification of 57.6% from 53.4% accuracy in multiclass score evaluation of knee osteoarthritis [28]. Similarly, there was 70.5% improvement in cytopathology picture was also observed using the DL CNN method [29].
- Object classification
  Object classification focuses on the smaller interesting bits that are contained inside the medical image. It is possible to project these portions into two or more different classes. Both the local knowledge of these chunks and the global conceptual information are particularly significant for achieving a higher level of precision. Researchers have also used this classification technique to get precision results. In one of the studies, three CNN methods of DL were used together to patch the image at a different scale of objects. These three methods ultimately produced results that reflected the features matrix of the overall image qualities [30].

Detection: organ and region
The phase that comes to the following classification is the one in which objects are found and their locations are determined. It is a key step in the segmentation process

in which we can extract the relevance of each object and focus solely on the object of interest while ignoring the noise. A strategy known as 3D data parsing, which makes use of DL algorithms, is being utilized to tackle this problem. When creating the medical image, the author utilized three separate groupings of 2D and 3D MRI bits. It is utilized to locate the regions of several linked objects that focus on some specific disorders such as the heart, aortic arch, and descending aorta, among others [31,32].

Segmentation
To process the many organs and substructures present in medical images, the segmentation technique is utilized. Quantitative analysis of the clinical aspects can be performed with its help. An example of this would be a brain or cardiac exam. In CAD, functions are another application for the technology. The identification of certain pixels that compose the object of interest is the task at hand here. The up-sampling and down-sampling layers' architectures have been combined to form what is known as the U-net. The connections between layers' convolution and deconvolution samples were combined as a result [33].

Registration
The process of transforming various data sets into a single coordinate system is known as registration. To give a comparison or integration of the data received from diverse viewpoints, times, depths, sensors, etc., this phase is required in medical pictures. It is a prerequisite for the process. During this stage of the iterative process, we will choose a certain category of parameters to use as a benchmark. Calculating the similarity parameters of two photos using DL algorithms is one of its many applications. The registration is utilized in the medical field, particularly in computer tomography (CT) and nuclear magnetic resonance (NMR) data. This is of great use in acquiring patient information, monitoring the development of the tumor, determining whether or not the patient has been cured, and comparing the patient's data with anatomical figures [34].

6.7   Medical diagnosis of various diseases using ML

The process of disease diagnosis has been explored by a substantial number of researchers and physicians from the standpoint of ML. The many forms of ML-based disease diagnosis (MLBDD), which have drawn a lot of attention in recent years because of the importance and complexity of the ailments they represent, are described in this section. For example, as a result of COVID-19's importance on a global scale, a number of studies have focused on understanding COVID-19 as a disease by utilizing ML between the years 2020 and the present day. ML has been utilized in a number of these studies. We will now discuss various severe diseases and the use of ML for the diagnosis of these diseases.

6.7.1   Heart disease
When it comes to diagnosing cardiac issues, the vast majority of academics and practitioners turn to diagnostic approaches that are supported by ML [35,36].

Ansari and his coworkers described a neurofuzzy integrated systems-based system for the automated diagnosis of coronary heart disease in 2011. The system's results revealed an accuracy of roughly 89% [36]. Researchers who developed the system did not provide detailed descriptions of a number of possible use cases, including multiclass classification, massive data analysis, and unequal class distribution. There is also no explanation of how the model arrived at its results, which is becoming increasingly recommended in the medical domains, especially to help users who are not from the medical domains understand the approach. However, later in 2017, Rubin and his colleagues made use of methods that were derived from deep convolutional neural networks (DCNN) to recognize aberrant heart sounds, and thus, they work in overcoming the drawback of the above-discussed method. The alteration of the loss function to improve the sensitivity as well as the specificity of the training dataset was introduced in this study. This was accomplished by increasing the size of the training dataset. At the PhysioNet computing competition in 2016, the above-mentioned model was put through its paces. They had a final forecast that had a specificity of 0.95 and a sensitivity of 0.73, which brought them to second place overall in the competition [37]. Aside from that, there has been a significant rise in interest in the use of algorithms that are powered by DL in the process of diagnosing conditions related to the heart. Similarly in 2018, based on a multiclass morphologic pattern, Miao developed a DL-based method for detecting cardiotocographic fetal health. In this method, the fetal heart rate is used. In this approach, the morphologic pattern is comprised of a large number of classes. The model that was built is put to use to differentiate and classify the morphologic pattern of persons who are experiencing issues connected to pregnancy. These individuals can be identified by the fact that they have a history of having complications during pregnancy. The first results of their calculations show that they are 88.2% accurate, 85.1% precise, and have an *F*-score of 0.85 [38]. In the course of that research, they implemented a number of dropout mechanisms to address overfitting concerns, which led to an increase in the amount of time spent training in the end. They did admit, however, that this was a necessary compromise to reach a higher level of precision. Despite the widespread use of ML applications in cardiac diagnosis, there has been no investigation into the challenges presented by multiclass categorization and data asymmetry.

6.7.2   Kidney disease

Renal disease can refer to either nephropathy or injury to the kidneys. Patients who are experiencing renal sickness have reduced renal functional motion, which, if not addressed as quickly as possible can lead to kidney failure. According to statistics provided by the National Kidney Foundation, 10% of the world's population is affected by chronic kidney disease (CKD), and each year, millions of individuals pass away as a direct result of insufficient care for their condition. Recent advances in artificial learning based on kidney disease diagnosis could be a chance for countries that can't handle the diagnostic tests that are linked to renal disease [39]. In 2016, Charleonnann and coworkers evaluated four distinct machine-learning techniques by using datasets that were freely available to the public. Logistic regression (LR), K-nearest neighbors (KNN), decision tree classifiers, and SVM were among the algorithms used. The researchers were able to achieve an accuracy of 98.1% with the KNN classifier, 98.3% with the SVM classifier, 96.55% with the LR classifier, and 94.8% with the decision tree classifier [40]. Moreover, in 2018, Aljaaf and colleagues conducted a study that was quite similar to the previous one, and they found very similar results. The authors evaluated a wide variety of ML methods, including RPART, SVM, and LOGR. They came to the conclusion that MLP was the method that was most accurate in detecting chronic renal disease (97.8% accuracy) [41]. Later, to make a diagnosis of chronic renal disease, Ma and coworkers made use of a combination of datasets, each of which contains data compiled from a different set of sources [42]. The heterogeneous modified ANN (HMANN) model that they proposed achieved an accuracy of between 87% and 99%.

6.7.3 Breast cancer

Several scholars who are active in the field of medicine have proposed the possibility that an evaluation of breast cancer based on ML could be a workable alternative for the diagnosis of the disease in its earlier stages. Therefore, in 2015, Miranda and Felipe proposed computer-aided diagnostic approaches for the classification of breast cancer that were based on fuzzy logic. Fuzzy logic has an advantage over more traditional approaches to ML in the sense that it may reduce the amount of computational complexity. They simultaneously imitate the thinking and approach of an experienced radiologist. This advantage gives fuzzy logic an advantage over more traditional approaches to ML. When an input is entered, parameters such as contour, form, and density, the algorithm generates a cancer category based on the technique selected by the user [43]. The proposed model showed an accuracy of 83.4%. The authors of the study carried out the experiment multiple times, and each time utilized around the same number of photos. However, the outcomes of the experiment were not enough accurate but also more objective. Unfortunately, because their data interpretation was not explored in an explicable manner throughout the investigation, it could be challenging to conclude that accuracy, in general, demonstrates genuine accuracy for both benign and malignant categories. In addition, there is no presentation of a confusion matrix to highlight the actual forecast that the models provide for each class. In contrast, Zheng and coworkers developed a hybrid method in 2014 that combines K-means clustering (KMC) and SVM for diagnosing breast cancer. Using the Wisconsin Diagnostic Breast Cancer (WDBC) dataset, their proposed model significantly reduced the dimensional difficulties and achieved an accuracy of 97.38% [44]. The dataset comprises 32 features split into 10 categories and is normally distributed. It is difficult to get to the conclusion that their planned prototypical would perform better in a dataset that contains a missing value and may also have an uneven class ratio. Similarly, Asri and his colleagues utilized a variety of ML methods on the Wisconsin Breast Cancer (WBC) datasets in 2016, including SVM, DT (C4.5), NB, and KNN. This was done to determine which ML models worked the best. According to the findings of their investigation, the SVM performed far better than any other approach to ML, with an accuracy of 97.13% [45]. A feedforward neural network was used by Bhattacherjee and colleagues in their 2020 project for the diagnosis of breast cancer (BNN). The trial was conducted with the use of the WBC dataset, and it included nine different features; the results demonstrated that it was accurate for about 99.27% [46]. Later, in 2021, using the datasets of WBCD and WDBI, Alshayeji with coworkers constructed a shallow ANN model for classifying breast cancer tumors. This model was used to classify breast cancer tumors. The authors demonstrated that the proposed model was capable of accurately classifying tumors at a rate of up to 99.85% without selecting features or adjusting the algorithms [47]. Furthermore, Sultan and his colleagues were effective in detecting breast cancer in 2021 by employing a novel ANN design on the WBC dataset. They used neural network architectures such as the probabilistic neural network (PNN), the SVM neural network, and the recurrent neural network (RNN). The PNN, which has an accuracy of 98.24%, is superior to the other NN models that were utilized in that study, according to the conclusive computational conclusion that they attained [48]. However, the interpretability of this study is not on par with that of a great many other investigations because it does not propose which features are most significant when it comes to the prediction phase of the process. Another strategy that Ghosh and his colleagues utilized was known as DL in 2021. The WBC dataset was used by the researchers to read seven different DL models. ANN, CNN, and gated recurrent unit (GRU), long short-term memory (LSTM), MLP, and RNN were some of the models that were utilized here. Among all DL models, the LSTM and GRU performed the best, with an accuracy of about 99% [49].

6.7.4   Diabetes

Based on the International Diabetes Federation (IDF), there are currently more than 382 million people living with diabetes worldwide, with that figure expected to rise to 629 million by the year 2045 [50]. There have been a significant number of studies that have presented algorithms that are based on ML for the diagnosis of diabetes patients. In 2015, Kandhasamy and Balamurali conducted an experiment to classify patients who had diabetes mellitus using a variety of ML classifiers, such as J48 DT, KNN, RF, and SVM. The UCI Diabetes dataset was used in the experiment, and the findings revealed that the KNN ($K = 1$) and RF classifiers attained an accuracy that was extremely near to being perfect [51]. In contrast, one of the limitations of this work was that it was carried out using a simplified Diabetes dataset that consisted of only eight features that were binary-classified. This was one of the ways in which the work was limited. It is not anything that should come as a surprise to anyone that it is possible to obtain a precision of one hundred percent utilizing a dataset that presents fewer difficulties. In addition, there is no description of in what manner the algorithms affect the final output or how the result should be interpreted from a perspective that is not technical. These two topics are noticeably absent from the essay's discussion. Clinical Decision Support

System, often known as CDSS, is a system that was proposed by Yahyaoui and associates in 2019. Its purpose was to provide assistance to medical professionals who were attempting to diagnose diabetes. To accomplish this purpose, the research made use of a number of ML methods, such as SVM, RFs, and DCNNs. RF outperformed all of the other algorithms in their computations by achieving an accuracy of 83.67%, whilst DL and SVM only achieved an accuracy of 76.81% and 65.38%, respectively [52]. The PIMA Diabetes datasets, which are available to the public, were analyzed by Naz and Ahuja in 2020 using a variety of ML techniques. ANN, neural bias, decision trees, and DL were some of these methods. According to their findings, DL is the method with the highest level of precision for detecting diabetes progression, with a precision of approximately 98.07% [50]. The PIMA dataset is one of the most thoroughly examined major datasets, making it simple to run both classic and advanced ML-based algorithms. The fact that we were able to improve our accuracy by utilizing the PIMA Indian dataset is not something that should come as a surprise to anyone. In addition, the publication does not cover any of the challenges associated with interpretability or how the model would fare when applied to a dataset that was either unbalanced or lacking a significant number of variables. In the field of healthcare, it is common knowledge that numerous types of data may be generated, some of which may not necessarily adhere to the same standards of labeling, categorization, and preprocessing as the PIMA Indian data-set. The PIMA Indian dataset follows some of these guidelines. Overfitting is a problem that has been studied in relation to diabetes datasets, and, in 2017, Ashiquzzaman and colleagues presented a deep-learning technique to address this issue. The PIMA Indian dataset was used in the experiment, and the findings revealed that it provided accurate results 88.41% of the time. The authors claimed that once the dropout approaches were adopted and the overfitting difficulties were controlled, there was a significant improvement in the performance [53]. On the other hand, excessive use of the dropout approach will make the overall amount of time necessary to complete the training for longer. It is difficult to evaluate whether or not their proposed model is the most efficient in terms of the amount of pro-cessing time it requires as a result of the fact that they did not address these chal-lenges in their research.

6.7.5   *Parkinson's disease*

Parkinson's disease is another critical disease that is taking everyone's attention. However, a considerable amount of research and discussion has taken place on the disease in published medical articles. It is a persistent neurological disorder that moves at a slow but steady pace from stage to stage. Disruption or death of dopamine-producing neurons in certain brain regions leads to difficulties with communication, motor control, and other basic skills [54]. Because of this, people have difficulties with other fundamental activities as well. Alternative approaches that make use of ML have been proposed on multiple occasions as possible answers. In 2013, Sriram and his coworkers built intelligent Parkinson's disease diagnostic systems by utilizing KNN, SVM, NB, and RF algorithms. These algorithms were used to analyze patient data. The conclusion that can be derived from their computations is that, in comparison to all of the other algorithms, the performance of RF is the best (90.26% accuracy), while the performance of NB is the worst (69.23% accuracy) [55]. Similarly, in 2018, Esmaeilzadeh and associates proposed using a deep CNN-based model to diagnose Parkinson's disease, and they reached an accuracy of nearly 100% on both the train and test sets [56]. Despite this, there was no reference made during the trial of any potential overfitting concerns that may have taken place. In addition, the results of the experiments do not provide an acceptable interpretation of the final classification and regression, which is something that is now usually anticipated, in particular in CDSS. This is the case because the experiments were conducted to investigate CDSS. Further in 2018, Grover and his teammates utilized DL-based methods on the Parkinson's tele-monitoring speech dataset that was provided by the University of California, Irvine. During this study, when attempting to identify people with Parkinson's disease symptoms through the use of DNN, the researchers were successful in reaching an accuracy rate of approximately 81.67% in their trial (54). The efficiency of the ML-based approach in decision support systems that are able to diagnose Parkinson's patients, as well as brain tumors, was the subject of an extensive study by Warjurkar and Ridhorkar in 2021. They discovered that the technique worked well in both of these scenarios. The results of the study made it plainly evident that boosted logistic regression was superior to all other algorithms and models, obtaining an accuracy rate of 97.15% in the identification of people with Parkinson's disease. This conclusion was reached as a direct result of the researchers' findings. The Markov random technique, on the other hand, performed exceptionally well when it came to the segmentation of tumors, with an accuracy of 97.4% [57].

6.7.6   COVID-19

The present pandemic, which is also known as COVID-19 and was caused by the new severe acute respiratory syndrome coronavirus 2 (SARS-CoV-2), has become the most significant challenge that humanity has encountered in recent history. In spite of the fact that the manufacturing of a vaccine had been sped up in response to the global emergency, the vast majority of people were unable to obtain it for the duration of the crisis [58]. As a result of the high transmission rates and vaccine-related resistance displayed by the recently found COVID-19 Omicron strain, a further layer of concern has been added to the situation. Real-time reverse transcription-polymerase chain reaction, often known as RT-PCR, is the diagnostic approach that is currently regarded to be the method of choice for COVID-19 infection [59,60]. Throughout the course of the epidemic, the researcher advocated for the implementation of supplementary diagnostic methods, such as chest X-rays and computed tomography (CT), in conjunction with Artificial Intelligence and ML, to facilitate the early identification of individuals who are at risk of contracting the disease. In 2020, Chen and his coworkers projected a UNet++ model that utilizes CT scans from 51 COVID-19 patients as well as 82 patients who did not have COVID-19, and they achieved an accuracy of 98.5% [61]. Using a limited dataset that included 108 COVID-19 patients and 86 non-COVID-19 patients, Ardakani and coworkers in 2020 examined ten distinct DL models. The dataset was used to test the models. They were successful in accomplishing their goal of having a total accuracy of 99% [62]. Similarly, in 2020 Wang and his colleagues created an inception-based model by making use of a large dataset that had 453 CT scan pictures. As a result of their efforts, they achieved an accuracy rate of 73.1% with their work. On the other hand, neither the model's region of interest nor its network activity was effectively explained [63]. The COVNet model was proposed by Li and his coworkers in 2020, and it was able to achieve an accuracy rate of 96% by leveraging a large dataset consisting of 4,356 chest CT scans of patients with pneumonia, of which 1,296 were confirmed instances of COVID-19 [64]. In addition, the model was able to achieve this accuracy rate by leveraging a large dataset consisting of 4,356 chest CT scans of patients with pneumonia.

6.7.7 Alzheimer's disease

It is thought that between 60% and 70% of persons who are diagnosed with dementia have Alzheimer's disease [65]. Alzheimer's disease is a brain disease that frequently begins slowly but worsens over time. Alzheimer's disease can be recognized by a number of symptoms, some of which include difficulty communicating, disorientation, fluctuations in mood, and a variety of behavioral and emotional concerns. The life expectancy of the patient at the time of diagnosis is typically between three and nine years, and the patient's body functions have steadily deteriorated. A correct diagnosis made in a timely manner, on the other hand, can be of assistance in avoiding and taking the necessary activities to enter into proper treatment as quickly as possible. This will not only increase the probability of a longer life expectancy but it will also increase the life expectancy itself. Over the course of the past few years, the use of ML and DL has produced some promising findings in the diagnosis of people suffering from Alzheimer's disease. In 2020, Neelaveni and Devasana developed a model that makes use of SVM and DT to diagnose Alzheimer's disease in patients. They were able to achieve a precision of 85% for the former and 83.3% for the latter [66]. In addition, Collij and coworkers, in 2016, used SVM to diagnose Alzheimer's disease as well as moderate cognitive impairment (MCI) in a single individual, and they achieved an accuracy of 82% [67]. During the process of developing a diagnosis for Alzheimer's disease that is based on ML, a large number of algorithms have been adopted and analyzed. For instance, Vidushi and Shrivastava in 2019 carried out research utilizing logistic regression (LR), SVMs, decision trees (DT), ensemble RF, and Boosting Adaboost, and they obtained an accuracy of 78.95%, 81.58%, 81.58%, and 84.21%, respectively [68]. Because CNN achieves superior outcomes in image processing in comparison to other algorithms that are now in use, a great number of researchers have utilized a method that is based on CNN to identify Alzheimer's disease sufferers. Because of this, Ahmed *et al.* in 2020 proposed the use of a CNN model as a method of early Alzheimer's disease identification as well as classification. After being applied to the dataset that consists of 6,628 MRI photos, the planned prototype achieved a level of accuracy that was 99% [69].

6.7.8   Other diseases

In addition to the problem that was just covered, ML and DL have been utilized in the diagnostic process for an extensive variety of other conditions as well. The proliferation of vast volumes of data and the development in the capabilities of computers to process that data are two key causes that are primarily responsible for this surge in utilization. In 2020, Mao with his coworkers utilized DT and RF to categorize diseases according to eye movement [70]. Nosseir and Shawky in 2019 examined KNN and SVM in an effort to build an autonomous skin disease classification system for systems. They found that KNN was superior to SVM in all cases. They discovered that the KNN algorithm had the best performance, as it was able to obtain an accuracy of 98.22% [71]. Using CNN-based approaches like VGG16 and VGG19, Khan and coworkers in 2020 were successful in classifying multimodal brain tumors. The experiment was carried out utilizing the BraTs2015, BraTs2017, and BraTs2018 photo datasets, all of which are openly accessible to the general public. The findings demonstrated an accuracy of 97.8%, 96.9%, and 92.5% [72]. In 2018, Amin and coworkers conducted an analysis that was quite similar to this one and used the RF classifier as a method for segmenting tumors. An accuracy of 98.7% was achieved using the BRATS 2012 dataset; 98.7% was achieved using the BRATS 2013 dataset; 98.4% was achieved using the BRATS 2014 dataset; and 90.2% was achieved using the ISLES 2015 dataset [73]. In 2019, Dai and coworkers presented a model that was based on CNN with the intention of designing an application to identify skin cancer. The authors of the study conducted their experiments using a dataset known as HAM10000 that was easily accessible to the general public, and they were able to achieve an accuracy of 75.2% [74]. In 2019, Daghrir and partners investigated how well KNN, SVM, CNN, and majority voting performed on the dataset provided by the International Skin Imaging Collaboration (ISIC) for the purpose of making a diagnosis of melanoma, a kind of skin cancer [75].

6.8   Conclusion

Diagnostics and monitoring based on imaging in medicine face numerous challenges across the technological, scientific, and societal spectrums. As a result of technological advancements in the sector, imaging now has a higher degree of precision than in the past. However, each imaging approach has certain limitations in terms of its practical applications, which are further constrained by the underlying compositional components of the organ and tissue structures. Also, the conventional method of reading results from medical images by medical care providers is prone to error, and it takes a significant amount of time to make accurate predictions based on the outcomes of such images. In the event of a medical emergency, early diagnosis of any ailment will result in rapid treatment, and effective time management is also an essential component of the procedure. Over the past few years, the capabilities of ML have improved. At the moment, methods of ML are extremely robust to practical settings, and the structures really take use of the learning process. It was utilized in the practice of medical imaging in the past, and it is anticipated that its development in the next years will occur at a rapid pace. The application of ML to medical imaging has substantial implications for the treatment being administered. It is of the utmost importance that this line of study leads to improved medical care for patients. To ensure that ML techniques are put to use in the most effective manner possible, it is essential to first establish their capabilities. DL algorithms are utilized in medical image analysis. These algorithms assist in the categorization, classification, and enumeration of disease patterns derived from image processing. In addition to this, it enables the extension of analytical goals and the generation of therapy prediction models for patients. These difficulties are being considered by researchers in medical imaging, and DL is being applied to study in the field of health care, where it is continuing to thrive.

References

[1] Baldi P and Pollastri G. The principled design of large-scale recursive neural network architectures-DAG-RNNs and the protein structure prediction problem. *Journal of Machine Learning Research.* 2004;4(4):575–602.

[2] Mirowski P, Madhavan D, LeCun Y, and Kuzniecky R. Classification of patterns of EEG synchronization for seizure prediction. *Clinical Neurophysiology.* 2009;120(11):1927–40.

[3] Lee S, Choi M, Choi HS, Park MS, and Yoon S. FingerNet: deep learning-based robust finger joint detection from radiographs. In: *IEEE Biomedical Circuits and Systems Conference: Engineering for Healthy Minds and Able Bodies, BioCAS 2015 – Proceedings.* 2015;7348440.

[4] Denas O and Taylor J. Deep modeling of gene expression regulation in an Erythropoiesis model. 2013. https://api.semanticscholar.org/CorpusID: 15361904.

[5] Schoepf UJ and Costello P.CT angiography for diagnosis of pulmonary embolism: state of the art. *Radiology.* 2004;230(2):329–37.

[6] Schoepf UJ, Schneider AC, Das M, Wood SA, Cheema JI, and Costello P. Pulmonary embolism: computer-aided detection at multidetector row spiral computed tomography. *Journal of Thoracic Imaging.* 2007;22(4):319–23.

[7] Rana A, Dumka A, Singh R, Rashid M, Ahmad N, and Panda MK. An efficient machine learning approach for diagnosing Parkinson's disease by utilizing voice features. *Electronics.* 2022;11(22):3782.

[8] Kaur A, Rashid M, Bashir AK, and Parah SA. Detection of breast cancer masses in mammogram images with watershed segmentation and machine learning approach. In: *Artificial Intelligence for Innovative Healthcare Informatics* (pp. 35–60). Cham: Springer International Publishing; 2022.

[9] Flach P. *Machine Learning: The Art and Science of Algorithms that Make Sense of Data.* Cambridge University Press; 2012.

[10]   Hornik K, Stinchcombe M, and White H. Multilayer feedforward networks are universal approximators. *Neural Networks*. 1989;2(5):359–66.

[11]   Dueck D and Frey BJ. Non-metric affinity propagation for unsupervised image categorization. In: *Proceedings of the IEEE International Conference on Computer Vision*. 2007.

[12]   Ghayvat H, Awais M, Bashir AK, *et al.* AI-enabled radiologist in the loop: novel AI-based framework to augment radiologist performance for COVID-19 chest CT medical image annotation and classification from pneumonia. *Neural Computing and Applications*. 2022;1–19.

[13]   Rashid M, Singh H, and Goyal V. The use of machine learning and deep learning algorithms in functional magnetic resonance imaging—a systematic review. *Expert Systems*. 2020;37(6):e12644.

[14]   Verma AK, Singh TN, and Maheshwar S. Comparative study of intelligent prediction models for pressure wave velocity. *Journal of Geosciences and Geomatics*. 2014;2(3):130–8.

[15]   Holzinger A. Data mining with decision trees: theory and applications. *Online Information Review*. 2015;39(3):437–8.

[16]   Breiman L. Bagging predictors. *Machine Learning*. 1996;24(2):123–40.

[17]   Duda RO and Hart PE. *Pattern Classification*. John Wiley & Sons; 2006.

[18]   Hand DJ and Yu K, Idiot's Bayes—not so stupid after all? *International Statistical Review*. 2007;69(3):385–98.

[19]   Madan P, Singh V, Chaudhari V, *et al.* An optimization-based diabetes prediction model using CNN and Bi-directional LSTM in real-time environment. *Applied Sciences*, 2022;12(8):3989.

[20]   Thandapani S, Mahaboob MI, Iwendi C, *et al.* IoMT with deep CNN: AI-based intelligent support system for pandemic diseases. *Electronics*. 2023;12 (2):424.

[21]   Mondal S, Agarwal K, and Rashid M. Deep learning approach for automatic classification of x-ray images using convolutional neural network. In: *2019 Fifth International Conference on Image Information Processing (ICIIP)* (pp. 326–331). IEEE. 2019.

[22]   Bianchi FM, Maiorino E, Kampffmeyer MC, Rizzi A, and Jenssen R. An overview and comparative analysis of recurrent neural networks for short term load forecasting. *arXiv preprint*, https://arXiv:1705.04378. 2017.

[23]   Suzuki K. Pixel-based machine learning in medical imaging. *Journal of Biomedical Imaging*. 2012;2012:1.

[24]   Agarwal TK, Tiwari M, and Lamba SS. Modified histogram based contrast enhancement using homomorphic filtering for medical images. In: *Souvenir of the 2014 IEEE International Advance Computing Conference, IACC 2014*. 2014;964–8.

[25]   Alanazi HO, Abdullah AH, and Qureshi KN. A critical review for developing accurate and dynamic predictive models using machine learning methods in medicine and health care. *Journal of Medical Systems*. 2017;41(4).

[26]   Narasimhamurthy A. An overview of machine learning in medical image analysis: trends in health informatics. In: *Medical Imaging: Concepts,*

Methodologies, Tools, and Applications, IGI Global, 2017. https://services.igi-global.com/resolvedoi/resolve.aspx?doi=104018/978-1-5225-0140-4.ch002.

[27] Prasoon A, Petersen K, Igel C, Lauze F, Dam E, and Nielsen M. Deep feature learning for knee cartilage segmentation using a triplanar convolutional neural network. *Lecture Notes in Computer Science (including subseries Lecture Notes in Artificial Intelligence and Lecture Notes in Bioinformatics)*, 2013;8150LNCS(PART 2):246–53.

[28] Antony J, McGuinness K, O'Connor NE, and Moran K. Quantifying radiographic knee osteoarthritis severity using deep convolutional neural networks. In: *Proceedings – International Conference on Pattern Recognition.* 2016 Jan 1;0:1195–200.

[29] Kim E, Corte-Real M, and Baloch Z. A deep semantic mobile application for thyroid cytopathology. In: *Medical Imaging 2016: PACS and Imaging Informatics: Next Generation and Innovations.* 2016;9789:97890A.

[30] Shen W, Zhou M, Yang F, Yang C, and Tian J. Multi-scale convolutional neural networks for lung nodule classification. *Lecture Notes in Computer Science (including subseries Lecture Notes in Artificial Intelligence and Lecture Notes in Bioinformatics).* 2015;9123:588–99.

[31] Wang CW, Huang CT, Hsieh MC, *et al.* Evaluation and comparison of anatomical landmark detection methods for cephalometric X-ray images: a grand challenge. *IEEE Transactions on Medical Imaging.* 2015;34(9):1890–900.

[32] de Vos BD, Wolterink JM, de Jong PA, Viergever MA, and Išgum I. 2D image classification for 3D anatomy localization: employing deep convolutional neural networks. *SPIE.* 2016;9784:97841Y.

[33] Çiçek Ö, Abdulkadir A, Lienkamp SS, Brox T, and Ronneberger O. 3D U-Net: learning dense volumetric segmentation from sparse annotation. *Lecture Notes in Computer Science (including subseries Lecture Notes in Artificial Intelligence and Lecture Notes in Bioinformatics).* 2016 Jun 21;9901LNCS:424–32.

[34] Wu G, Kim M, Wang Q, Gao Y, Liao S, and Shen D. Unsupervised deep feature learning for deformable registration of MR brain images. *Medical Image Computing and Computer-Assisted Intervention.* 2013;16(Pt 2):649–56.

[35] Ahsan MM, Mahmud MAP, Saha PK, Gupta KD, and Siddique Z. Effect of data scaling methods on machine learning algorithms and model performance. *Technologies.* 20219:52.

[36] Ansari AQ and Gupta NK. Automated diagnosis of coronary heart disease using neuro-fuzzy integrated system. *2011 World Congress on Information and Communication Technologies*, Mumbai, India, 2011, pp. 1379–84.

[37] Rubin J, Abreu R, Ganguli A, Nelaturi S, Matei I, and Sricharan K. Recognizing abnormal heart sounds using deep learning. In: *CEUR Workshop Proceedings.* 2017;1891:13–19.

[38] Miao JH and Miao KH. Cardiotocographic diagnosis of fetal health based on multiclass morphologic pattern predictions using deep learning classification. *International Journal of Advanced Computer Science and Applications.* 2018;9(5):1–11.

[39]   Levey AS and Coresh J. Chronic kidney disease. *Lancet.* 2012;379(9811): 165–80.
[40]   Charleonnan A, Fufaung T, Niyomwong T, Chokchueypattanakit W, Suwannawach S, and Ninchawee N. Predictive analytics for chronic kidney disease using machine learning techniques. *2016 Management and Innovation Technology International Conference (MITicon)*, Bang-San, Thailand, 2016, pp. MIT-80–MIT-83.
[41]   Aljaaf AJ, Al-Jumeily D, Haglan HM, *et al.* Early prediction of chronic kidney disease using machine learning supported by predictive analytics. *2018 IEEE Congress on Evolutionary Computation (CEC)*, Rio de Janeiro, Brazil, 2018, pp. 1–9.
[42]   Ma F, Sun T, Liu L, and Jing H. Detection and diagnosis of chronic kidney disease using deep learning-based heterogeneous modified artificial neural network. *Future Generation Computer Systems.* 2020;111:17–26.
[43]   Miranda GHB and Felipe JC. Computer-aided diagnosis system based on fuzzy logic for breast cancer categorization. *Computers in Biology and Medicine.* 2015;64:334–46.
[44]   Zheng B, Yoon SW, and Lam SS. Breast cancer diagnosis based on feature extraction using a hybrid of K-means and support vector machine algorithms. *Expert Systems with Applications.* 2014;41(4):1476–82.
[45]   Asri H, Mousannif H, Al Moatassime H, and Noel T. Using machine learning algorithms for breast cancer risk prediction and diagnosis. *Procedia Computer Science.* 2016;83:1064–9.
[46]   Bhattacherjee A, Roy S, Paul S, Roy P, Kausar N, and Dey N. Classification approach for breast cancer detection using back propagation neural network. *Deep Learning and Neural Networks.* 2019;1410–21.
[47]   Alshayeji MH, Ellethy H, Abed S, and Gupta R. Computer-aided detection of breast cancer on the Wisconsin dataset: an artificial neural networks approach. *Biomedical Signal Processing and Control.* 2022;71:103141.
[48]   Sultana Z, Khan MdAR, Jahan N, Sultana Z, Khan MdAR, and Jahan N. Early breast cancer detection utilizing artificial neural network. *WSEAS Transactions on Biology and Biomedicine.* 2021;18:32–42.
[49]   Ghosh P, Azam S, Hasib KM, Karim A, Jonkman M, and Anwar A. A performance based study on deep learning algorithms in the effective prediction of breast cancer. In: *Proceedings of the International Joint Conference on Neural Networks.* 2021 18, July.
[50]   Naz H and Ahuja S. Deep learning approach for diabetes prediction using PIMA Indian dataset. *Journal of Diabetes and Metabolic Disorders.* 2020;19 (1):391–403.
[51]   Kandhasamy JP and Balamurali S. Performance analysis of classifier models to predict diabetes mellitus. *Procedia Computer Science.* 2015;47(C):45–51.
[52]   Yahyaoui A, Jamil A, Rasheed J, and Yesiltepe M. A decision support system for diabetes prediction using machine learning and deep learning techniques. *2019 1st International Informatics and Software Engineering Conference (UBMYK)*, Ankara, Turkey, 2019, pp. 1–4.

[53] Ashiquzzaman A, Tushar AK, Islam MR, *et al.* Reduction of overfitting in diabetes prediction using deep learning neural network. *Lecture Notes in Electrical Engineering.* 2017;449:35–43.

[54] Grover S, Bhartia S, Akshama, Yadav A, and Seeja KR. Predicting severity of Parkinson's disease using deep learning. *Procedia Computer Science.* 2018;132:1788–94.

[55] Sriram T, Rao M, Narayana G, Vital T, and Dowluru K. Intelligent Parkinson disease prediction using machine learning algorithms. *International Journal of Engineering and Innovative Technology.* 2013;3: 212–215.

[56] Esmaeilzadeh S, Yang Y, and Adeli E. End-to-end Parkinson disease diagnosis using brain MR-images by 3D-CNN. *arXiv preprint*, arXiv:1806. 05233.2018.

[57] Warjurkar S and Ridhorkar S. A study on brain tumor and Parkinson's disease diagnosis and detection using deep learning. In: *Proceedings of the 3rd International Conference on Integrated Intelligent Computing Communication & Security (ICIIC 2021) [Internet].* 2021;4:356–64. https://www.atlantis-press.com/proceedings/iciic-21/125960845

[58] Ahsan MM, Nazim R, Siddique Z, and Huebner P. Detection of COVID-19 patients from CT scan and chest X-ray data using modified MobileNetV2 and LIME. *Healthcare* [Internet]. 2021;9(9). /pmc/articles/PMC8465084/

[59] Kumar S, Nagar R, Bhatnagar S, *et al.* Chest X ray and cough sample based deep learning framework for accurate diagnosis of COVID-19. *Computers and Electrical Engineering.* 2022;103:108391.

[60] Haghanifar A, Majdabadi MM, Choi Y, Deivalakshmi S, and Ko S. COVID-CXNet: detecting COVID-19 in frontal chest X-ray images using deep learning. *Multimedia Tools and Applications* [Internet]. https://arxiv.org/abs/2006.13807v2

[61] Kumar I, Alshamrani SS, Kumar A, *et al.* Deep learning approach for analysis and characterization of COVID-19. *Computers, Materials and Continua*, 2021;70(1):451–68.

[62] Jha N, Prashar D, Rashid M, *et al.* Deep learning approach for discovery of in silico drugs for combating COVID-19. *Journal of Healthcare Engineering.* 2021:1–13.

[63] Wang L, Lin ZQ, and Wong A. COVID-Net: a tailored deep convolutional neural network design for detection of COVID-19 cases from chest X-ray images. *Scientific Reports*, 2020 10:1 [Internet]. 2020;10(1):1–12. https://www.nature.com/articles/s41598-020-76550-z

[64] Li L, Qin L, Xu Z, *et al.* Artificial Intelligence distinguishes COVID-19 from community acquired pneumonia on chest CT. *Radiology* [Internet]. 2020;296(2):E65–71. /pmc/articles/PMC7233473/

[65] Graham N and Warner J. *Alzheimer's Disease and Other Dementias.* Northampton, UK: Family Doctor Publications Limited; 2009.

[66] Neelaveni J and Devasana MSG. Alzheimer disease prediction using machine learning algorithms. *2020 6th International Conference on*

Advanced Computing and Communication Systems (ICACCS), Coimbatore, India, 2020, pp. 101–104.

[67] Zhang J, Dong Q, Shi J, *et al.* Predicting future cognitive decline with hyperbolic stochastic coding. *Medical Image Analysis* [Internet]. 2021;70:102009. /pmc/articles/PMC8049149/

[68] Vidushi ARAKS. Diagnosis of Alzheimer disease using machine learning approaches. *International Journal of Advanced Science and Technology* [Internet]. 2020;29(04):7062–73. http://sersc.org/journals/index.php/IJAST/article/view/28115

[69] Ahmed S, Kim BC, Lee KH, and Jung HY. Ensemble of ROI-based convolutional neural network classifiers for staging the Alzheimer disease spectrum from magnetic resonance imaging. *PLoS One*. 2020;15(12): e0242712. https://journals.plos.org/plosone/article?id=10.1371/journal.pone.0242712

[70] Mao Y, He Y, Liu L, and Chen X. Disease classification based on eye movement features with decision tree and random forest. *Frontiers in Neuroscience*. 2020;14:798.

[71] Nosseir A and Shawky MA. Automatic classifier for skin disease using k-NN and SVM. In: *ACM International Conference Proceeding Series*. 2019 Apr 9;259–62.

[72] Khan MA, Ashraf I, Alhaisoni M, *et al.* Multimodal brain tumor classification using deep learning and robust feature selection: a machine learning application for radiologists. *Diagnostics*. 2020;10:565. https://www.mdpi.com/2075-4418/10/8/565/htm

[73] Amin J, Sharif M, Haldorai A, Yasmin M, and Nayak RS. Brain tumor detection and classification using machine learning: a comprehensive survey. *Complex & Intelligent Systems*. 2021;8:4 [Internet]. https://link.springer.com/article/10.1007/s40747-021-00563-y

[74] Dai X, Spasic I, Meyer B, Chapman S, and Andres F. Machine learning on mobile: an on-device inference app for skin cancer detection. In: *2019 4th International Conference on Fog and Mobile Edge Computing, FMEC 2019*. 2019 Jun1;301–5.

[75] Daghrir J, Tlig L, Bouchouicha M, and Sayadi M. Melanoma skin cancer detection using deep learning and classical machine learning techniques: a hybrid approach. In: *2020 International Conference on Advanced Technologies for Signal and Image Processing, ATSIP 2020*. 2020 Sep 1.

Chapter 7

Deep learning approach for the prediction of diseases in medical images

Sabeena Hussain[1] and Sonali Powar[2]

The categorization of medical images is an important component of clinical practice; this helps medical experts to analyze the root causes of a problem. However, the traditional methods are not appropriate to get measurable performance. In addition, when we use them, we will need to spend a significant amount of time and effort extracting and choosing categorization characteristics. The deep neural network is an emerging technique of machine learning that has a lot of potential for classification tasks. A deep learning (DL) approach-based convolutional neural network (CNN) consistently achieves the highest results on varying image classification tasks. Therefore, this research studies how to apply CNN-based algorithm on magnetic resonance imaging (MRI) dataset to classify brain tumor detection. DL technique has been evaluated through experiments to identify the features from inputted MRI images using the CNN model. The findings of the studies reveal that adding more information to the dataset is an efficient method to increase their overall performance.

7.1 Introduction

The brain is the most complex and an essential organ of the human body. It assists with decision-making and governs the whole performance of the body's other organs. It basically serves as the central nervous system's command and control center and is in charge of carrying out all of the daily actions that occur in the human body, both voluntarily and involuntarily. The tumor is a fibrous mesh of undesired tissue development that is occurring inside our brain and is expanding in an unrestricted manner [1]. A proper knowledge of brain tumors and the stages they progress through is a necessary step in the process of both preventing the sickness and treating it after it has shown itself. Magnetic resonance imaging, often referred to as MRI, is frequently used by radiologists for diagnosing and evaluating brain malignancies [2]. The outcome of the investigation that was carried out for the

[1]Department of Pharmacy, Vishwakarma University, Pune, India
[2]Department of Computer Science, Vishwakarma University, Pune, India

purpose of this research discloses, via the use of the deep learning (DL) methodologies, whether the brain in question is healthy or ill.

Convolutional neural network (CNN) is utilized in this study for the purpose of differentiating between normal and tumorous brain tissue [3]. It functions similarly to the nervous system of a human being, and a digital computer is interconnected and networked extensively on the basis of this. As a result, a neural network can be trained using basic processing units that are implemented into the training set, and it can also store experience-based knowledge. It has multiple layers of neurons that are all linked to one another. A data set on the learning process is used by the neural network to enable learning. There may be any number of hidden layers, but there will only be one input and output layer. During the process of learning, the weight and bias of the neurons of each layer are adjusted based on the input characteristics as well as the layers that came before them (for hidden layers and output layers). Training a model involves applying an activation function not just to the visible features but also to the hidden layers, which are the locations of additional learning that must take place to produce the desired output [4].

As a result of the tremendous growth of the economy, people's health has emerged as the primary concern that determines their level of living. Brain disorders are extremely prevalent and have a negative impact on human health. These conditions are ranked according to the degree of impairment they cause. There is no doubt that brain tumors are the form of brain illness that presents the greatest danger to the health of humans. Tissue in the brain is a functional organization characterized by a sophisticated structure and an uneven form. The precise segmentation of brain pictures yields an abundance of information that is both rich and beneficial for therapeutic operations. However, "images of brain tissues are typically prone to interference, such as noises, uneven grayscale, local volume effects, and artefacts." These types of problems can be difficult to diagnose and treat. In the meanwhile, there are significant challenges involved in detecting and segmenting brain pictures as a result of the lack of contrast in the image borders as well as the intricate structure of brain tissue [5].

Artificial intelligence (AI) technologies like Internet of Things, Big Data Analytics, and DL have been broadly recognized in a variety of disciplines; consequently, intelligent development in the medical field becomes increasingly crucial for monitoring people's health state. The accurate processing of medical pictures that have been distorted geometrically and disrupted by powerful noises is essential for accurate clinical diagnosis and therapy. DL methods have made tremendous progress in the detection and segmentation of picture resolution. In spite of this, actual medical photographs with a low quality are murky and difficult to understand. Deep neural network (DNN) is an effective mechanism to find the pattern and study medical images. DNN does not take into consideration blurring while training the data. DNN mechanisms can work effectively on blurring images while training the data. The fuzzy theory challenges the conventional "either/or" viewpoint, which results in the picture information being utilized in a more comprehensive manner. The fuzzy system, which is an unsupervised classification model, on the other hand, does not call for any kind of user involvement since its process of segmentation is carried out entirely automatically. It is possible to successfully process the image's unpredictability and ambiguity. Therefore, the proper interpretation of brain pictures can have a highly practical value for the purposes of identifying and treating brain illnesses [6].

The techniques of nuclear magnetic resonance (NMR) can effectively work on various degrees of noise, weak borders, and artifacts found in MRI pictures, enabling the study of the intricacies of human brain tissues. As a result, the analysis of brain images for the purpose of predicting brain diseases offers an exceptionally important value for minimizing the risks associated with therapeutic therapy. The novel aspects of this research include the improvements that were made to fuzzy clustering in regard to noises, weak boundaries, and artifacts in brain images [7].

7.2 Literature review

According to [1], the two categories of major brain tumors that are most common right now are malignant and benign. It is believed that both children and adults can suffer from brain cancer. When brain tissue develops in an abnormal manner, this might lead to the formation of a brain tumor. The abnormal tissues grow faster than the healthy cells, resulting in the creation of a cellular mass that can eventually evolve into tumors.

According to [2], early and precise detection of a brain tumor is essential for successful treatment of the tumor. It is dependent on the knowledge and experience of the attending physician, as well as the treatment approach that is chosen for the patient to facilitate a speedy recovery. In the early stages, it can be difficult to identify the specific type of brain tumor that a patient has; yet, this information is essential for the doctors so that they can treat the patient appropriately.

According to [3], the most prevalent kind of cancer that is diagnosed is gastrointestinal cancer. It stimulates the polyps that are found in the digestive tract. Video endoscopy is the technique that is used to diagnose polyps in the digestive tract. A little camera is inserted into the patient's body and then maneuvered through the digestive system to detect and remove polyps. On the other hand, some polyps are thought to be unnoticed and might develop into cancerous tumors at some point. "A computer-aided polyp identification method" ought to be utilized to cut down on the rate of incorrect polyp detection.

According to [4], glioma is the form of brain tumor that occurs most frequently. In most cases, MRI scans will divide glioma into areas of necrotic tissue, active tumor, and edematous surrounding tissue (ED). The manual segmentation of tumors is a laborious process that is time consuming and requires the assistance of a qualified medical professional. To properly segment gliomas, computerized instruments are an absolute necessity. The methods used to categorize glooms may often be broken down into two categories: standard machine learning and DL. The 3D Dense Unit CNN DL algorithm was reportedly suggested in research to categorize the output in the total tumor (WT), tumor core (TC), and boosting tumor (ET).

The analysis of medical photographs is shown to play an important part in supporting human beings in the diagnosis of a variety of illnesses in [5]. Two techniques that are frequently used for examining the anomalies in brain tissues related to the size, position, or form of cells that can aid in the early detection of tumors are computed tomography (CT) and MRI. These two methods are categorized as imaging methods.

Robust machine learning algorithms improve the accuracy of identification, which aids doctors in the treatment process, as described in [6]. To attain the highest possible level of productivity, it is essential to categorize the tumor using an efficient algorithm that possesses a unique set of traits and descriptors. In comparison to the more common practice of manually categorizing data, categorization by algorithms is both more efficient and accurate.

According to [7], DL simulates the function of the brain in terms of the processing of data, the recognition of patterns, and the creation of decisions. The ability to learn unsupervised from unstructured material is one of the capabilities of deep neural networks. In the field of DL, the CNN performs remarkably well, particularly in the detection and categorization of images, sounds, or text. The conventional structure of a convolutional network consists of an inner layer, a resultant layer, and several layers that have not yet been identified. Within the unknown layers is a chain of convolutional layers that are connected together. The RELU layer is incorporated into the beginning function, and the backpropagation is wrapped up in the final convolution.

Researchers identified a mechanism in [8] that might be used to identify brain cancers in their early stages. Images obtained through MRI have been examined to identify areas that contain tumors and to categorize these tumor-containing areas according to a variety of tumor types. When it comes to image classification jobs, DL produces results that are rather efficient. As a result, the CNNs approach was chosen for this investigation, and its implementation was carried out with the help of the TensorFlow framework. It has been demonstrated that the quicker CNN approach may result in an accuracy that is 91.66%, which is greater than the work that is linked to this topic.

Researchers presented a model in reference number [9] that would allow MRI scans to determine the sort of brain tumor present. The classification was carried out using a 2D CNN of 91.3% accuracy for recognizing pituitary, glioma, and meningioma tumors. The data collection that was used for the research project included information on the top three most prevalent types of brain tumors.

Researchers suggested a brain tumor segmentation approach that was both flexible and successful in [10]. This technique reduces the amount of time spent calculating and eliminates the overfitting issues that occur in DL techniques. This CNN model utilizes two distinct paths, each of which mines either local or global features. In addition to this, the accuracy of segmenting brain tumors is increased in comparison to models that are considered to be state of the art. A mean WT score of 0.9203, a mean enhancing tumor score of 0.9113, and a mean tumor core dice score of 0.8726 may be accomplished with the strategy that has been suggested.

Using MRI, researchers constructed a model to diagnose brain cancers in [11]. The methodology includes three steps: finding the tumor, diagnosing it in terms of grade and sort, and pinpointing its position. To organize brain MRI data, this method used one model rather than a different model for each categorization task. The tasks that were being classified were distinct. The multitask classification that is based on a CNN has the capability to both categorize and identify cancers. Using a CNN-based model, it is also possible to identify the location of a brain tumor. This is accomplished by reaching an accuracy of 92% when segmenting the brain tumor.

Researchers used the brain tumor division in [12] by merging the "Regularized Extreme Learning Machine" with other computational methods (RELM). The photographs were initially preprocessed by the approach to make it simpler for the system to read them. The min–max strategy was utilized by the system throughout the preprocessing phase. The min–max preprocessing method was really helpful in bringing out more contrast in the photos that were being read in.

Researchers were able to detect and divide brain tumors using a combination of the two procedures described in [13]. The first method put out was the local binary pattern (LBP), also known as nLBP, which was based on the neighbor distance relation. The second approach, known as LBP, put a lot of emphasis on the angle that existed between the neighbors. These two methods were utilized in the preprocessing of the MRIs of the three types of brain tumors that are the most common: gliomas, meningiomas, and pituitary. The evolution of the characters was determined by using the histograms of the preprocessed photos. The redesigned model performed significantly better as compared to the conventional methods of feature extraction.

Researchers proposed a strategy to enhance the Whale Optimization Algorithm that was based on a Multilayer Perceptron (MLP) neural network. The article can be found here (WOA). With the hybrid model, we achieved an improved version of WOA that enabled more interesting character evolution and division. In a more advanced version, the Median Filter was used to clean the images of noise. The enhanced WOA was utilized to choose characteristics from among those that had been retrieved. When used for tumor classification, the MLP-IWOA-based classifier showed significantly improved results compared to other current classification approaches.

Researchers developed a method for the division of brain tumors using a combination of statistical characteristics and algorithms based on neural networks, as described in [14]. For the extraction of tumor features, classification of brain tumors was carried out using a backpropagation neural network (BPNN). To do this, a sizable image database of tumors was utilized.

CNN was employed in this study effort [15], which generates an overall accuracy of 91.3% and a recall of 88%, 81%, and 99% correspondingly in the identification of pituitary, glioma, and meningioma tumor, respectively. For the purpose of classifying the various kinds of brain tumors based on MRI image slices, a DL architecture that makes use of 2D CNNs has been utilized. Methods such as data gathering, data preprocessing, pre-modeling, model optimization, and hyperparameter tweaking are utilized in this article. In addition, the generalizability of the model was evaluated using a 10-fold cross-validation procedure that was carried out on the whole dataset.

In [16], the researcher explains that the approach used in this research is based on Hough voting, which is a strategy that enables entirely automated localization and segmentation of the relevant anatomies. In addition to that, it employed a segmentation approach that was based on learning techniques. This method is robust, multi-regional, versatile, and easily adaptable to a variety of modalities. When it comes to the prediction of the final outcomes, different amounts of training data as well as different data dimensionalities were used.

In [17], researchers elaborated the brain as an essential component of the human body that controls and coordinates the functions carried out by the many other bodily parts. All of the daily actions that take place in the human body, both freely and involuntarily, are generally carried out by the brain, which also acts as the central nervous system's command and control center. The tumor is a fibrous mesh of undesired tissue development that is occurring inside of our brain and is expanding in an unrestricted manner. Radiologists routinely use magnetic resonance imaging, also known as MRI, to evaluate the various stages of brain tumors to both prevent and treat the disease. This analysis reveals that there is a tumor present in the patient's brain as a result of its findings.

The application of information technology within the healthcare industry has contributed to a heightened rate of evolution in this sector in recent years. The goal of integrating information technology into healthcare is to make living a more comfortable and cheap life for individuals, much to how cell phones have made living easier [18].

Making healthcare more intelligent might make this goal attainable; for instance, there could be an intelligent ambulance and good medical facilities that provide assistance to patients and medical professionals in a variety of different ways [19].

After doing a study on patients in a certain area who suffer from chronic illnesses every year, it was found that there is actually very little gender discrepancy among the patients. In addition, it was found that many patients were hospitalized in 2014 with the purpose of treating chronic illnesses. Results are substantially more accurate when both structured and unstructured data are used than when only structured data is used. It is preferable to combine unstructured data with structured data, which includes patient data, disease details, lifestyle, and results of laboratory tests [20,21], which also includes patient symptoms and grievances described by them and doctor's records on patients with diseases, is advantageous.

The diagnosis process for uncommon illnesses can be challenging. Therefore, the utilization of data on the individuals' own self-reported behaviors is helpful in distinguishing between persons who have uncommon diseases and those who have common chronic conditions. It is considered that the identification of uncommon diseases is highly achievable [22] if questionnaires and methods of machine learning are used in conjunction with one another.

In the past 10 years, a number of cutting-edge technologies have been developed and put into use to expedite the process of data collection. These technologies include readouts from MRI, ultrasonography, data gained from social media, data generated through electronic devices, behavioral, and clinical data. These high-dimensional huge healthcare data sets suggest that the number of recordable attributes per observation may exceed the total number of observations. They have a high noise level, a low sample size, a cross-sectional design, and a lack of statistical power. The challenges presented by the high-dimensional data sets can be conquered by the application of machine learning techniques [23]. The use of machine learning has increased contributions in a number of fields. While we are on the cusp of a significant paradigm change in healthcare epidemiology [24], many of the more complicated models make use of already existing, bigger data sets for training. These data can help improve patient risk stratification, minimize healthcare-associated infections, and uncover ways to spread infectious illnesses [25]. They can also increase the amount of knowledge gained about the risk factors of diseases, which helps reduce such infections. The early diagnosis of illnesses can be aided by the application of machine learning, which can make the interpretation of test findings and other patient details more efficient. The low-level data in the database may be transformed into high-level knowledge through the process of knowledge discovery, enabling the collection of knowledge about sickness patterns to aid early detection [26]. To accurately predict a disease, only the most important characteristics should be selected from the data that have been collected for the purpose of creating a data set after any missing values have been preprocessed out. This is done to improve the accuracy of disease prediction while simultaneously reducing the amount of time needed for model training [27].

Nowadays, with the Internet and advanced technology, people do not worry about their lives or their health. Because everyone is preoccupied with activities related to surfing the web and using social media, they neglect to go to hospitals for their annual checkups. Using this practice as a benefit, a machine learning model should be created [28] that takes the symptoms supplied as input and utilizes those symptoms to forecast the likelihood and risk of the illness being impacted or the onset of such diseases in a person based on those symptoms. Among the most prevalent chronic diseases include cardiovascular disease, cancer, diabetes, arthritis, strokes, and hepatitis C. The identification of such diseases is of utmost significance in the field of healthcare due to the fact that such conditions last for an extended period of time and have a high death rate. The condition may be anticipated, which can help people take preventative measures and avoid becoming afflicted with it. Additionally, early discovery of the disease can aid in improving therapy [29]. Machine learning encompasses a wide range of methodologies, including supervised, semi-supervised, and unsupervised learning, as well as reinforcement, evolutionary, and DL. The issue stems from the processing of vectorized representations of vectorized characteristics that have been derived from actual data [30].

The proper technique in which the vectors are mixed determines the processing's quality. The huge dimension of the vector or the inconsistent nature of the data, however, is typically to blame for the issue. Therefore, to make the data set a very suitable dimension, it is imperative to decrease the date set dimensionality. Even if certain features are lost as a result, this should still be done.

This decreases the data set complexity and enhances the effectiveness of the model [31].

A management system that may help those with chronic diseases who require adequate medical evaluation and treatment information [32] is desperately needed. Additionally, those who require self-care to enhance their existing level of health may find this technique useful. This is due to the fact that self-management has been proven to be the most effective type of care for persons with chronic diseases and is seen as a key factor in the recovery process. Patients' health information may be recorded with the use of mobile applications, and these apps are also a more effective tool for enabling patients to take charge of their own care [33]. Information such as a narrative about the symptoms that patients are experiencing, the specifics of their consultations with medical professionals, the outcomes of laboratory examinations, and pictures obtained from computed tomography and X-rays are necessary for accurate disease prediction [34]. When it comes to the diagnosis of illnesses, relatively little research is done to determine the accuracy and predictive capacity of constructing a machine learning model using just the findings of laboratory examinations as the only source of information. Additionally, DL and ensemble machine learning models may be used to boost performance [35,36]. AI plays a crucial role in the process of automating the tasks involved in illness diagnosis and therapy recommendation in the realm of medicine. AI also plays a role in scheduling the perfect timing for medical professionals to carry out a variety of responsibilities that cannot be automated [37].

Using a method based on machine learning, the suggested system's primary goal is to detect and make accurate predictions regarding the occurrence of chronic illness in an individual. The data set includes both structured and unstructured information about the patient, such as the condition of the patient, sex, tallness, weight, and other demographics—absent personal data like name and ID—as well as the patient's symptoms, details of any doctor consultations regarding the illness, and details about the patient's lifestyle. These data have been preprocessed to locate the values that are missing. They are then rebuilt to improve the overall quality of the model, which in turn improves the accuracy of the predictions. Algorithms based on machine learning, like CNN and KNN, are utilized for the purpose of prediction [38,39].

7.3   Materials and methods

7.3.1   Dataset

The dataset is obtained from the Kaggle site [38]. The MRI images of a brain tumor may be found in this collection. There are two folders: one represents normal brain images, and the other represents tumor images. One folder contains normal brain photos, while the other contains tumor images. These two folders contain a combined total of 400 photos in their entirety. In all, 230 photos of

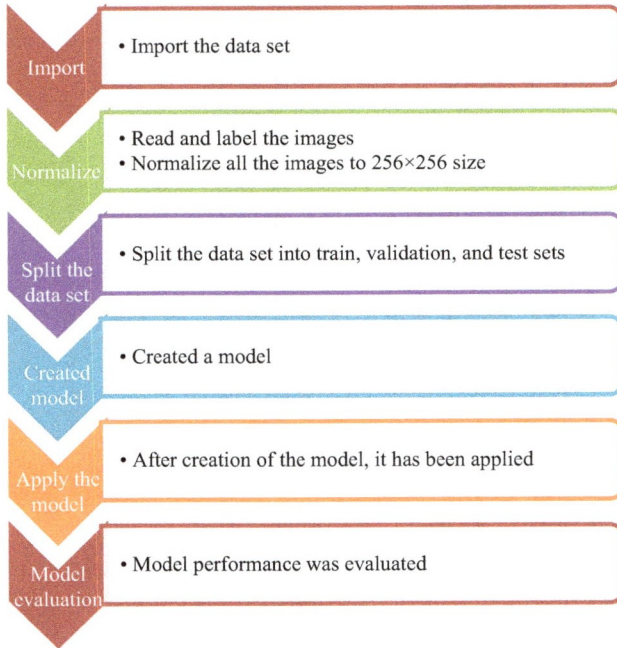

Figure 7.1   Proposed model

tumors and 170 images of normal tissue are captured. The images take on a variety of various forms.

7.3.2   Proposed model

On the dataset including brain tumor images, the CNN approach was employed, and their performance in categorizing the images was assessed. Figure 7.1 shows the procedure carried out to apply CNN to the dataset including brain tumors.

7.4   Results and analysis

7.4.1   Model validation and accuracy

During the validation of model, it was applied to the training dataset for a total of 10 iterations, the highest level of validation accuracy that can be achieved is 91%. The ratio of validation accuracy to training accuracy, as well as the training loss and the validation loss, is shown in the graph in Figure 7.2.

When we consider the accuracy, recall, and F1 score of CNN and compare it to its effectiveness in determining the existence of a brain tumor, we find that

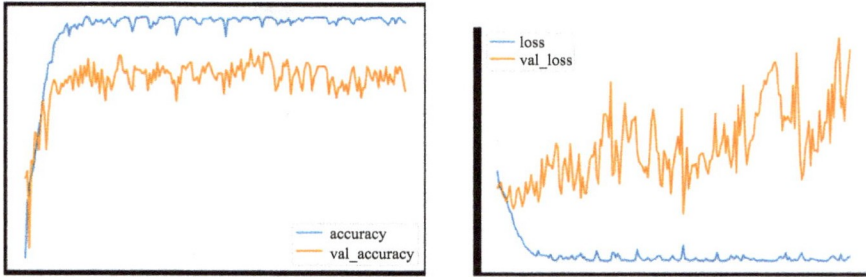

Figure 7.2   Training and validation accuracy and loss of proposed CNN method

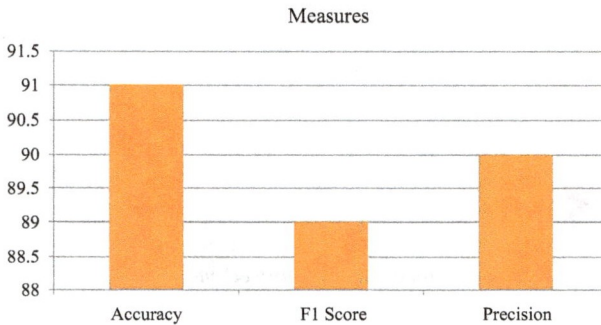

Figure 7.3   Accuracy measures

CNN is the most effective supporting approach since it has the highest precision value.

The CNN model's accuracy when applied to testing data was 91%. Figure 7.3 shows accuracy measures.

7.5   Conclusion

In the field of image analysis, CNN is often regarded as one of the most effective methods. By decreasing the size of the image while maintaining all of the information that is necessary for generating predictions, CNN is able to make its predictions in an efficient manner. The approach of trial and error was used to construct the model that was built for this purpose. Future optimization methods could be used to calculate the maximum number of layers and filters that could be included in a model. It has been determined that the CNN is the method that is most effective in determining whether or not a patient has a brain tumor based on the data that has been provided.

References

[1] L. A. J. Prabhu and A. Jayachandran, "Mixture model segmentation system for parasagittal meningioma brain tumor classification based on hybrid feature vector," *Journal of Medical Systems*, vol. 42, no. 12, pp. 1–6, 2018.

[2] N. Sengupta, C. B. McNabb, N. Kasabov, and B. R. Russell, "Integrating space, time, and orientation in spiking neural networks: a case study on multimodal brain data modeling," *IEEE Transactions on Neural Networks and Learning Systems*, vol. 29, no. 11, pp. 5249–5263, 2018.

[3] S. Mondal, K. Agarwal, and M. Rashid, "Deep learning approach for automatic classification of X-ray images using convolutional neural network," in: *2019 Fifth International Conference on Image Information Processing (ICIIP)*, Shimla, India, 2019, pp. 326–331, doi:10.1109/ICIIP47207.2019.8985687.

[4] C. G. B. Yogananda, B. R. Shah, M. Vejdani-Jahromi, *et al.*, "A fully automated deep learning network for brain tumor segmentation," *Tomography*, vol. 6, no. 2, pp. 186–193, 2020.

[5] A. Tiwari, S. Srivastava, and M. Pant, "Brain tumor segmentation and classification from magnetic resonance images: review of selected methods from 2014 to 2019," *Pattern Recognition Letters*, vol. 131, pp. 244–260, 2020.

[6] G. Mohan and M. M. Subashini, "MRI based medical image analysis: survey on brain tumor grade classification," *Biomedical Signal Processing and Control*, vol. 39, pp. 139–161, 2018.

[7] I. M. Dheir, A. S. A. Mettleq, A. A. Elsharif, and S. S. Abu-Naser, "Classifying nuts types using convolutional neural network," *International Journal of Academic Information Systems Research (IJAISR)*, vol. 3, no. 12, 2020.

[8] K. Salçin, "Detection and classification of brain tumours from MRI images using faster R-CNN," *Tehnički glasnik*, vol. 13, no. 4, pp. 337–342, 2019.

[9] S. Sarkar, A. Kumar, S. Chakraborty, S. Aich, J. S. Sim, and H. C. Kim, "A CNN based approach for the detection of brain tumours using MRI scans," *Test Engineering and Management*, vol. 83, pp. 16580–16586, 2020.

[10] R. Ranjbarzadeh, A. B. Kasgari, S. J. Ghoushchi, S. Anari, M. Naseri, and M. Bendechache, "Brain tumor segmentation based on deep learning and an attention mechanism using MRI multi-modalities brain images," *Scientific Reports*, vol. 11, no. 1, pp. 1–17, 2021.

[11] B. Kokila, M. S. Devadharshini, A. Anitha, and S. A. Sankar, "Brain tumor detection and classification using deep learning techniques based on MRI images," *Proceedings of the Journal of Physics: Conference Series*, vol. 1916, no. 1, p. 012226, 2021.

[12] A. Gumaei, M. M. Hassan, M. R. Hassan, A. Alelaiwi, and G. Fortino, "A hybrid feature extraction method with regularised extreme learning machine for brain tumor classification," *IEEE Access*, vol. 7, pp. 36266–36273, 2019.

[13]   A. S. Belhe, J. A. Pagariya, V. V. Ganthade, M. Rashid, and P. S. Uravane, "An efficient deep learning based approach for the detection of brain tumors," in: *2022 5th International Conference on Contemporary Computing and Informatics (IC3I)*, Uttar Pradesh, India, pp. 417–421, 2022.

[14]   M. R. Ismael and I. Abdel-Qader, "Brain tumor classification via statistical features and backpropagation neural network," in: *Proceedings of the 2018 IEEE International Conference on Electro/Information Technology (EIT)*, pp. 0252–0257, IEEE, Rochester, MI, USA, May 2018.

[15]   R. Hashemzehi, S. J. S. Mahdavi, M. Kheirabadi, and S. R. Kamel, "Detection of brain tumors from MRI images base on deep learning using hybrid model CNN and NADE," *Biocybernetics and Biomedical Engineering*, vol. 40, pp. 1225–1232, 2020.

[16]   F. Özyurt, E. Sert, E. Avci, and E. Dogantekin, "Brain tumor detection based on Convolutional Neural Network with neutrosophic expert maximum fuzzy sure entropy," *Measurement*, vol. 147, p. 106830, 2019.

[17]   F. Milletari, S. A. Ahmadi, C. Kroll, *et al.*, "Hough-CNN: Deep learning for segmentation of deep brain regions in MRI and ultrasound," *Computer Vision and Image Understanding*, vol. 164, pp. 92–102, 2017.

[18]   S. Swaminathan, K. Qirko, T. Smith, *et al.*, "A machine learning approach to triaging patients with chronic obstructive pulmonary disease," *PLoS One*, vol. 12, no. 11, Article ID e0188532, 2017.

[19]   Z. Wang, J. W. Chung, X. Jiang, Y. Cui, M. Wang, and A. Zheng, "Machine learning-based prediction system for chronic kidney disease using associative classification technique," *International Journal of Engineering & Technology*, vol. 7, pp. 1161–1167, 2018.

[20]   A. Kumar and A. Pathak, "A machine learning model for early prediction of multiple diseases to cure lives," *Turkish Journal of Computer and Mathematics Education (TURCOMAT)*, vol. 12, no. 6, pp. 4013–4023, 2021.

[21]   C. Kalaiselvi, "Diagnosing of heart diseases using average K-nearest neighbor algorithm of data mining," in *Proceedings of the 2016 3rd International Conference on Computing for Sustainable Global Development (INDIACom)*, pp. 3099–3103, IEEE, New Delhi, India, March 2016.

[22]   D. Jain and V. Singh, "Feature selection and classification systems for chronic disease prediction: a review," *Egyptian Informatics Journal*, vol. 19, no. 3, pp. 179–189, 2018.

[23]   R. Mamoon, H. Singh, and V. Goyal, "The use of machine learning and deep learning algorithms in functional magnetic resonance imaging—a systematic review," *Expert Systems*, vol. 37, no. 6, e12644, 2020.

[24]   M. Rashid, H. Singh, and V. Goyal, "Efficient feature selection technique based on Fast Fourier transform with PSO-GA for functional magnetic resonance imaging," in *2021 2nd International Conference on Computation,*

Automation and Knowledge Management (ICCAKM), Dubai, United Arab Emirates, pp. 238–242, 2021.

[25] P. Ghosh, S. Azam, A. Karim, M. Jonkman, and M. D. Z. Hasan, "Use of efficient machine learning techniques in the identification of patients with heart diseases," in *Proceedings of the 2021 the 5th International Conference on Information System and Data Mining*, pp. 14–20, Silicon Valley, USA, May 2021.

[26] Y. Chang and X. Chen, "Estimation of chronic illness severity based on machine learning methods," *Wireless Communications and Mobile Computing*, vol. 2021, Article ID 1999284, 13 pages, 2021.

[27] T. H. H. Aldhyani, A S Alshebami, and M. Y. Alzahrani, "Soft clustering for enhancing the diagnosis of chronic diseases over machine learning algorithms," *Journal of Healthcare Engineering*, vol. 2020, Article ID 4984967, 16 pages, 2020.

[28] H. Fröhlich, R. Balling, N. Beerenwinkel, *et al.*, "From hype to reality: data science enabling personalised medicine," *BMC Medicine*, vol. 16, no. 1, pp. 1–15, 2018.

[29] S. Ganiger and K. M. M. Rajashekharaiah, "Chronic diseases diagnosis using machine learning," in *Proceedings of the 2018 International Conference on Circuits and Systems in Digital Enterprise Technology (ICCSDET)*, pp. 1–6, IEEE, Kottayam, India, December 2018.

[30] S. S. Kumar, N. Malaiyappan, R. Ramalingam, S. Basheer, M. Rashid, and N. Ahmad, "Predicting Alzheimer's disease using deep neuro-functional networks with resting-state fMRI," *Electronics*, vol. 12, no. 4, 1031, 2023.

[31] J. Mishra and S. Tarar, "Chronic disease prediction using deep learning," in *Proceedings of the International Conference on Advances in Computing and Data Sciences*, pp. 201–11, Springer, Valletta, Malta, April 2020.

[32] E. Jeong, S. Osmundson, C. Gao, D. R. V. Edwards, M. Bradley, and Y. Chen, "Learning the impact of acute and chronic diseases on forecasting neonatal encephalopathy," *Computer Methods and Programs in Biomedicine*, vol. 211, Article ID 106397, 2021.

[33] F. Ceccarelli, M. Sciandrone, C. Perricone, *et al.*, "Prediction of chronic damage in systemic lupus erythematosus by using machine-learning models," *PLoS One*, vol. 12, no. 3, Article ID e0174200, 2017.

[34] Md M. Mottalib, J. C. Jones-Smith, B. Sheridan, and R. Beheshti, "Identifying the risks of chronic diseases using BMI trajectories," 2021, https://arxiv.org/abs/2111.05385.

[35] S. Agarwal, C. Prabha, and M. Gupta, "Chronic diseases prediction using machine learning–a review," *Annals of the Romanian Society for Cell Biology*, vol. 25, pp. 3495–3511, 2021.

[36] G. Hemant, M. Awais, A. K. Bashir, S. Pandya, M. Zuhair, M. Rashid, and J. Nebhen, "AI-enabled radiologist in the loop: novel AI-based framework to augment radiologist performance for COVID-19 chest CT medical image annotation and classification from pneumonia," *Neural Computing and Applications*, pp. 1–19, 2022.

[37] D. Zufferey, T. Hofer, H. Jean, M. Schumacher, R. Ingold, and S. Bromuri, "Performance comparison of multi-label learning algorithms on clinical data for chronic diseases," *Computers in Biology and Medicine*, vol. 65, pp. 34–43, 2015.

[38] https://www.kaggle.com/datasets/mhantor/mri-based-brain-tumor-images

[39] B. Yin, C. Wang, and F. Abza, "New brain tumor classification method based on an improved version of whale optimisation algorithm," *Biomedical Signal Processing and Control*, vol. 56, Article ID 101728, 2020.

Chapter 8

Detection of food allergy using deep learning

Abdul Majid Soomro[1], Sanjoy Kumar Debnath[2],
Awad Bin Naeem[3], Susama Bagchi[2], Neha Sharma[2],
Kamal Saluja[2] and Sunil Gupta[2]

Consuming an excessive number of calories can lead to obesity. It is a manageable medical condition marked by an abnormal growth in body fat. It has a wide range of implications. The most prevalent conditions are high blood pressure, colon cancer, and prostate cancer, although diabetes, high cholesterol, and heart attacks are all dietary-related conditions. Computer-based methods are mostly employed to address such problems. In this study, we develop a system to recognize and detect food allergies using photographs of food. To conclude, after training, the model obtained an accuracy of 95% to recognize the food label using modern computer methods, such as transfer learning (ResNET-50). The study involved teaching a system to recognize various food types by analyzing labels from the Food-101 dataset and extracting nutritional information. The primary objective of this research was to develop a framework capable of efficiently managing the complex process of identifying, locating, and categorizing food hypersensitivity (allergies). Furthermore, the study explored enhanced weight parameter optimization using datasets containing images of both healthy and allergenic foods, with a focus on comparing the performance of Adam and RMSProp optimizers. The ResNET-50 trained to get the highest mean average precision compared to the other transfer learning meta-architectures. It achieved an accuracy of 95% with best identifying results by utilizing an Adam optimizer. The proposed method was determined to be novel since it will identify every food type before providing the food's nutrients from a different dataset. In real life, a transfer learning approach to food allergy identification could help to reduce the negative impact of diet management difficulties.

[1]Department of Computer Science, University Tun Hussein Onn Malaysia (UTHM), Johor, Malaysia
[2]Department of Computer Science and Engineering, Chitkara University Institute of Engineering & Technology, Chitkara University, Rajpura, India
[3]Department of Computer Science, National College of Business Administration & Economics, Multan, Pakistan

8.1   Introduction

When the body's immune system reacts improperly to a certain food, a food allergy develops. Food intolerance has grown into an unexpected "second wave" representation of hypersensitivity (allergy), resulting in a sharp rise in allergy diseases in babies and young children [1]. In certain highly industrialized locations, food allergy rates among youngsters have surpassed 10%. Furthermore, there is already evidence that these rates in nations with high economic growth correspond to the abrupt gradient of economic change [2]. Despite the fact that international epidemiological studies, such as the ISAAC study, have thoroughly demonstrated the rising global burden of asthma [3], there is no publicly available data on food aversions that are similar across the globe. Some foods that trigger allergies include eggs, tree nuts, shellfish, cow's milk, peanuts, wheat, fish, and soy. Young children typically experience egg and cow's milk allergies, whereas older kids are more prone to experience allergies to shellfish, peanuts, tree nuts, and seafood [4]. Create a technique in this study to identify and categorize food allergies using food photos. Using state-of-the-art computer techniques, such as a deep neural network (CNN) that has been trained to identify and classify food sensitivities among youngsters, two of the most prevalent chronic non-communicable disorders are eczema and food allergies, but data on their prevalence, particularly in developing countries, is lacking [5]. To gather evidence to support the data currently accessible on global trends and incidences of food aversion, this study was carried out in 2012. All of the World Allergy Organization's national member societies were questioned, along with some of their neighboring countries [6]. Gathering data from 89 different countries, statistics were collected on changes in the cost of food and health care, along with other relevant factors. Data on the prevalence of food allergies were unavailable for 52 out of the 89 countries examined [7]. Based on oral food challenges (OFCs), only 9 out of 89 (10%) provided dependable information on food aversions. The information from various countries, estimated at 25 out of 91, is primarily based on parents' reported diagnoses or signs of food hypersensitivity (allergies). This method is understood to potentially inflate the frequency of reported food hypersensitivity (allergies) [8]. To establish more reliable benchmarks, researchers examined the prevalence of medically certified (OFC certified) food aversions in toddlers. In some nations, this incidence has reached up to 10%. For instance, in China, approximately 7% of preschoolers now consume food certified by the OFC, a rate comparable to that observed in Europe. The phenomenon of food aversion has been on the rise in the vast and rapidly growing societies of Asia. It appears that there is an increase in dietary aversions in both demographic groups. There have not been many high-quality comparative statistics between industrialized and developing countries in the past 11–16 years. The differences in pediatric aversion facilities are also brought to light by this survey [9]. National epinephrine standards and auto-injectors are easily accessible. Finally, there is still a need for more trustworthy information on the frequency of foodborne illness. To better anticipate and address the expanding societal and health problems, allergies are being studied in several industrialized and developing nations. The service system is heavily burdened by food aversion [10]. Anxious food hypersensitivity (allergies) may result in responses and a loss of self-esteem. Food intolerances are more common than they used to be in numerous locations around the globe in the last decades. About 178 foods have been identified as having the potential to induce allergies. There are regional variations in food aversion, and only a small number of them actually cause the majority of the symptoms [11]. The best course of action for a food allergy is complete abstinence from the offending food. Even though medications can help with disease symptoms, there is no cure for dietary aversions at the moment.

The major contributions of this chapter are: (1) to classify the nutrients included in food and (2) to determine the type of food allergy.

The key contribution is handling the difficult process of recognizing, detecting, and categorizing food allergies. Due to the wide variety of food allergies, it can be challenging to classify nutrients in food and identify the type of allergy in current circumstances. The identification of food allergies might be advantageous for the prevention of disease in youngsters. Using reinforcement learning, the type of hypersensitivity (allergy) is identified once a food image has been recorded and the item has been divided into a number of nutrients.

Following is how this research is structured: the literature review is divided into two sections. The methodology of the investigation is presented in Section 8.3. A discussion of the findings is presented in Section 8.4. Section 8.5 describes the conclusion and upcoming work.

8.2 Literature review

Due to the high levels of vitamin C in the plants like tomatoes and potatoes, these are nutritious. Additionally significant nutrients included in a healthy diet are potassium, niacin, folate, vitamin B6, pantothenic acid, thiamin, riboflavin fiber, glycemic, carbohydrates, non-glycemic sugars, calcium, magnesium, phosphorus, copper, fiber, and various chemical substances [12]. The plants like tomatoes and potatoes have no fat and are a good source of food which is free from cholesterol. Fresh fruit is a vital food option for those worried about gaining weight due to its low average calorie value [13]. An orange, for example, has 62–82 calories of energy. A grapefruit contains 90 calories, while a tablespoon of lemon juice only has 4 calories. Fruit is also beneficial in the prevention of many organ and organ system disorders, heart attacks, birth defects, lungs, liver, and skin cancers, which are just a few of the illnesses that can occur in people. Furthermore, it offers healthy and well-balanced nutrition [14]. Good food pulp and peel are fed to animals directly and processed to make animal forage. Food has a variety of therapeutic properties [15]. Good fruits provide constipation relief, and the oils and juices extracted from them are used to make medicinal and cosmetic products. The harvest time is signaled by the maturity of the Good Food tree. The Brix/acid ratio serves as a method for assessing the maturity of Good Food [16]. In a study presented by Kenta Itakura, the fluorescence spectrum will be analyzed using a similar methodology, incorporating CNN regression alongside the Brix/acid method [17]. Their research demonstrates that the machine learning technique's calculated absolute error is roughly 2.48, which is less than the absolute error calculated by other techniques [18].

Public health is impacted by nutritional quality, particularly the consumption of orange juice, but further by eating fresh fruit. It has been demonstrated that the consumption of foods high in vitamins like flavonoids dietary fibers, phenols minerals, carotenoids, and other bioactive substances lowers the risk of obesity, cancer, and savvier heart-related problems [19]. A study was carried out to examine modifications in organic acids, vitamin C, and sugars. Cultivar and rootstock types were shown to affect ascorbic and organic acid concentrations in addition to the fruit maturity stage [20]. Researchers examined the nutritional and antioxidant content of four good food species. Pests and insects reduce fruit and vegetable yield. Pesticides are detrimental to these fruits and vegetables. Insect infestations must be discovered as soon as possible [21]. A review of non-destructive methods for detecting insect infestations was conducted. This study also looks at the limitations, benefits, principles, and protocols of these techniques. Longjing tea is a geographically significant product [22]. The geographical origin of Longjing tea is an important consideration in conducting a study using hyperspectral imaging systems to identify geographical regions.

This chapter also goes over terminology, specifications, proper implementation examples, eligibility, and restrictions for several post-harvest fruit harvesting techniques [23]. Among the revised approaches are spectroscopy, ultrasound, acoustic sensing, and chemical reactions, with a focus on non-invasive methods [24]. This investigation delves deeper into the study's current limitations as well as additional testing recommendations for the use of non-destructive techniques to detect and distinguish fruit and vegetable diseases [25]. Levels of TSS are represented through TSS: TA ratio, and ascorbic acid rose with potassium addition, which also reduced the amount of juice acidity. Potassium additions of 760, 1,600, 2,350, and 4,000 g/tree were made; the 2,260 g/tree potassium level considerably increased the layer thickness of the good food fruit. [26]. KNO3 was applied to "Clementine" mandarins, which resulted in an increase in the rise in the levels of TA and ascorbic acid in the fruits during the on year and a decrease in the maturity index during the on year. (K2O) Nwaru (0, 50, 75, 100 kg ha^{-1}) K was found to increase the size and weight of delicious orange fruit when administered to K-deficient crops in four Punjab areas together with P and N [27]. It has also been demonstrated that adding micronutrients enhances the quality of good food fruit. Fruit weight in Kinnow mandarins was boosted by foliar application of boron. Zn, however, boosted juice volume. In general, fruits' exterior and inside are affected by macronutrients and micronutrients [28]. Yet, there has not been a lot of nutritional research done.

8.2.1   *Management in young plants*

Because young trees require different amounts of nutrients than older trees do, young orchards may have low fruit quality [29]. To create fertilizer management plans for newly planted orchards, endogenous nutrient concentrations in various age groups must be compared. When homocysteine levels in the blood exceed normal, the vascular wall becomes a toxin, increasing the risk of cardiovascular disease [30]. A lack of nutritional folate raises plasma homocysteine levels, which contribute to a decrease in plasma folate. Fruit and vegetable consumption lowers plasma homocysteine levels. Consumption of oranges and their juice lowers homocysteine levels, resulting in an increase in plasma folate levels. Homocysteine levels in the elderly have been linked to cognitive dysfunction. Consumption of vegetables, fruits, folate, and vitamin C regularly has been demonstrated to enhance cognition tests, and 0.1% to shellfish [31].

Eating citrus fruits can help prevent a number of common ailments, such as heart disease, cancer, obesity, and type 2 diabetes. Because citrus fruits have several therapeutic properties, they are used to treat scurvy [32]. The consumption of lemon, lime, and orange helps to prevent the formation of kidney stones. Grapefruit was ingested by hypertensive persons to block the calcium-blocking channel and reduce blood pressure. Kumquat peel polyphenols are used as antioxidants. Orange juice is highly recommended for reducing inflammation [33]. Grapefruit juice is high in anti-genotoxic compounds. Food aversion has emerged as an unexpected new allergy trend, and increasing the prevalence of allergic disorders has increased considerably in young children and newborns. In some highly industrialized places, the prevalence of childhood food allergies has reached 10%, and there are already signs that rates in rapidly developing countries will follow the abrupt economic change.

8.2.2   Gradient

The rising global burden of asthma, rhinitis, and eczema has been well documented in recent decades in international epidemiology studies like the ISAAC Study (International Study of Asthma and Asthma Control). Similar data on dietary aversions have not been made public globally [33].

The work proposes that pathological medical images be synthesized to get over the problems of uneven and limited datasets. To create fake chest X-rays using a minimal collection of labeled data, they used Deep Convolutional Generative Adversarial Network (DCGAN) [34,35]. Deep convolutional neural networks were trained to find pathology in five chest radiograph categories using a mix of actual and fake images (DCNNs). Comparing trained DCNN networks on actual and synthetic images reveals that these networks outperform comparable trained networks in the classification of pathology in real instances [36].

8.3   Materials and methods

8.3.1   Proposed framework

Algorithm: for Route discovery in the improved hybrid approach
The research technique is provided in this section. The introduction of the food allergy classification and the three components that follow:

- Obtaining the Kaggle image.
- Extraction of features.
- Non-destructive analysis for food allergy prediction.

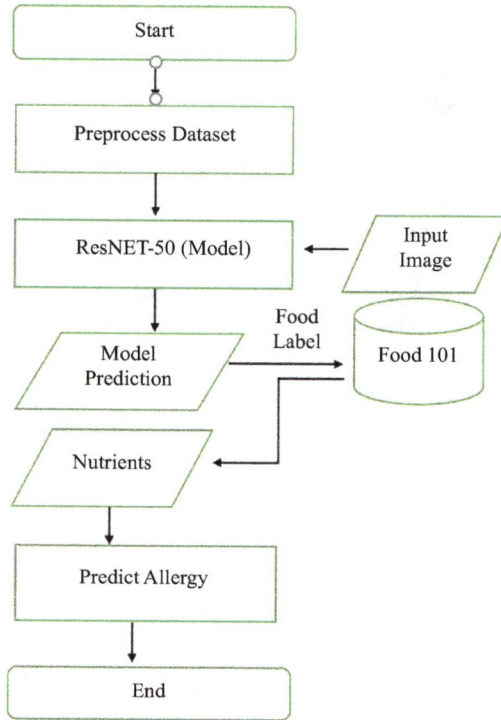

Figure 8.1   Proposed flowchart of work

Phase I involves collecting a data set from Kaggle and preparing it. Food allergy classification is accomplished in phase II using COLAB and ResNET-50. Step III involves developing a model for uniform food allergy prediction using non-destructive analyses. The suggested work's methodology is depicted in Figure 8.1.

8.3.2 Dataset collection

The images for the food allergy dataset were acquired from Kaggle. There were more than 15,000 high-resolution pictures showing food allergies. The food allergy variety dataset is split into 70–30% with 3,300 images as test-size and 11,700 images as training size. Figure 8.2 shows the sample images of the dataset.

8.3.2.1 Training and validation

Algorithm 8.1 lists the steps of the proposed model in which images are trained and validation process is implemented in Python to produce the desired results.

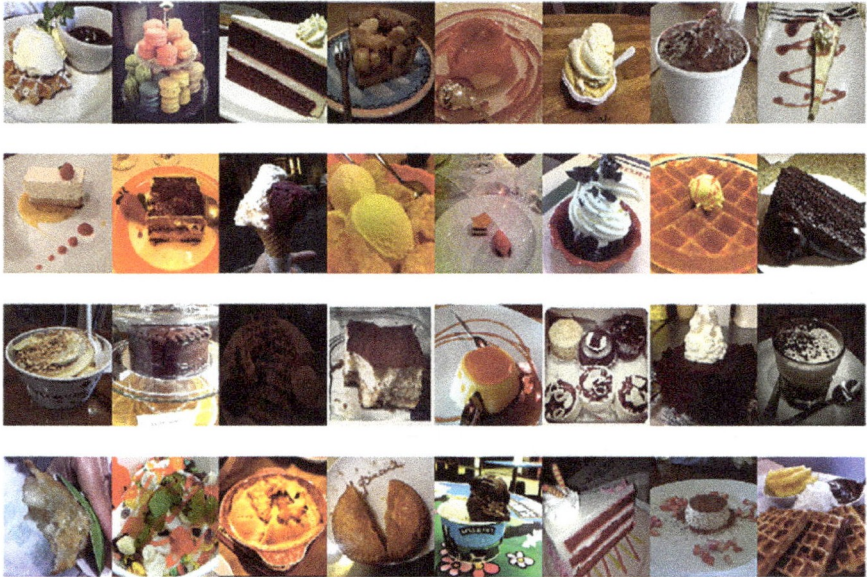

Figure 8.2   Sample images of the dataset

Algorithm 8.1 Training and validation

---

1. Start
2. Pass data set of images
3. Classified data set of images
4. Label of data
5. Train data
6. Test data
7. End

8.3.2.2   Predicting images

Algorithm 8.2 lists the steps involved in predicting images.

Algorithm 8.2 Predicting images

---

1. Start
2. Test Image data
3. Predict image data
4. Predict image data by preprocess input image

5. Print the test image
6. Print shape of the image
7. Probability list is the model
8. Print probability list
9. Max probability list
10. Duplicate list is listprobability
11. Index duplicate list
12. Print of original class
13. Print predicted class
14. nutrients data
15. Nutrients list
16. Print all result
17. End

8.3.2.3   Transfer learning model code and text

Algorithm 8.3 lists the steps which explain the transfer learning of the model.

Algorithm 8.3 Transfer learning model code and text

1. Start
2. Load model ResNET-50
3. Summarize the model
4. Import ResNET-50
5. Print train files result

    End

8.3.3   *Preprocessing and feature extraction*

Input images are frequently preprocessed in the input layer. A number of pre-processing steps, including size and normalization, may be required. However, ResNET-50 required less preprocessing than other neural networks. To remove unimportant distinctions, however, simple preprocessing is required. The ResNET-50 comprehensive transformation approach preserves pixel associations when used in image processing for feature recognition. It uses the appropriate convolution approach for the representation of kernel to identify a given feature. The convolution kernel rotates both horizontally and vertically in a single convolution process, treating columns sequentially. It effectively extracts features by carefully lowering dimensionality, producing an unrepeated data collection called an attribute map. Each attribute identifier (kernel) in convolution finds and eliminates characteristics of the veritable image. The outcome is presented in the form of a map, illustrating how these qualities are distributed based on altitude. Specific specialized general feature characterizing approaches must be used when processing images. Such convolution is limited in its ability to deconstruct the symbolic content of the images because it requires extensive preparation, such as image segmentation, for directly investigating the original data. CNN uses a convolution approach to automatically extract significant characteristics. The kernel parameters are constant throughout the identification process, and the convolution kernels are the modest in comparison to the input image. This leads to each receptive neuron's weight-sharing property.

8.3.3.1   Convolutional layer

Figure 8.3 shows that the first layer in the convolutional network is the neuron layer and is the key component of CNN. The image, represented as matrices, is fed into the convolutional layer and convolved with a corresponding filter or kernel matrix within this layer. The convolution technique produces a resultant matrix known as a feature map. The total of all feature maps is then computed, and each element of the resulting matrix is given a bias value.

8.3.3.2   Feature map

A matrix is obtained as the result of a convolution operation when the kernel slides over the input image. At every location of the input matrix, element-wise multiplication with kernel matrix is performed: left to right, top to bottom. The kernel is applied methodically to each overlapped area of the input matrix. The total results from the element-by-element multiplications of the kernel with the corresponding patch of the input matrix, which is always treated as a single value. Finally, this single value sum of the dot product goes into the feature map. Figure 8.4 shows the convolution of 5 × 5 matrixes multiplied with a 3 × 3 filter matrix to produce a feature map.

The size of the kernel (set of weights) always remains smaller than the input matrix because it enables the kernel needs to be several times multiplied by the input matrix. at different locations on the input matrix. In the convolutional layer, more than one kernel is employed; in fact, to learn various features from the input matrix, a convolutional layer typically uses 32–512 kernels for parallel learning.

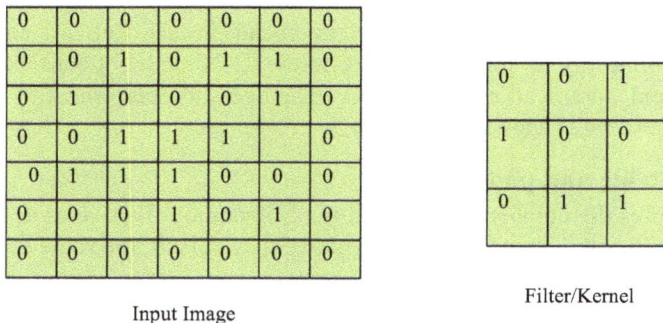

Input Image

Filter/Kernel

Figure 8.3   Kernel matrix

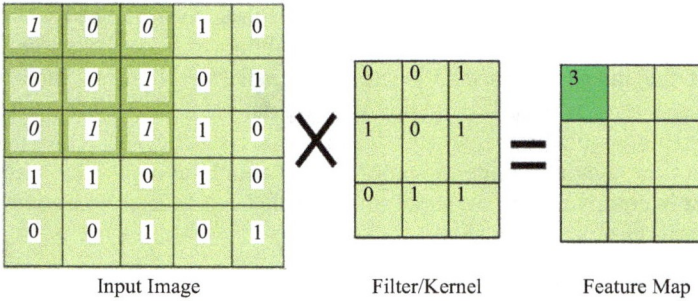

Input Image   Filter/Kernel   Feature Map

Figure 8.4   Feature map kernel layer

Transform Function

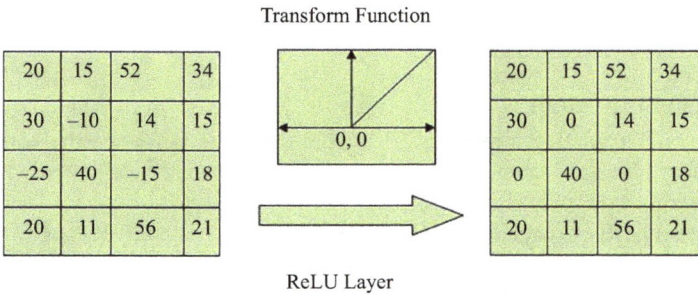

ReLU Layer

Figure 8.5   ReLU operation

8.3.3.3   Non-linearity (ReLU)

After the feature map creation, the next step is to remove non-linearity by passing each value in the feature map through activation function ReLU (short for rectified linear unit) $f(y) = \max(0, y)$. ReLU function has been applied to them and the final feature maps are not actually the sums. There are also several other non-linear functions, such as the hyperbolic tangent function $f(y) = \tanh(y)$ and sigmoid function $f(y) = 1/(1 + e-y)$. Why ReLU is crucial; in fact, ReLU is employed to provide non-linearity to our CNN model. In the CNN model, it enhances learning efficiency and classification performance. The operation performed by the ReLU activation function is shown in Figure 8.5.

8.3.3.4   Stride and padding

Stride specifies the number of steps that the convolution filter takes to move next individually in both horizontal and vertical axes. By default, the value of stride is 1. Figure 8.6 shows the feature map demonstration with a stride of 1.

Figure 8.6 shows that the number of pixels shifts over the input matrix. As stride is 1, move the filters to 1 pixel at a time. The overlap between the Over the input matrix and the number of pixels changes. As stride is 1, set the filters to 1

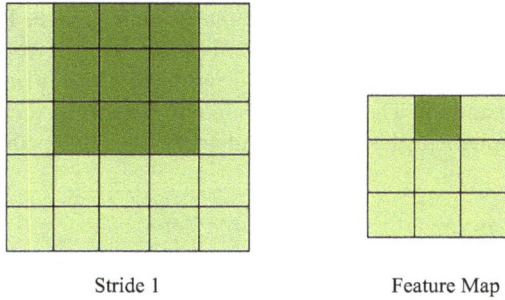

Stride 1   Feature Map

Figure 8.6   Feature map demonstrates a stride of 1

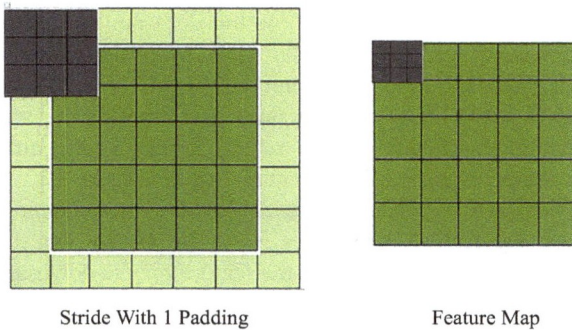

Stride With 1 Padding   Feature Map

Figure 8.7   Stride padding and feature map

pixel at a time. The receptive fields can be reduced by increasing the value of stride. Due to the reduction in overlap, the potential location in convolution is also skipped which makes the smaller size of feature map. Suppose we choose a stride of 2 and reduce the size of the feature map by moving the filters 2 pixels at a time, as shown in Figure 8.10. Input: $n \times n$; Padding: p; Stride: s are the dimensions for stride. $f \times f$, filter size output: $[(n+2p-f)/s+1] \times [(n+2p-f)/s+1]$. Stride is a beneficial function because it allows you to shrink the size of the image.

8.3.3.5   Padding

When an input matrix is used, the feature map's dimensionality is decreased and convolved with the smaller size of the kernel and it would be shrinking at each layer, which is not desirable. Figure 8.7 shows that when the input of 5×5 convolved with a kernel of 3×3, then the resultant feature map is obtained of 3×3.

Input: $n \times n$; filter size: $f \times f$; output: $(n-f+1) \times (n-f+1)$

By maintaining the size of the feature maps, padding is frequently utilized to resolve these problems. When padding is used, the image 1.8 input is a pad with an additional one-pixel border around the edges. As a result, the input matrix is 67 by 7 (instead of a 5×5 matrix). Now, the 5×5 matrix feature map created by the convolution of 3 × 3 is the same size as the original image. Padding: p; input: $n \times n$; sof filter: $f \times f$; output: $(n+2p-f+1) \times (n+2p-f+1)$. Two different kinds of padding exist: valid: when correct padding is used, the result is $(n-f+1) \times (n-f+1)$, which signifies no padding. The output size in our instance is the same as the input size because we implement the VGG 16 and apply the same padding. $n+2p-f+1 = n$. So, $p = (f-1)/2$.

8.3.3.6 Pooling layer

To decrease the dimensionality of the input image and accelerate the calculation, the next layer of CNN pooling is carried out after the convolution processes. This reduction in parameters is useful to shorten the training time and combats overfitting. Max pooling, which removes the maximum from the pooling window, is the most popular type of pooling. Average pooling can also be employed, which uses the median value rather than the maximum. Pooling does not use the padding idea in contrast to convolution. Just like convolution, it takes the maximum value after sliding the kernel across the input. Convolution in CNN architectures is carried out using a 3 × 3 kernel, stride 1, and padding. Stride 2 and no padding are utilized in this case; however, pooling is often done with a 2 × 2 kernel. Max pooling is applied on the 4 × 4 matrix which results in a 2 × 2 feature map. In Figure 8.8, each color shows the different window of 2 × 2 size with stride 2, without overlapping.

In Figure 8.8, the feature map's size is cut in half by the stride and kernel settings, but the crucial data is kept while the feature map is downsampled thanks to pooling. The following formula shows the effect of pooling layer on the input size of nh × nw × nc, then the output will be $[\{(nh - f)/s + 1\} \times \{(nw - f)/s + 1\} \times nc]$.

8.3.3.7 Fully connected layer

The last layer of CNN is the fully connected layer. As a result of operations from earlier layers (convolution and pooling), the size of the input image was reduced in this layer so that the classification's useful characteristics could be preserved as 3D matrices. But a one-dimensional vector of numbers is needed for a layer that is completely connected. Therefore, the output of the feature map of the last pooling layer needs to be flattened here.

Flattening is simply converting the input pooled feature map of the 3D matrices into a 1D vector as shown in Figure 8.9. The resultant flatten output becomes the input to the fully connected layer to choose the corresponding

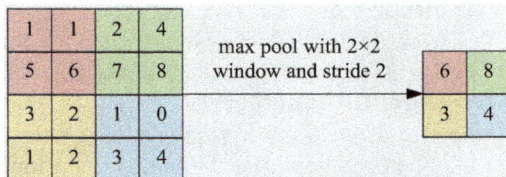

Figure 8.8 Downsampling the feature map

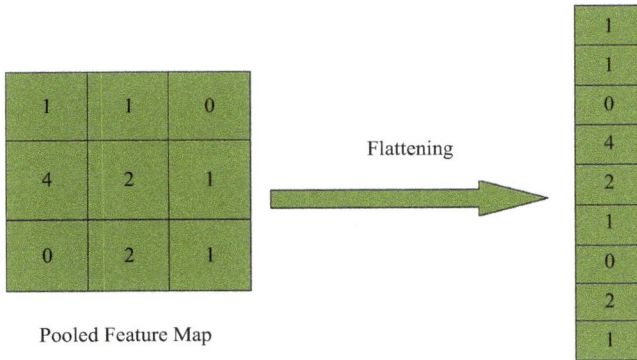

Figure 8.9   Pooled feature map of the 3D matrices

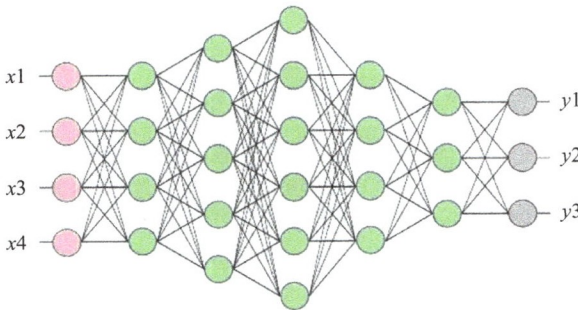

Figure 8.10   Values of flatten vector (×1, ×2, ×3, …)

category with regard to those feature maps. The fully connected layer is a way of learning nonlinear combinations of the feature map.

In Figure 8.10, values of flattening vector (×1, ×2, ×3, …) are combined together to create a model. Finally, an activation function softmax was applied to classify the outputs as food allergy.

8.3.3.8   ResNET-50

Unlike AlexNet, VGGNet, the architecture of ResNET is based on building block modules (network-in-network architectures). Building blocks (convolution, ReLU, pooling) are used to construct the network that leads to macro-architecture. As global average pooling is used in ResNET through the use of this technique, the model's size was decreased to 102 MB from completely connected layers.

Another feature of this architecture is that all 150 levels periodically stack, the number of filters is doubled with stride 2, and the classes are finally produced by the completely linked layer. In this architecture, hyperparameters include batch normalization at each convolution layer. Weight decay is 1e−5, the learning rate is

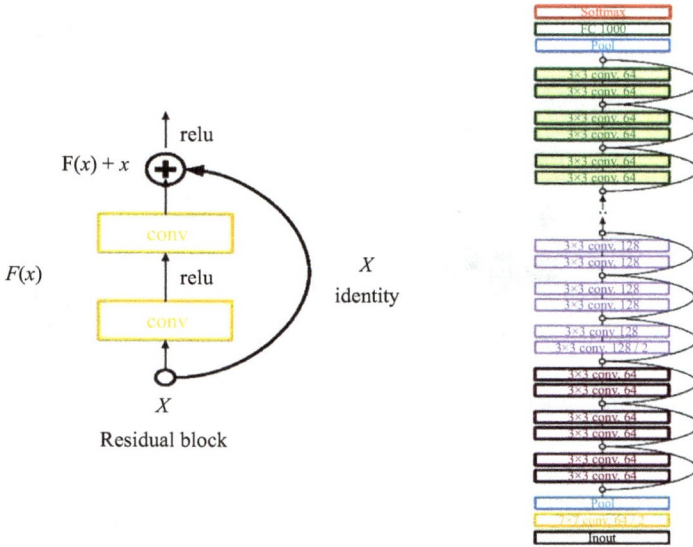

Figure 8.11   Architecture of ResNET-50

0.1, and the batch size is 256; one important point is that there is no dropout that is used in ResNET. The architecture of ResNET-50 is shown in Figure 8.11.

8.3.4   Recognition process

The ResNET-50 convolutional neural network has a multilayer neural network with numerous layers. CNN's three primary function layers are: (1) convolution, (2) pooling, and (3) fully connected. Some of the symmetric and asymmetric building elements in inception include: (a) convolutions, (b) average pooling, (c) max pooling, and (d) drop-out and fully connected layers. To decrease the amount of computing needed, a bottleneck layer that is 11 convolutions is utilized. In one network module, 12, 34, and 56 convolutions are calculated. The inception design serves as a multi-level feature extractor.

We graded the four most prevalent types of food allergies in Pakistan using Inception v3. The ResNET-50 model analyzes a picture of food allergy classes, assigns it to the proper food allergy class, and then classifies it. In this case, the CNN model is fed an image of a food allergy. It is then fed into fully linked layers after passing through a sequence of convolution and pooling layer procedures. Finally, in multiclass classification, the softmax is used to take output.

8.4   Results and discussion

To achieve the best results, the specified methodology is implemented. A comparison analysis with several models is performed, using the help of the suggested technique,

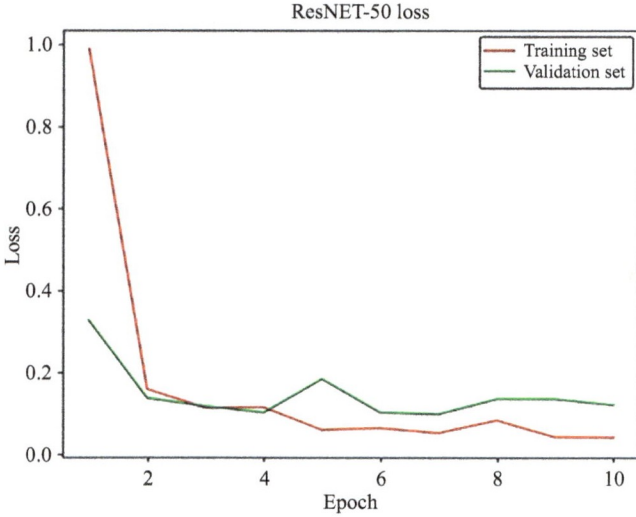

Figure 8.12   Training and validation loss of ResNET-50: ROC curve

graphs, and tables, the results are obtained and reported. The dataset is split into training and testing datasets with proportions of 70% and 30%, respectively, to get the results. In the dataset distribution model, ResNET-50 follows a general principle: a larger training dataset with high quality tends to result in better performance. The aforementioned dataset distribution is implemented in the proposed work to prevent the model from underfitting due to a small training dataset. Additionally, several key terms are defined here to enhance your understanding of the outcome analysis. The model for detecting food allergies is shown in Figure 8.12 for training and validation loss. The findings reveal that the model's training loss decreases continually as the training goes, and we end training at the ideal loss.

8.4.1   Accuracy of model

The percentage of instances that are correctly classified out of all instances is called accuracy. The accuracy of predictive models is critical for correctly determining the quality of forecasts to create scientific evidence that can be used to support policies and decision-making. Observed and expected values are differentiated by the prediction accuracy evaluation. Using predicted and observed values, predictability differences between anticipated values and values from fresh data usually correspond to values modeled from training samples. The training and validation set of the food allergy detection model's accuracy is shown in Figure 8.13:

$$\text{Accuracy} = \frac{\text{Number of correct prediction}}{\text{Total number of prediction}}$$

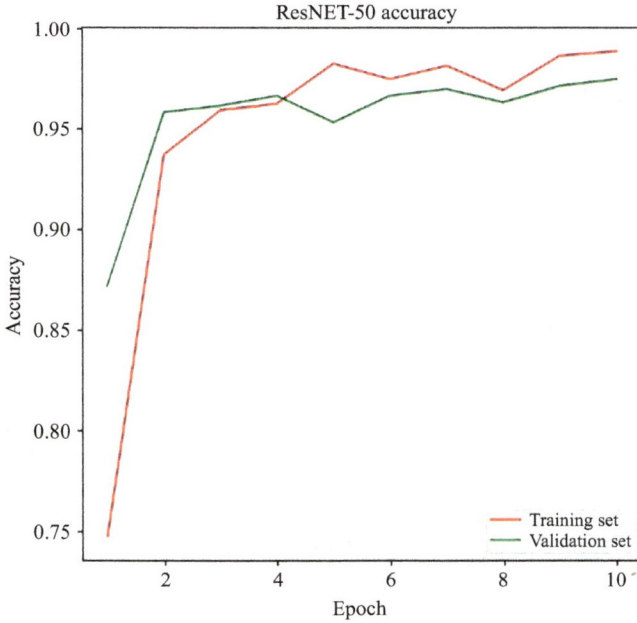

Figure 8.13   ROC curve accuracy on training and validation set

Table 8.1   Comparative analysis of current state of the art methods

S. no.	Algorithm used	Model	Accuracy
1	Detection of food allergy using deep learning	CNN	95.00%
2	A comparison of new deep learning and ensemble learning models to predict food protein allergen city	SVM, K-NN, and NB	74.18%, 77.22%, and 72.03%
3	Using hospital safety event reports to develop and validate a deep learning model for detecting allergic reactions	DNN	93.00%
4	Machine learning and XAI approaches for allergy diagnosis	DT, SVM, and RF	81.62%, 81.05%, and 83.07%
5	Using lengthy short-term memory, protein allergen detection using deep learning	LSTM, extra tree classifier, and quadratic discriminant analysis	91.5%, 90%, and 76.13%

Based on multiple past works, Table 8.1 compares various algorithms and methodologies of the state of the art.

8.5 Conclusion and future work

The results show that ResNET-50 and transfer learning have been a great solution for our needs. As a result, there is no need to manually extract picture categorization characteristics in resent. To extract original features, it employs kernel matrices as local feature extractors. Tuning the model involves adjusting hyperparameters to identify a set of kernels that effectively extract discriminative features. However, transfer learning has proven to be the most effective strategy for categorizing (food) images and discovering nutrients, achieving a remarkable 95% accuracy. This research presents a logical and non-invasive approach to addressing food allergies, potentially offering advantages in disease detection in young individuals. The early diagnosis of food allergies will help to keep kids healthy. In the future, we can create a mobile application with the help of our qualified personnel for users so they can use their phones to identify allergenic foods and stay healthy.

References

[1] P. M. Shanthappa and R. Kumar, "ProAll-D: protein allergen detection using long short-term memory – a deep learning approach," *Admet dmpk*, vol. 10, no. 3, pp. 231–240, 2022, doi:10.5599/admet.1335.

[2] S. Manzoor, M. Habib-ur-Rahman, G. Haider, *et al.*, "Biochar and slow-releasing nitrogen fertilizers improved growth, nitrogen use, yield, and fiber quality of cotton under arid climatic conditions," *Environ Sci Pollut Res Int*, vol. 29, no. 9, pp. 13742–13755, 2022, doi:10.1007/s11356-021-16576-6.

[3] L. Wang, D. Niu, X. Zhao, X. Wang, M. Hao, and H. Che, "A comparative analysis of novel deep learning and ensemble learning models to predict the allergenicity of food proteins," *Foods*, vol. 10, no. 4, p. 809, 2021, doi:10.3390/foods10040809.

[4] M. Sufyan Tahir, A. Latif, S. Bashir, *et al.*, "Transformation and evaluation of broad-spectrum insect and weedicide resistant genes in *Gossypium arboreum* (Desi Cotton)," *GM Crops Food*, vol. 12, no. 1, pp. 292–302, 2021, doi:10.1080/21645698.2021.1885288.

[5] R. Kavya, J. Christopher, S. Panda, and Y. B. Lazarus, "Machine learning and XAI approaches for allergy diagnosis," *Biomed Signal Process Control*, vol. 69, p. 102681, 2021, https://doi.org/10.1016/j.bspc.2021.102681.

[6] S. Halken, A. Muraro, D. de Silva, *et al.*, "EAACI guideline: preventing the development of food allergy in infants and young children (2020 update)," *Pediatr Allergy Immunol*, vol. 32, no. 5, pp. 843–858, 2021, doi:10.1111/pai.13496.

[7] R. X. Foong, J. A. Dantzer, R. A. Wood, and A. F. Santos, "Improving diagnostic accuracy in food allergy," *J Allergy Clin Immunol Pract*, vol. 9, no. 1, pp. 71–80, 2021, doi:10.1016/j.jaip.2020.09.037.

[8] D. M. Fleischer, E. S. Chan, C. Venter, *et al.*, "A consensus approach to the primary prevention of food allergy through nutrition: guidance from the

American Academy of Allergy, Asthma, and Immunology; American College of Allergy, Asthma, and Immunology; and the Canadian Society for Allergy and Clinical Immunology," *J Allergy Clin Immunol: In Pract*, vol. 9, no. 1, pp. 22–43. e4, 2021/01/01/ 2021, https://doi.org/10.1016/j.jaip. 2020.11.002.

[9]   H. S. Ahmad, M. Imran, F. Ahmad, *et al.*, "Improving water use efficiency through reduced irrigation for sustainable cotton production," *Sustainability*, vol. 13, no. 7, p. 4044, 2021. [Online]. Available: https://www.mdpi.com/ 2071-1050/13/7/4044.

[10] E. Lee, K. Jeong, Y.-S. Shin, *et al.*, "Causes of food allergy according to age and severity: a recent 10-year retrospective study from a single tertiary hospital," *Allergy, Asthma & Respiratory Disease*, vol. 8, pp. 80–88, 2020.

[11] A. Khan, D. Khan, and F. Akbar, "Bibliometric analysis of publications on research into cotton leaf curl disease," *Discoveries (Craiova)*, vol. 8, no. 2, p. e109, 2020, doi:10.15190/d.2020.6.

[12] B. Iqbal, F. Kong, I. Ullah, *et al.*, "Phosphorus application improves the cotton yield by enhancing reproductive organ biomass and nutrient accumulation in two cotton cultivars with different phosphorus sensitivity," *Agronomy*, vol. 10, no. 2, p. 153, 2020. [Online]. Available: https://www. mdpi.com/2073-4395/10/2/153.

[13] R. Yunus, O. Arif, H. Afzal, *et al.*, "A framework to estimate the nutritional value of food in real time using deep learning techniques," *IEEE Access*, vol. 7, pp. 2643–2652, 2019.

[14] M. Volpicella, C. Leoni, M. C. G. Dileo, and L. R. Ceci, "Progress in the analysis of food allergens through molecular biology approaches," *Cells*, vol. 8, no. 9, 2019, doi:10.3390/cells8091073.

[15] P. Satitsuksanoa, K. Jansen, A. Głobińska, W. van de Veen, and M. Akdis, "Regulatory immune mechanisms in tolerance to food allergy," *Front Immunol*, vol. 9, p. 2939, 2018, doi:10.3389/fimmu.2018.02939.

[16] N. Mitselou, J. Hallberg, O. Stephansson, C. Almqvist, E. Melén, and J. F. Ludvigsson, "Cesarean delivery, preterm birth, and risk of food allergy: nationwide Swedish cohort study of more than 1 million children," *J Allergy Clin Immunol*, vol. 142, no. 5, pp. 1510–1514, 2018, doi:10.1016/j. jaci.2018.06.044.

[17] W. Loh and M. L. K. Tang, "The epidemiology of food allergy in the global context," *Int J Environ Res Public Health*, vol. 15, no. 9, p. 2043, 2018, doi:10.3390/ijerph15092043.

[18] M. Zubair, S. S. Zaidi, S. Shakir, I. Amin, and S. Mansoor, "An insight into cotton leaf curl Multan betasatellite, the most important component of cotton leaf curl disease complex," *Viruses*, vol. 9, no. 10, p. 280, 2017, doi:10.3390/ v9100280.

[19] P. Krithika and S. Veni, "Leaf disease detection on cucumber leaves using multiclass support vector machine," in *2017 International Conference on Wireless Communications, Signal Processing and Networking (WiSPNET)*, pp. 1276–1281, 2017.

[20]   J. Amara, B. Bouaziz, and A. Algergawy, "A deep learning-based approach for banana leaf diseases classification," in BTW, 2017.

[21]   A. Ahmad, M. Zia-Ur-Rehman, U. Hameed, *et al.*, "Engineered disease resistance in cotton using RNA-interference to knock down cotton leaf curl Kokhran virus-Burewala and cotton leaf curl Multan betasatellite expression," *Viruses*, vol. 9, no. 9, p. 257, 2017, doi:10.3390/v9090257.

[22]   C. Lozoya-Ibáñez, S. Morgado-Nunes, A. Rodrigues, C. Lobo, and L. Taborda-Barata, "Prevalence and clinical features of adverse food reactions in Portuguese adults," *Allergy Asthma Clin Immunol*, vol. 12, p. 36, 2016, doi:10.1186/s13223-016-0139-8.

[23]   D. Doğruel, G. Bingöl, M. Yılmaz, and D. U. Altıntaş, "The ADAPAR Birth Cohort Study: food allergy results at five years and new insights," *Int Arch Allergy Immunol*, vol. 169, no. 1, pp. 57–61, 2016, doi:10.1159/000443831.

[24]   A. Wassmann and T. Werfel, "Atopic eczema and food allergy," *Chem Immunol Allergy*, vol. 101, pp. 181–90, 2015, doi:10.1159/000371701.

[25]   F. E. Simons, L. Rf Ardusso, M. B. Bilò, *et al.*, "International consensus on (ICON) anaphylaxis," *World Allergy Organ J*, vol. 7, no. 1, p. 9, 2014, doi:10.1186/1939-4551-7-9.

[26]   M. F. Munsell, B. L. Sprague, D. A. Berry, G. Chisholm, and A. Trentham-Dietz, "Body mass index and breast cancer risk according to postmenopausal estrogen-progestin use and hormone receptor status," *Epidemiol Rev*, vol. 36, no. 1, pp. 114–36, 2014, doi:10.1093/epirev/mxt010.

[27]   S. L. Prescott, R. Pawankar, K. J. Allen, *et al.*, "A global survey of changing patterns of food allergy burden in children," *World Allergy Organ J*, vol. 6, no. 1, p. 21, 2013, doi:10.1186/1939-4551-6-21.

[28]   B. I. Nwaru, L. Hickstein, S. S. Panesar, *et al.*, "The epidemiology of food allergy in Europe: protocol for a systematic review," *Clin Transl Allergy*, vol. 3, no. 1, p. 13, 2013, doi:10.1186/2045-7022-3-13.

[29]   L. Bolier, M. Haverman, G. J. Westerhof, H. Riper, F. Smit, and E. Bohlmeijer, "Positive psychology interventions: a meta-analysis of randomized controlled studies," *BMC Public Health*, vol. 13, p. 119, 2013, doi: 10.1186/1471-2458-13-119.

[30]   H. Chen, N. Qian, W. Guo, *et al.*, "Using three overlapped RILs to dissect genetically clustered QTL for fiber strength on Chro.D8 in Upland cotton," *Theor Appl Genet*, vol. 119, no. 4, pp. 605–12, 2009, doi:10.1007/s00122-009-1070-x.

[31]   M. Kebede, D. Ehrich, P. Taberlet, S. Nemomissa, and C. Brochmann, "Phylogeography and conservation genetics of a giant lobelia (*Lobelia giberroa*) in Ethiopian and Tropical East African mountains," *Mol Ecol*, vol. 16, no. 6, pp. 1233–43, 2007, doi: 10.1111/j.1365-294X.2007.03232.x.

[32]   A. Kumar, J. Rawat, I. Kumar, *et al.*, "Computer-aided deep learning model for identification of lymphoblast cell using microscopic leukocyte images," *Expert Syst*, vol. 39, no. 4, p. e12894, 2022.

[33]   R. C. Cronn, R. L. Small, T. Haselkorn, and J. F. Wendel, "Rapid diversification of the cotton genus (Gossypium: Malvaceae) revealed by analysis of

sixteen nuclear and chloroplast genes," *Am J Bot*, vol. 89, no. 4, pp. 707–25, 2002, doi:10.3732/ajb.89.4.707.

[34]   Li, Peng, Asif Ali Laghari, M. Rashid, *et al.*, "A deep multimodal adversarial cycle-consistent network for smart enterprise system," *IEEE Trans Ind Inf*, vol. 19, no. 1, pp. 693–702, 2022.

[35]   S. Bagchi, K. G. Tay, A. Huong, and S. Debnath, "Image processing and machine learning techniques used in computer-aided detection system for mammogram screening-A review," *Int J Electr Comput Eng*, vol. 10, no. 3, p. 2336, 2020.

[36]   Y. Bao and N. Ishii, "Combining multiple K-nearest neighbor classifiers for text classification by reducts," in *Discovery Science*, 2002.

Section 2

Use of AI-enabled IoT in healthcare

Chapter 9

Design and development of Internet of Things and artificial intelligence-based medical imaging system

Rupali A. Mahajan[1], Smita Chavan[2], Prajakta Ajay Khadkikar[3], Gayatri Mahendra Bhandari[4] and Jyoti Manish Shinde[5]

The Internet of Things (IoT) and artificial intelligence (AI) are interrelated research areas that have gained a huge impact in designing and customizing the healthcare systems. Smart healthcare is termed as an imperative factor of connected living. Healthcare is termed as a fundamental pillar of human requirements and smart healthcare helps to generate many dollars in revenue. The current evolutions in AI and IoT have exposed emerging possibilities in healthcare applications. AI has powered medical technologies and is quickly growing into applicable solutions for clinical usage. The execution of augmented medicines is awaited by patients and thus it permits huge autonomy and customized diagnosis. This chapter elaborates on various studies and techniques based on AI considering IoT-based medical imaging. The IoT-based medical imaging is carried out by executing various types of AI-based techniques. Furthermore, the applications and challenges of the IoT-based medical imaging are included. Here, the efforts of various researchers in executing the AI techniques are described for carrying out the IoT-based medical imaging. In addition, the current chapter highlights methodological, theoretical, and empirical concepts considering instances based on healthcare applications. Moreover, the details on several advancements in the IoT and available wearable and smart devices that targets healthcare applications and assessment of standard protocols of AI for predictions of health-based issues are discussed. In addition, the nomenclature of different mechanisms is elaborated. Thus, by concentrating on discerning criteria, the methods are classified and illustrated in this chapter.

[1]Department of Computer Engineering, Vishwakarma Institute of Information Technology, Pune, India
[2]Department of Information Technology, Government College of Engineering, Aurangabad, India
[3]Department of Computer Engineering, SCTR's Pune Institute of Computer Technology, Pune, India
[4]Department of Computer Engineering, JSPM's Bhivarabai Sawant Institute of Technology and Research, Wagholi Pune, India
[5]JMS Brilliance Infotech, Pimpri, India

Moreover, the past, present, and future scores of the IoT-based medical imaging using AI are focused and research scope for analyzing different types of IoT-based medical imaging techniques is described.

9.1 Introduction

Internet of Things (IoT), artificial intelligence (AI), and big data are the inter-related research area that contains the pertinent impact factor on the modeling and progression of improved personalized healthcare models. IoT provides the pervasive and ubiquitous performance for sensing and communication abilities. IoT is generally utilized in various domains like noise pollution supervision, agriculture, monitoring of indoor quality, and other various applications of improved living atmospheres and endorse health. IoT is normally converted into hospital settings and the generated a new model is termed as Internet of Medical Things (IoMT) [1]. IoMT offers several advantages to most of the patients who utilize the wearable sensors for improving their well-being and health that closely dependent on mHealth and eHealth. There are various kinds of sensors that have been utilized by the people for monitoring their health. Nowadays, most of the people normally utilize mobile sensors due to its availability, accessibility, and low cost. In addition, the personalized healthcare schemes are also used to support the healthcare monitoring [2,3].

Generally, the personalized healthcare schemes gather the significant biological information for supporting the clinical diagnostics as well as decisions. The wearable medical sensors offer the functioning of constant monitoring by gathering the huge quantity of medical information through the sensors to predict the information of patients by doctors. The data assessment and knowledge mining are complex methods that ensure the performance of security approaches [4]. In IoT, the AI-based medical imaging approaches provide the improved monitoring performance.

9.1.1 Medical imaging

Some of the preliminary development in computer vision depend on the photographic images of various objects like houses, cars, fruits, and so on. One of the familiar competitions in medical imaging is ImageNet large-scale visual recognition challenge that was established in 2010 using the training set that contains greater than 1.2 million Joint Photographic Expert Group (JPEG) photographic color images dispersed in 1,000 classes. Generally, the medical images are saved in digital imaging and communications in medicine (DICOM) format that are characteristically distinct from the ImageNet dataset [5].

The DICOM standard was formed to establish several secure processes in clinical imaging, which are accountable for a numerous progression in the area specifically in the radiology digitization. Moreover, the DICOM format permits the images with distinct resolution and the bit-depth allocation. Generally, the medical images have been captured by various medical imaging modalities, such as computerized tomography (CT), magnetic resonance imaging (MRI), Doppler ultrasound, and so on [6,7].

Most of the medical imaging equipment generally creates the gray-scale images, and the equipment, such as PET, CT, secondary capture objects, and Doppler ultrasound, produce color images. The way of capturing medical images is distinct from the different photographic image equipment. For instance, in radiographic study, it requires larger than one view for determining the three-dimensional structure of organ within the body. Likewise, the cross-sectional modalities, like CT and MRI, gather the image-based data in a volumetric form [8,9].

Moreover, the multi-sequence modalities, like MRI, provide the multiple kinds of images for the same body portion to mine the particular features of the specific tissue. The image comparison concept is a significant feature in medical imaging, which is utilized to evaluate the variations in the health status of patients. Moreover, this technique is not applicable in nonmedical usages. Furthermore, medical imaging discoveries are often not precise in a single disease entity and it is recognized in a diversity of diseases [10].

9.1.2 AI

AI is signaled as the most troublesome method of health services in the 21st century. Numerous commentary articles distributed in the common public as well as health areas identify that the medical imaging is at the forefront of these variations due to the huge digital data outline. Radiomics is converting the clinical images into mineable high-dimensional information to improve the clinical decision-making [11].

9.1.2.1 AI in healthcare

AI techniques provide various chances to the IoT-based healthcare systems that can suggestively progress the global public health. The discovery of AI technology in healthcare significantly reduces the global cost of avoidance of chronic illnesses. Besides, the gathered real-time health information used in AI systems can help to assist the patients while performing the self-administration therapies.

Mobile devices utilize the mobile applications for health monitoring through AI by integrating the application installed mobile devices with mHealth and telemedicine [12]. The consequences of assessing the medical data from IoMT systems can progress the significance of data interpretations and reduce the time to assess the data outcome. Nowadays, the newly modeled healthcare system, namely "Personalized Preventative Health Coaches," is introduced, which sustains the experiences, and it is used in explaining and understanding the health as well as well-being information. Figure 9.1 shows the AI in healthcare systems.

9.1.2.2 AI in medical imaging

Medical imaging area greatly perceives the advantages from AI as most of the gathered medical information is difficult to process and uncertain in nature,

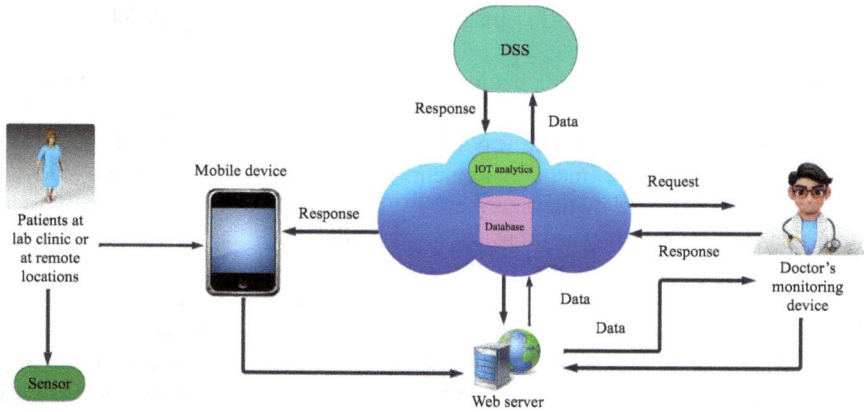

Figure 9.1   AI in healthcare systems

and it is complex to identify the significant features. Deep learning (DL) is discovered from machine learning (ML) that is the subdomain of computer science and is termed as AI. The main goal of AI is to take the decision based on the environment without utilizing any program to recognize any of their particular patterns.

The AI system transforms the diagnosis of healthcare sector in the medical imaging domain. Moreover, the AI-based health prevention, management, and precision is done by integrating the various format of medical data, like proteomics, demographics, and genomics with radiomics. In medical imaging, the AI tools have been utilized at a local level for reducing the labor-intensive and repetitive processes, such as medical image assessment [13].

9.1.2.3   AI in medical diagnosis

"Medical imaging and diagnosis drive by AI that witness greater than 40% of its growth to surpass USD 2.5 billion by 2024." Based on the adaptation of DL and neural network schemes, AI transforms the image diagnosis area in medicine to resolve the complex assessment of MRI scan that makes the process based on AI as simple.

- MRI scans are very complex to assess owing to the presence of medical information. The standard MRI assessment consumes several hours to process; however, the researchers consume a few hours for formulating an outcome from the huge datasets to produce the scan.
- Large-sized and complex dataset can be assessed by the neural networks that consider excess quantities of MRI scans for training the dataset.
- The neural network takes the input data that undergoes the transformation process throughout the network until generating the desired outcome by considering the principles of bias and weights.

9.1.2.4 AI in medical assistance

As increasing the requirement for medical assistance, the AI-based virtual nurses have been progressed. Based on the survey taken recently, the virtual nursing assistants based on the value of highest near-term is USD 20 billion by 2027. One of the examples of widely used virtual nurse is Sensely that executes the natural language processing, ML, speech recognition, and wireless incorporation with medicinal devices, like blood pressure cuffs to offer the medical assistance to patients [14]. Some of the benefits provided by the virtual nurse include the following:

- Clinical advice
- Self-care
- Scheduling an appointment
- ER direction
- Nurse line

9.1.2.5 AI in decision-making

AI acts as a significant function in decision-making. AI is not only used in the medical field but also widely used in various domains, such as businesses by observing the customer needs and computing any complex tasks. The more significant and powerful tool of AI in decision-making is the usage of surgical robots that significantly reduce the errors and discrepancies for helping to improve the accuracy of surgeons. One of the surgical robots is named as Da Vinci, that is a familiar professional surgeon to handle the complex surgeries with better elasticity and control than conservative approaches. Moreover, the special features of Da Vinci are given in the following:

- It helps the surgeons by handling the advanced instruments set.
- The hand movement of the surgeon is translated at the console in real time.
- It produced the magnified, clear, and 3D high-resolution image of the surgical portion. Moreover, the surgical robots are not only used in making the decision but used to progress the overall efficiency of the system.

9.2 IoT system

In healthcare application, the IoT perceives more attention as they help in facilitating the remote observation of patients. Recently, IoT system in healthcare receives more attention as the IoT systems offer more significant features that establish the remote observation of patients. A Personal Healthcare Device (PHD) acts as an indispensable part of monitoring the medical system when the healthcare applications in IoT schemes are deliberated. PHD is an efficient electronic healthcare device that makes sense and computes the biomedical signals of users. In IoT, the PHD devices are processed by linking the devices to the main healthcare servers. The system failure problem arose due to the malfunctioning of hardware, environmental hazards, software bugs, and power shortages. As utilizing the increasing usage of multiple nodes in large-scale IoT system, the occurrence of a fault on the nodes increases such that the entire systems function inappropriately. Furthermore, some PHD information is too valuable to drop due to the failure of the system with u-healthcare atmospheres [15].

9.2.1   IoT

IoT is referred to as the interconnection of multiple devices including sensors, actuators, and other communication devices. A sensing device is a sensor that significantly admits the intelligent device as well as converts the exterior physical signal into the signal, which can be identified by the intelligent device. Generally, the sensing instrument converts the physical information into digital information format, and then forwards the physical information to the intelligent devices through the bus. In other words, a sensing device is termed as a sensor network that can gather and transfer the information through the desired path to the intelligent devices. Moreover, the executing devices perceive the control signals, whereas the intelligent devices are responsible to transfer and control the control things' behaviors that rely on control signals. Figure 9.2 shows the various applications of IoT. The IoT system contains the intelligent device layer that gathers the information of things that are directly connected to the Internet. The intelligent devices are categorized into computer, LAN, and IoT terminal. IoT terminal is referred to as an embedded system that contains the general-purpose computer, intelligent chip, personal mobile devices or industrial computer, and control equipment for providing the information of things.

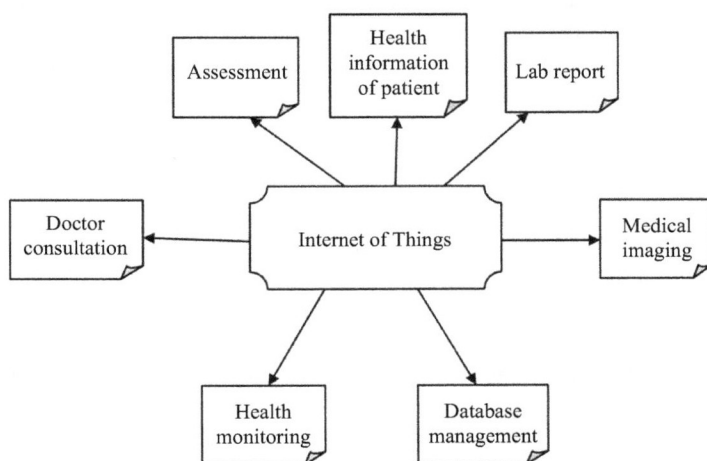

Figure 9.2   Applications of IoT

Moreover, the device layer provides the physical information, whereas the logical information layer provides the logical information of things. In addition, the basic service layer is the critical layer in connecting things as well as the Internet. The fundamental services offered by the things linked to the Internet are categorized into three types:

- Things identification
- Data assortment of things
- Things performance control

The multiple numbers of sensors used in IoT are as follows:

- Image sensor
- Temperature sensor
- Pressure sensor
- Gyrometer sensors
- Level sensor
- IR sensor
- Motion detection sensors
- Gyrometer sensors
- Optical sensors
- Humidity sensors, and so on.

9.2.2   IoT image sensor

It is also termed as "eyes of machines" that is considered as a core device for numerous applications. The applications of IoT sensors vary from robotics to drones that require the image sensor to provide distinct aspects and features. Image sensors are considered as significant sensors in various developing applications of IoT. They offer the comprehensive environment information through the big array of photodiodes and have a high market price because of their standardization. The commonly used application of IoT image sensor is the camera system, which is used for supervising and observing the location using video streaming. Moreover, they can be protracted when they are joined with image processing practices. In IoT, image sensors are widely used in various domains wherein the image sensors are utilized for surveillance video schemes in smart cities, personalized healthcare schemes, understanding and identifying the human activities, and video streaming schemes in vehicular IoT [16].

9.2.3   IoT imagery

The utilization of IoT technology in healthcare applications assures the healthcare industries of improving the quality of care and reduces the cost with automation and resource optimization offered by it. The IoT imagery helps to establish the identification and remedial measures in real time by auto-analyzing the parameters of imaging apparatus. The advantage of considering the IoT imagery is that it provides reduced waiting time and reduces the vexation of patients and doctors [17].

9.2.4   IoT medical imaging system

The process of gathering the medical images of patients having the interior structure of the human body is termed as medical imaging. The medical imaging is helpful in diagnosing and treating the disease of patients. The medical imaging is considered as one of the important necessities in the hospital. IoT medical imaging establishes the diagnosis, sharing, and information retrieval in real time and evades the issue of recurring investigations, consultation problems, and misdiagnosing. The machine-to-machine interrelation offered by the IoT helps the medical imaging equipment for improving the quality and reduces the cost of operations.

9.2.4.1   MRI

MRI utilizes a powerful magnetic field and the pulses of radio frequency for generating the clear picture of tissues within the human body, like soft tissues, bones, and interior structure of the human body. Moreover, the MRI is useful in diagnosing various diseases, such as brain or head trauma, spinal issues, brain tumor, abdomen, brain, and liver abnormalities. Figure 9.3 shows the image of the MRI scanner.

9.2.4.2   X-ray (X-radiation)

X-ray is utilized for capturing an accurate and clear picture using the radiation. The X-ray setup utilizes the electromagnetic radiation for capturing the picture of the body structure by penetrating the radiation within the body. Moreover, the X-ray is helpful in detecting and identifying the irregularities within the body. An X-ray is a rapid and simple test that creates the inner structures of images in the body, especially in bones. Here, the X-ray beams are passed through the body and the beams are absorbed in dissimilar amounts based on the density of material they permit through. Figure 9.4 shows the X-ray machine block diagram.

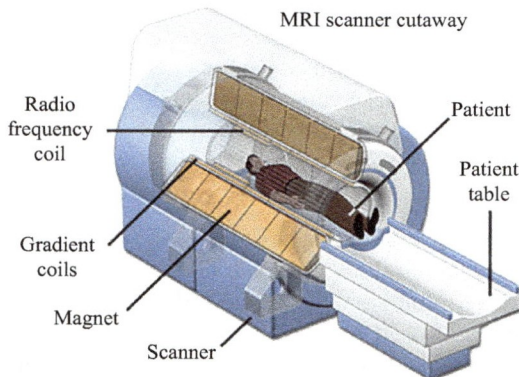

Figure 9.3   MRI scanner

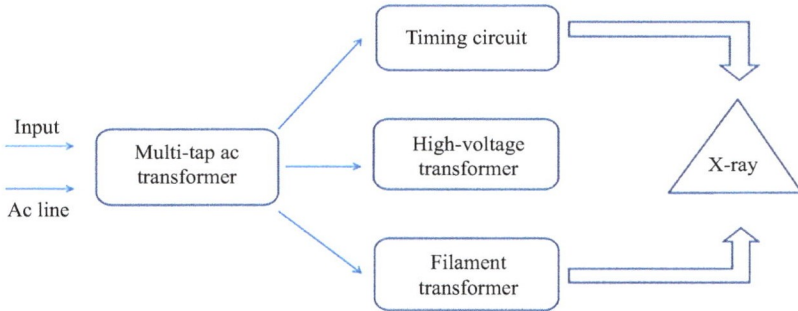

Figure 9.4   X-ray machine block diagram

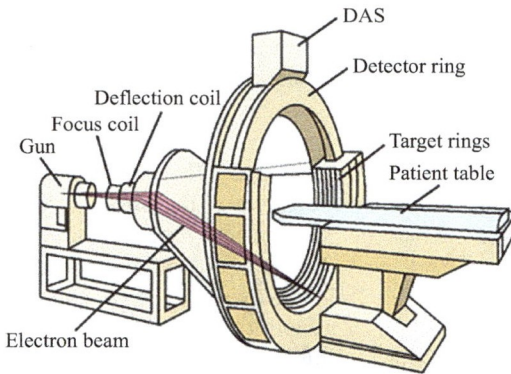

Figure 9.5   Electron beam CT scanner configuration

9.2.4.3   Computed tomography

Computed tomography (CT) scan is a beneficial diagnostic tool for sensing diseases and damages. It practices a sequence of X-rays and a processor to create a 3D image of soft bones and tissues. CT is an easy, painless, and non-invasive method for diagnosing the conditions. The CT scanning is generally available at an imaging center or at a hospital. In CT scanning setup, it exploits the X-rays to take the comprehensive image of organs within the human body in the form of very thin slices. The medical professionals utilize the CT scan for examining the inner structure of the human body. Moreover, the CT scan considers the X-rays to generate the cross-sectional image of body, like blood vessels, muscles, and organs, and the captured image is in very thin slices [18]. Figure 9.5 shows the electron beam CT scanner configuration.

9.2.4.4   Ultrasound

The ultrasound imaging (sonography) is a kind of medical imaging equipment that is used for observing the inner structure of the body. The ultrasounds are the

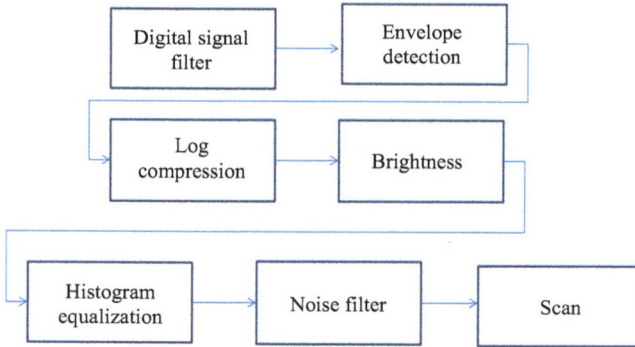

Figure 9.6   Ultrasound flow diagram

acoustic energy in wave form with the frequencies higher than the human hearing range. Moreover, it is widely used in assessing the interior structure of the human body. This kind of medical imaging is generally used in diagnosing the abdominal issues, uterus issues, kidney problems, and recognizing the growth of a baby in the fetus. Figure 9.6 shows the ultrasound flow. The ultrasound imaging utilizes the high-frequency sound waves for observing the inner structure of the body. Moreover, the ultrasounds are gathered in real time, and they are used to observe the inner movement of organs and blood flow via the vessels. An ultrasound scan practices sound waves with high frequency to create an image of the structure of the inner body. Doctors usually utilize the ultrasound to monitor the developing fetus (unborn baby), pelvic organs, abdominal organs, muscles, and heart and blood vessels.

9.2.5   Merits and demerits IoT in medical field

Nowadays, IoT is considered as an important area in the medical field. The IoT in the medical industry basically offers the visualization of material supervision, digitization of medical data, and the digitization of the therapeutic process. The IoT with the radio frequency recognition assures the evading of healthcare difficulties by assisting the distribution, production, and tracking of medicines and the medical gadgets with the upsurge in the quality of diagnosis and reduction in the management cost. Moreover, the integration of RFID with the IoT provides the advantages in various areas, such as medical waste and emergency management, pharmaceutical anti-counterfeiting, drug identification, medical equipment, medical record, and drug storage. The IoT in medical field assists the physicians for monitoring the disease spread and suggests the real-time advice and the protections to be taken. Moreover, it also permits the faster access of the patient information by the physician. The IoT in the medical field provides several advantages, such as it provides as smarter, remote real-time monitoring, and a healthier environment. In addition, the IoT-driven medical imaging systems gather and identify the changes in the human body periodically for providing the potential impact to the clinicians and diagnostic approaches. However, the IoT-permitted medical field offers certain limitations in real-time monitoring. The limitations include complications in the management of node mobility, data compression, data completeness, data security, and so on [19].

9.3 IoT medical images

IoT is acknowledged as one of the hopeful research theme in an area of health-care, especially in medical image processing. With a development of medical IoT devices, the volumes and categories of medical images have increased significantly. Owing to IoT in medical images, it is feasible to detect the issues and take preventive measures in actual time. It also performs an automatic assessment of imaging device parameters in effortless manner and minimizes the time for waiting, which annoys doctor as well as patient [20]. However, medical images play a crucial part in disease identification in IoT-based healthcare applications, the medical images transmission over the network as well as cloud storage-based services has become very significant. Several healthcare applications based on IoT consist of numerous count of medical images and visualized electronic healthiness reports, which are conveyed by means of Internet each day. Therefore, it is very important to construct an effectual system for assuring the confidentiality and reliability of patient medical images that are transmitted and stored up in IoT atmosphere.

Several medical imaging modalities achieved a burst through in detecting various diseases. Some of the medical modalities are enlisted [21,22]. Figure 9.7 shows the block diagram of various modalities.

9.3.1 X-ray

The X-ray is utilized on high density or hardest tissues such as bones and is also employed for capturing precise and clear images using radiation. It is less contrast with decreased capability and some information within the image owing to high amount of penetration, blurring, and radiations. X-ray utilizes electromagnetic radiation for penetrating through the structure to generate images of the structure and thus helpful in identifying and diagnosing the irregularity or abnormal conditions inside the body.

9.3.2 CT scan

The CT images have higher contrast of narrow range grayscale characteristics for an elaborate categorization of tissues. These images give an excessive foreground of organs, vessels, and so on, which also suffers from inexact edges among organs and vessels. CT is the most significant equipment utilized for acquiring these images owing to its accessibility in about every emergency condition and its fastest attainment of outcomes. Moreover, CT has gained ever-increasing significance as the diagnosis of a disease is lesser invasive than other methods and provides exact results. Additionally, it can be utilized for acquiring the images of bones, brain, heart, lung, and arteries. CT employs X-rays to have complete image of human

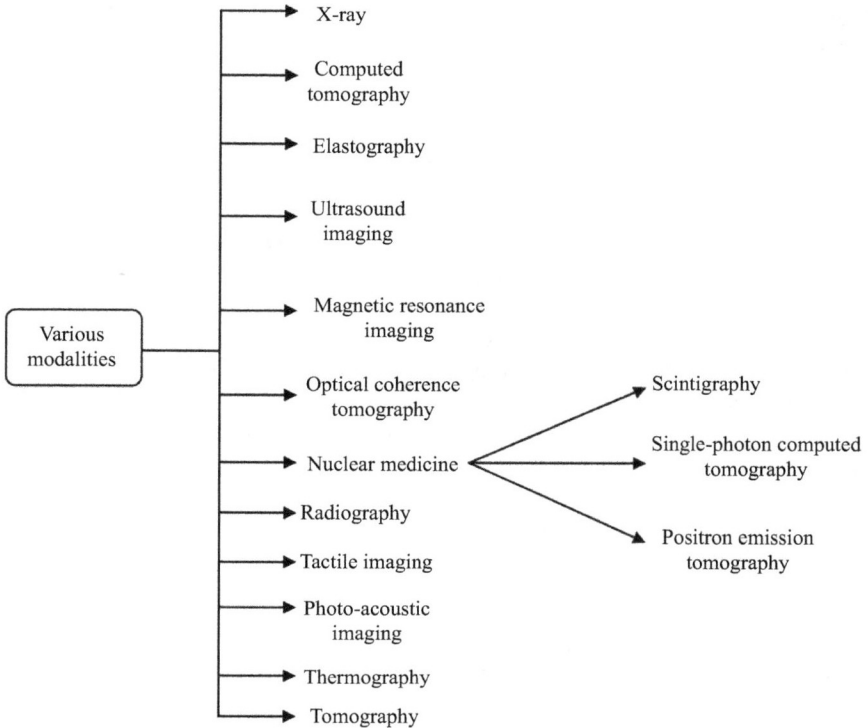

Figure 9.7   Block diagram of various modalities

organs in much thinned slices. As CT tests correspond to a critical reason for radiation exposure for public from diagnosing process of medical imaging, the development of low-dose CT imaging process is most preferable.

9.3.3   Elastography

The medical imaging modality, which maps the elasticity feature of soft tissues, is known as elastography. The information about an occurrence or condition of diseases is diagnosed on the basis of hard tissue or soft tissue.

9.3.4   Ultrasound imaging

The sound waves having high frequency than audio frequency is known as ultrasound. The ultrasound scans are medical imaging modality, which is utilized for looking on inside the body. It is an acoustic energy in a formation of waves having a frequency more than the hearing level of a human. Ultrasound imaging is an accessible and convenient tool for testing as it is comparatively low cost and quick.

Medical ultrasound, which is also known as ultrasonography or diagnostic sonography, is an analytic imaging method for analyzing the internal structures of the human body based upon ultrasound application. The images of ultrasound or sonograms are developed by passing ultrasound pulses into the tissues with an assist of probes. The benefits of ultrasound are actual time image and low cost.

9.3.5 Magnetic resonance imaging (MRI)

MRI is a medical imaging method utilized in the radiology field for producing anatomy images and physiological processes of body. It employs the powerful magnetic field and radio frequency pulses for generating clear images of human body organs like soft tissues, bones and structure of internal body. It is a powerful tool for giving information about the internal structure of the body in a detailed manner. It also confronts a few disadvantages of time acquirement and spatial motion that degrade the image superiority by introducing the noise at processing time. It offers more elaborated information regarding soft tissues as also more sharp identification [23].

9.3.6 Optical coherence tomography (OCT)

OCT has become an essential imaging modality in ophthalmology, which can be utilized in diagnosing various retinal diseases like age-related macular degeneration, glaucoma, and diabetic retinopathy. These scan images provide a complete view of the retinal structure and it permits non-invasive and higher-resolution image of interior cell layers of the retina.

9.3.7 Nuclear medicine

It is an extraordinary medical modality in which the radioactive substance applications are discovered for diagnosing and providing treatment for the diseases. Some properties of isotopes and an emitted strong particle from radioactive material are utilized in nuclear medicine for diagnosing several pathologies. Other than various medical imaging modalities, the nuclear medicine examinations reveal the investigated physiological function of system. This modality is also called molecular imaging and therapeutic or molecular medicine.

9.3.7.1 Scintigraphy

In this type of diagnostic examination, radio nuclides are internally governed and thereafter the emitted radiation from radio nuclides are pictured utilizing gamma cameras, also known as external detectors and thus images are obtained.

9.3.7.2 Single-photon CT (SPECT)

For generating 3D representation, the nuclear medicine method known as SPECT is utilized, where the radio nuclides that generate a flowing emission of single photon are only detected by means of SPECT cameras. Here, the radioisotopes, namely Gallium, Iodine, Thallium, and Technetium, are fed into the body of patients.

9.3.7.3 Positron emission tomography (PET)

PET is a most powerful imaging method that facilitates in vivo investigations of human brain operations. In the previous decades, PET has been utilized in the research field because of more expensive and complications of support infra-structures like radio chemistry labs, PET scanners, and cyclotrons. It is highly utilized in clinical neurology for enhancing the understandability of disease pathogenesis to help diagnose and to check the progression of disease and come-back for treatment.

9.3.8   Radiography

Radiography is a medical imaging method, which makes utilization of X-rays. It is employed in the diagnostic process prior the consequences that were very injurious to humans because of discovering ionization radiation. X-ray penetration into the body and the absorption of radiation are disparity, which the depends on the density of the tissue.

9.3.9   Tactile imaging

In tactile imaging, the touching sense is transformed into a digitalized image. This imaging modality rebuilds the interior mechanical formation of tissue utilizing stress pattern data. It imitates the manual palpation as the equipment with an array of pressure sensor mounted on the face performs in an exact manner such as fingers of the human when examination. Tactile imager helps in counseling patients concerning the difficulties in childbirth and decision-making about a delivery organization.

9.3.10   Photo-acoustic imaging

The hybrid medical imaging technique based upon the effect of photo-acoustic is known as photo-acoustic imaging. There are two kinds of photo-acoustic imaging methods: the initial one is photo-acoustic tomography or thermo-acoustic CT that utilizes an unfocused ultrasound detector for acquiring the signals of photo-acoustic and second is known as photo-acoustic microscopy (PAM) in which photo-acoustic microscopy (PAM) along with two-dimensional point-by-point scanning is utilized.

9.3.11   Thermography

The emitted, reflected, and transmitted infrared energy by an object is known as thermograms or thermal images. Thermography is utilized by firefighters to view through the smoke by maintenance technicians to place over the heating joints concerning building technicians to observe thermal signatures, which signify the leaks of heat.

9.3.12   Tomography

In the tomography method, the tomographic optical scheme utilized for obtaining virtual slices of a particular cross-section of an object is viewed without cutting it practically. In advanced tomography, a projectional data from numerous directions are collected and subjected to an approach known as tomography reconstruction software, which is thereafter processed by computer.

Nowadays, the decision system for IoT medical images is very hard for physicians owing to a shortage of quantitative equipment. Generally, such a decision system permits the doctors to see the opinions and conflicting choices, thus assisting them to decrease the indecision related to diagnosis. It also lowers the diagnostic mistakes and enhances the caring quality. The health reports from patient's medical reports, which include images, charts, text, and so on, are correlated for the purpose of decision system. The decision system also analyzes various modalities to detect the reports of the same patient.

9.4 Decision support system for IoT-assisted medical images

A decision support system (DSS) is an informative system that is generated by employing the models, information, images, and gathered knowledge for assisting the doctors in resolving the detected as well as replicated issues. DSS are methods developed by approaches and equipment for supporting high-grade decisions. Among the major significant benefits of DSS, it is referred to rapid and effortless access the information, fast computation, simple to utilize, further interaction with health center, capability to provide complicated reports and store many information. It tries to provide speed and enhance the process among the persons who make decisions. For devising DSS, it is essential to be alert about the categorization of DSS and hence interactions for development methods are enhanced to aware and assist the decisions. DSS indicates the foremost move in medical healthcare as it encourages targeted decisions of medical, data of patients, and medical-related information. DSS is mentioned as a program devised for analyzing e-health data to directly help in making decision. It is observed to be a fast development from the initial day of its utilization.

DSS development increased highly as it is significantly utilized for medical care and expansively managed by means of e-medical reports. The major intention of DSS is to offer data to doctors, patients as well as others for making decision about healthcare at a specific time. It also decreases the cost, enhances the effectiveness, and decreases the difficulties for patients. IoT assisted to implement DSS as it gives the necessary information rapidly and cheaply as well as its capability to meet the necessities of a decision-making method in satisfactory, secure, and effectual manner. Even though the DSS is very complicated software method, it is functioning in the structure of e-health as well as the phases usually follow in its devise and development can be commonly busted down. The most vital process in DSS development is gathering information concerning the classes of diagnosis and categorizing of given criteria for diagnosing.

In the diagnosis process and treatment of disease, the doctor utilizes the networking abilities provided by DSS to recover data from the distributed e-health reports and consults other medical experts who are located at various locations. Though the doctor introduces suitable approaches for particular health conditions, there are a few issues concerning crucial functions that require DSS. The DSS is a typical portion of present healthcare that assesses data and supports providers of healthcare in taking clinical decisions [24]. IoT-based support system serves as a platform for internal and external interactions in healthcare and acts as a helpful tool for patients as well as medical employees. Ontology is utilized in DSS for supporting the medical specialists to provide proficient medicines. The DSS provides the functionalities to system that are elucidated as follows.

(a) Historical data

The IoT-based method maintains a collection of historical data regarding a patient's healthcare before beginning a new diagnosis. It compresses the diagnosis and reduces the difficulty in pointing out various problems. The initial phase of decision aid begins with medical employees and then the data related to health is stored in a similar platform for accessing everywhere. A crucial portion of this data frequently occurs to be routine data, which is also important too. The efficiency of IoT-based DSS is that the patient requires to not completely keep track of all previous medical history. Instead, all historical data is stored in an informative database for universal access.

(b) Predictive analytics

One of the major significant characteristics of DSS is that it gives the deepest grade of insights into health-based data of patients. The aim of predictive analytics is to execute statistical assessment and recognition of the pattern on the current pool of data for predicting a similar prospective trend. Additionally, the predictive analytics helps in earlier detection of diseases.

9.4.1 General block diagram of DSS

The general block diagram comprises patient medical sensors, IoT, server, and decision support healthcare system, which are expounded in below subsections [25]. Figure 9.8 reveals the general diagram of DSS.

(a) Patient medical sensors

An initial element is patient medical sensor equipment for measuring and sending the medical data. These medical sensors are arranged in the body of patients and are utilized for monitoring the physiological state of patients very intimately. It senses the important body signs of patients and transmits the sensed data in an appropriate way to other locations without the interference of humans. A physician can utilize these readings from medical sensors and gain an expanded analysis of a patient's physical condition. The significant signs of patients are temperature, blood pressure, movement, pulse rate, and so on.

(b) IoT

IoT augments as a potent area where the embedded sensors and devices can connect as well as swap information over Internet. It has a prolonged impact on the monitoring of health, management, and medical services to patients about physiological conditions. Patients connected with the sensors and data are linked with controlling devices, which are then forwarded to health monitoring units. Each sensor is signified as a collection unit, which collects the data of patients, aggregates it, executes fundamental processing, and then transmits it to the server for further processing.

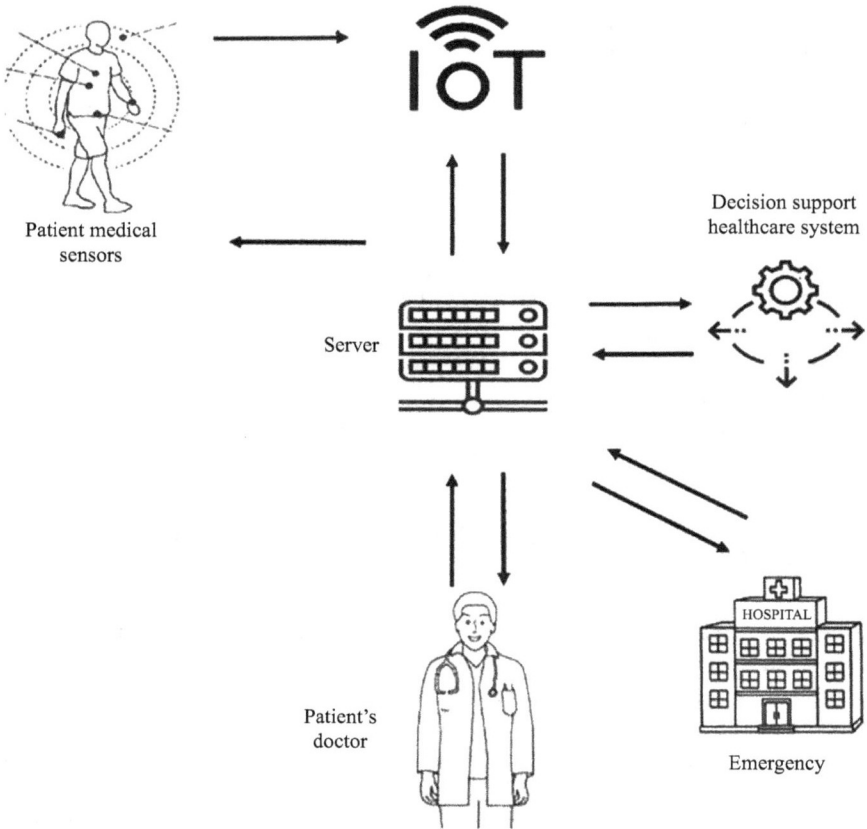

Figure 9.8   General diagram of DSS

(c) Server

The server stores all the medical information of patients stated by a user and also receives the flow of sensor data from sensors. It executes the fundamental data assessment and aggregation by developing obvious signals thus making data accessible to the person subscribed. Additionally, the server is able to receive a requisition for particular data from an end-user.

(d) Decision support healthcare system

The server of DSS has an approach for learning to assist medical experts for best decision-making systems. This decision support healthcare system delivers the data from the server and sends the decision to the physician, clinics, or hospital.

9.4.2   Advantages of DSS

- DSS has an ability to quickly examine the input data for validating the mode of decision and requires minimum time to attain the decision.

- In the medicinal field, DSS is utilized as clinical DSS that is employed for managing the complicated clinical data as the medicinal data has a broad level of flexible information.
- It decreases the repetition, duplication tests, and purchase of drugs, when these decision systems are utilized as cost-control system.
- DSS enhances the reliability of decision and provides solution for larger scale as well as complicated problems.
- It has a capability for processing the knowledge as well as information and proves the generation for supporting the decision.
- All the medical data will be secured for making decision about the health conditions of patient.
- The treatment process utilizing DSS is faster and provides effectual information in accordance with their diseases.
- DSS for IoT medical images assures a significant part in supporting to have good health conditions and secure commonly.

9.5   General architecture of the IoT-assisted DSS for medical images

In the field of healthcare, taking valuable and proficient differential medical diagnoses is highly crucial, as a single decision-making impacts the treatment plan and the prognosis of the disease. The process of decision-making in the healthcare field involves a widespread exploration of medical knowledge and complex mental workout. Further, the asymptotic or varied symptoms of the disease from one patient to another and the scale of infections complicate the process of decision-making. A major process in enhancing the efficiency of hospitals is to optimize the diagnosis considering the time period and count of the patients examined. Moreover, the process has to be carried out with high specificity, sensitivity, and accuracy for improving the doctor–patient relationship and also for minimizing the control costs, death rate, and morbidity. The process of diagnosis is highly complicated owing to several ambiguities. The patients may not be able to convey accurately how they feel or what happened, and the doctors may not comprehend the information observed or conveyed accurately. Further, obtaining medical reports may be time-consuming and may be erroneous; and the doctors may not characterize how exactly a disease changes the functionality of the human body. This challenge is compounded by the decreased ratio of medical practitioners in comparison to the patient influx. All these factors have fueled the development of accurate diagnostic systems, which are capable of detecting health issues accurately and in a timely manner, as the progression and mortality of any disease depend on its early detection and the treatment plan [26].

The availability of Internet access ubiquitously has paved the way for researchers in gathering advanced methods and datasets online for the development of enhanced healthcare systems. Recent development in IoT has garnered attention from industry and academics, especially in the field of healthcare. With the emerging trend of e-health systems comprising personalized systems for monitoring patient's health and electronic recording devices, conventional approaches to healthcare services have been reinstated by IoT-based systems which are capable of providing high-quality services. The rapid increase of wearable devices and smartphones has led to the evolution of traditional systems to customizable healthcare systems. The utilization of IoT in the field of medicine is known as medical IoT (mIoT), which provides the user with various benefits of recording the patient's data, its assessment, and using the accumulated data in diagnosing the condition of the patient. The innovations in mIoT have reshaped the healthcare field by providing various solutions based on advanced IoT-based systems. The traditional healthcare systems require physicians to perform various functions, such as monitoring and diagnosis, and these are replaced by the computation algorithms and techniques in the IoT-based healthcare system. The accuracy of the diagnosis systems can be improved by the application of DL networks. Further, the usage of DSS in the healthcare sector can effectively improve the quality of healthcare provided by constantly monitoring the patient's health and providing effective decisions based on the patients' detail, clinical knowledge, and other relevant health details [27].

The general architecture of the IoT-based DSS in the medical field is depicted in Figure 9.9. The basic architecture comprises various modules, such as the data collection module, sensor network, interface, decision layer, and advising module. These modules are briefed below.

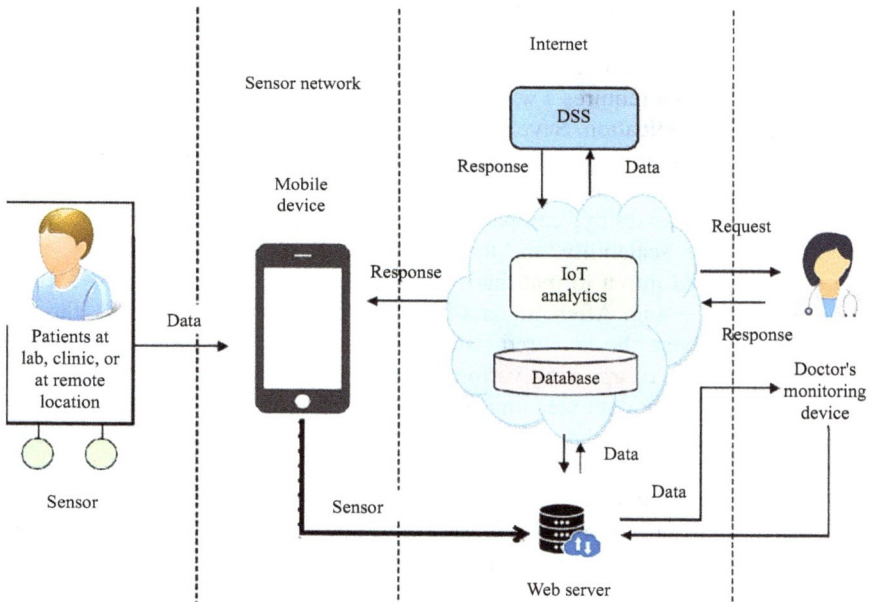

Figure 9.9   General architecture of the IoT-assisted DSS for medical purposes

9.5.1   Data collection module

The working of any automatic healthcare system requires the collection of input, which can be obtained from various sources [28]. Data collection in automated systems requires two kinds of inputs, such as the live images from the person for assessing the severity of the issues, and the inputs needed for creating decision rules. The decision rules are made by considering the already available data regarding the particular scenario, which are present in the case history of patients, surveys, opinions of medical experts, research publications, and so on. The images concerning the patient's condition are captured in a real-time environment by using various approaches, like MRI, X-ray, CT scans, ultrasound, mammogram, fluoroscopy, positron emission tomography (PET) scan, optical coherence tomography (OCT), single-photon emission CT (SPECT), confocal scanning laser ophthalmoscopy (CSLO), scanning laser polarimetry (SLP), etc.

9.5.2   Sensor network

Sensor network [29] comprises multiple sensors connected over the wireless network, which gathers the information collected from the various nodes or the sensors in the clinics/labs and transmits the data to the concerned persons over the Internet or to the servers for storage. The data collected by the sensors are transmitted over to the network by means of mobile devices. The sensor network may be USB-based connection, Wi-Fi application, or Bluetooth. The sensor network enables interaction between various nodes directly or through intermediate nodes. Among the numerous nodes, one, or more node acts as a sink(s) node, which is accountable for transmitting information directly to the user or over the available wired network.

Data transmission can happen by means of a single or multiple hops, wherein the multihop network requires a wireless medium, like optical, radio, or infrared for establishing communication. Several factors have to be considered while designing a sensor network, such as power consumption, overhead, data latency, Quality of Service (QoS), transmission media, hardware constraints, sensor network topology, data aggregation, flexibility, compatibility, security, operating environment, production costs, size, scalability, and fault tolerance. Before transmitting the data, it has to be converted into a format that is usable, and this is accomplished with the help of data processing. After the data is gathered from various sources, the next process is to convert the acquired data into a usable format. The input data is converted by means of applying various data mining tools based on the scenario. Various tools, such as data cleaning, data transformation, and data reduction, are employed for processing the data. Real-time monitoring of patients requires the collection of images using different sensors in the IoT-based circuits. During the real-time collection of data, the sensors may miss certain values; data may be inconsistent, and outliers may be present. Further, the images are captured in a noisy environment, thereby affecting the effectiveness of the diagnostic approaches. In real-time scenarios, a large amount of data is recorded by the sensors in a short time, which has to be reduced for minimizing the load.

Many techniques, such as tuples reduction and attribute values reduction, are employed for minimizing the data size. Moreover, the data gathered is normally of varying ranges, which requires conversion into a single range for enabling the system to deal with the data effectively. Thus, data transformation approaches, like discretization, generalization, aggregation, and normalization are required for converting the data into a single range.

9.5.3   Interface and decision layer

The data from the sensor network is forwarded to the interface and the decision layer, for enabling transmission of the data to the concerned health authorities for proper advice or for storage in the web servers. This module comprises the DSS, which provides effective decisions based on the input image received from the patient and the related data available. The ever-increasing amount of data generated can be effectively handled by the utilization of the cloud.

9.5.3.1   IoT interface

IoT enables the connection of various sensors present in the clinic/labs to remote locations for the purpose of data collection. The huge amount of data collected by the devices can be analyzed by using algorithms based on AI, and thus enabling the hospitals to analyze the data by connecting to a central unit. Further, it can be used as the medium of communication between the clinic and healthcare personnel present at any remote location. IoT also provisions users with easy viewing of real-time physiological images using mobile applications or web browsers irrespective of the time and place. Further, it enables medical professionals with the potential to perform effective monitoring of patients by increasing the interactions, thus effectively minimizing the duration of hospital stay and healthcare costs.

9.5.3.2   Web server

The medical records of any patient can be stored using three options, such as storing it physically, on a local server or on a remote server. The physical storage of medical records is ineffective and very hard to manage. Storage of the medical records in the local server implies that they are stored in the machine which generates the data, and this process requires dedicated hardware resources and hence is not economical. The remote server, on the other hand, signifies the utilization of dedicated servers at distant locations for storing the data. This method of storage can effectively function as a means of assessing the medical records anywhere, anytime. Further, they can be upgraded easily based on the requirements, and can effectively minimize the cost and time of maintenance. The medical data generated in real-time scenarios is bulky, which requires high storage space and this is addressed by the utilization of web servers.

9.5.3.3   DSS

DSS [10] has successfully enhanced the productivity of the healthcare systems by targeting enhanced quality and mitigating the risks associated. This has also led to a decrease in healthcare costs by enabling the medical practitioners in making optimal decisions. In the field of healthcare, there has been an evolution in the concept of DSS with an advent of technologies, like AI, ML, cloud computing, and dig data. This evolution has improved the intelligence of DSS, thus helping in decision-making by retrieving the most significant data. Decision-making is the process of choosing the optimal alternative among the several options available.

DSS helps in making targeted decisions by considering the patients' medical records available in the electronic format and the related information available. DSS refers to the program that is developed with the purpose of analyzing the medical data and the knowledge database, and then aiding in taking effective decisions. DSS utilizes algorithms based on AI and machine or DL for providing data to the medical practitioners, patients, and others in taking crucial decision regarding the treatment plan.

9.5.4   Advising module

The advising module comprises the medical practitioners, who may be present at remote locations. Whenever the system collects the data from the patient, it is forwarded to the DSS for analyzing the input data and producing treatment recommendations based on the analysis. The system generates a request which is forwarded to the healthcare providers. Upon receiving the request, the doctors/medical practitioners access the medical records of the patient from the web server and the treatments recommended by the DSS. After analyzing these details carefully, the healthcare providers respond to the request by suggesting the course of the treatment plan, which is then conveyed to those at the clinic, based on which the patient is treated.

9.6   Applications

The progress in IoT and AI has enabled the medical practitioners in enhancing the quality of life of patients by making effective decisions regarding the treatment planning in a short duration with high accuracy. The AI- and IoT-based systems have been effectively employed in healthcare for enhancing the accuracy of detection and for managing the innate complexity of the medical systems. In medical imaging, AI and IoT have been efficiently applied in the detection of several diseases, such as pulmonary cancer, and classification of chest X-rays, drug discovery, and wound monitoring and as such. The various applications of IoT and AI in the field of medical imaging are elaborated below.

9.6.1   Disease detection and prediction

The healthcare system mainly comes into the picture when an individual suffers from illness and requires efforts in restoring his/her physical state. Hence, disease detection plays a significant part in improving the well-being of any person. Disease detection should be performed accurately as it impacts the treatment plan and thus the prognosis of the disease. IoT and AI offer enhanced effectiveness in identifying various diseases and a few of these diseases are detailed here with an emphasis on medical imaging.

9.6.2   Pulmonary cancer

Pulmonary or lung cancer [30] is one of the most dangerous cancers with a high mortality of 70% and accounts for the death of one-fourth of overall cancer-affected persons. In the majority of cases, lung cancer is detected at a large stage resulting in an increased death rate. Early detection is highly challenging as the lesion grows inside the lung as a nodule. Pulmonary cancer is normally detected from CT images of the lungs. With the utilization of IoT, the sensors can transmit the data collected over the Internet, and using the AI systems, lung cancer can be accurately detected and classified by considering the CT images, sensor recordings, and the dataset available online, thus augmenting the identification accuracy.

9.6.3   Brain tumor classification

Similar to pulmonary cancer, brain tumor [31] is also a cause for serious concern in the current scenario. Brain tumors are identified by analyzing the MRI images of the brain. The brain tumor refers to the group of anomalous cells that poses the likelihood of turning fatal owing to its capability to attack adjacent cells and form metastases. IoT can be used in the process of brain tumor identification for gathering the brain tumor images from various IoT devices and transmitting and accepting them along the brain tumor-related information over the Internet. Further, the accuracy of identification can be enhanced by employing AI schemes in the detection process. DL approaches have been found to produce high detection accuracies and can effectively extract the relevant features.

9.6.4   Diabetic retinopathy (DR) detection

DR [32] is one of the major aftereffects of diabetes leading to blindness caused by the injury to the blood vessels in the light-sensitive cells of the retina. Taking into account the number of diabetic individuals globally, DR is highly significant. AI requires advanced algorithms for analyzing the huge clinical data available and it facilitates early diagnosis. Though DR is evaluated primarily by direct or indirect ophthalmoscopy, the application of AI in the eye care sector is based on fundus images of the patients. The fundus images offer crucial data in diagnosing various other eye diseases, like vascular abnormalities, age-related macular degeneration, and glaucoma. AI-based approaches have provided efficient results in ocular disease screening, with low cost and promising results.

9.6.5   Diabetic macular edema (DME)

Another ocular disease that can be easily identified by AI-assisted IoT-based systems is DME. DME is caused by the building up of extra fluid in the space outside the cells in the macular area of the retina. The DME can be identified by evaluating optical coherence tomography (OCT) images. With the fast progress of the graphics processing unit (GPU), AI utilizes DL for discriminating numerous images at a fast rate.

Though AI usually requires high-end GPU and expensive systems to do certain tasks, the usage of smartphones with minimum memory has effectively overcome the need for such sophisticated systems. Screening platforms, such as MobileNet [33], have been developed for analyzing the OCT images, and these platforms can be installed on mobiles and can be integrated into any healthcare system over the Internet.

9.6.6   Cardiovascular diseases (CVD)

AI-assisted IoT-based systems have also been devised for the detection of CVD, such as cardiomyopathy, rheumatic heart disease (RHD), coronary heart disease (CHD), strokes, and various heart ailments. CVDs have a major effect on the well-being of any individual, particularly elder people, and a majority of these diseases are chronic requiring continued treatment throughout their lifetime. Thus, pre-diagnosis of CVD can effectively enhance the quality of life of patients, and reduce the risks to life.

With the integration of AI and IoT, the conventional monitoring systems can be easily replaced and the patients' condition can be easily monitored. In medical imaging, CVD can be identified by analyzing cardiovascular magnetic resonance (CMR) and cardiac CT [34]. AI-assisted CMR has accelerated the process of image capturing and processing. The DL networks can easily reconstruct the data in low-resolution and under-sampled images.

9.6.7   Wound monitoring

Another major application of the IoT in healthcare is the monitoring of wounds. The individuals with surgical and nonsurgical wounds would need constant checking of the wounds to ensure timely healing. Various parameters, such as wound size, color, appearance, and environment, have to be verified during wound monitoring. Any minor wound can transform into a chronic one depending on various aspects, such as biological anomalies, autoimmune diseases, mechanical strain, aging, and diabetes mellitus, owing to impaired healing. Further, if the wound has been left uncovered for a long time, it will be prone to infections caused by various pathogens. Thus, the wound has to be constantly monitored to ensure that it is healed properly. The application of IoT and DSS can effectively reduce the number of hospital visits for monitoring the wound [35]. Though there are a variety of techniques that can be applied to do this task, the ones based on smartphones can be employed with ease and at a low cost. IoT can ensure remote monitoring of wounds with enhanced accuracy and provide a means of communication between the patient and medical practitioners, thus improving the convenience and pro-ductivity of the treatment.

9.6.8   Drug discovery

AI can be effectively employed in the process of discovering drugs [36], AI-enabled systems can easily detect the underlying chemical structure of the drugs. Drugs can be discovered by using the high-throughput (cell) imaging (HTI) of cells. HTI enables to capture the morphology of cells using a high-throughput micro-scope to understand the protein activity of the cell when exposed to drugs during testing. Prediction of biological activity is performed by analyzing the morphological character patterns present in the image.

9.6.9 X-ray classification

Chest X-ray [37] helps in diagnosing various diseases in the thorax region. Traditionally, X-rays are examined by the radiologist for identifying the diseases in the lungs and chest cavity, which is time-consuming. The automatic systems utilize AI for detecting diseases in a short duration with high accuracy. IoT provides a way for connecting X-ray machines in various clinics with the intent of gathering data. The amount of data collected by the IoT systems is overwhelming and requires AI approaches for evaluating them. Support vector machines (SVM) and DL models, such as Residual Network (ResNet)-18 and AlexNet, have been effectively employed in the classification of X-rays.

9.6.10 Bedsore assessment

Bedsore [38] is caused by the continuous pressure on the skin of individuals who are paraplegics, or bedridden. Any immobile person is prone to have bedsores due to the constant pressure caused by the person's weight. The presence of bedsores adversely affects the quality of life of the person and results in a greater risk of infection and expense. This also impacts the quality of healthcare provided by the clinics; further, the organizations are required to increase their workforce to deal with this issue. Thus, effective techniques are required to constantly monitor the bedsores by measuring, classifying, and tracing its origin, for enabling the creation of an efficient treatment plan. AI systems can help in creating DSS for assessing the nature of bedsores. These systems help the medical practitioners in classifying the sores and hence boosting the decision-making ability of the healthcare providers.

9.6.11 Spinal injuries

AI and IoT can be applied in the field of spine [39] for predicting the outcomes of surgeries or viability of individuals with spinal metastasis. AI can be utilized for segmenting the spinal structures, measuring different parameters of the spinal curve, classifying the disintegration of the disc, and identifying tumors or injuries in the spine.

9.6.12 Laparoscopic surgery

IoT can be utilized for implementing intraoperative events using IoT-enabled surgical devices. IoT along with AI can be employed for monitoring the control of various surgical equipment's during surgeries [40]. Further, they are used for managing surgical devices, like steel tools. During surgery, the visualization of the process is provided by using a rigid laparoscopic system for accumulating the data regarding the conduct of various surgical tools.

9.6.13 Other applications

The usage of IoT and AI can enhance the efficiency of various applications, like diagnosis of abdominal issues, pregnancy checkup, fracture detection, detection of liver abnormalities, for rehabilitation of paralyzed patients, chest radiology, and so on. The availability of sensors and the advent of Internet has revolutionized the healthcare system. In medical imaging, IoT enables the easy transfer of images, captured by various modalities, such as digital pathology, ultrasound, CT scan, MRI, and fundus photography, can be transmitted to the medical practitioners at remote locations, thereby enabling the provision of expert recommendations.

Echocardiogram and Doppler imaging of the heart can be used to create a visualization of the blood flow and various chambers in the heart. Various diseases, like metastatic bronchogenic carcinoma, Alzheimer's, glioma, and colon cancer, can be successively predicted by using the AI approaches with high accuracy. In pregnancy, the images can provide crucial information about the wellbeing of the unborn child and help in alleviating the complications of glioma, Alzheimer's, and metastatic bronchogenic carcinoma. Further, AI and IoT can provide individuals, especially the disabled to ascertain their surroundings by analyzing the non-diagnosing images of the environment, thus they can be used for creating the brain computer interface (BCI).

9.7   Conclusion

IoT and AI have revolutionized the field of healthcare systems by transforming the conventional medical system into a smart system. The recent advancements in AI and IoT have improvised the quality of life of individuals by promulgating a healthy lifestyle. AI-embedded systems, such as fitness trackers and smartwatches have sensors with the ability to screen, gather and detect illness based upon the symptoms. Further, the AI systems have been effectively able to monitor the health of a patient by using robotic nurses in the absence of healthcare providers.

Further, IoT has enabled smart healthcare systems competent to handle issues in a real-time scenario. In this chapter, the various researches carried out in the field of AI with IoT-based medical imaging is detailed. It also exemplifies different AI-based approaches devised for carting out IoT-based medical imaging. It also presents the concept of IoT and application of IoT in the field of healthcare is described. In recent years, DSS is utilized for enhancing the productivity of healthcare. Here, an elaborated study on the DSS in medical imaging is carried out along with a description of the general architecture of the IoT-assisted DSS for medical imaging. Moreover, the applications and issues encountered by IoT-based medical imaging are incorporated. It also highlights the efforts undertaken by numerous researchers in developed AI methods for performing IoT-based medical imaging. Furthermore, the various modalities utilized for capturing the images are also detailed elaborately.

References

[1]   Joyia, G.J., Liaqat, R.M., Farooq, A., and Rehman, S., 2017. Internet of medical things (IoMT): applications, benefits and future challenges in healthcare domain. *J. Commun.*, 12(4), pp. 240–247.

[2] Thandapani, S., Mahaboob, M.I., Iwendi, C., *et al.*, 2023. IoMT with deep CNN: AI-based intelligent support system for pandemic diseases. *Electronics*, 12(2), p. 424.

[3] Rathour, N., Alshamrani, S.S., Singh, R., *et al.*, 2021. IoMT based facial emotion recognition system using deep convolution neural networks. *Electronics*, 10(11), p. 1289.

[4] Oniani, S., Marques, G., Barnovi, S., Pires, I.M., and Bhoi, A.K., 2021. Artificial intelligence for Internet of Things and enhanced medical systems. In: *Bio-inspired Neurocomputing*, Springer, New York, NY, pp. 43–59.

[5] Singh, K.U., Abu-Hamatta, H.S., Kumar, A., Singhal, A., Rashid, M. and Bashir, A.K., 2021. Secure watermarking scheme for color DICOM images in telemedicine applications. *Computers, Materials and Continua*, 70(2), pp. 2525–2542.

[6] Geethanath, S. and Vaughan Jr, J.T., 2019. Accessible magnetic resonance imaging: a review. *Journal of Magnetic Resonance Imaging*, 49(7), pp. e65–e77.

[7] Withers, P.J., Bouman, C., Carmignato, S., *et al.*, 2021. X-ray computed tomography. *Nature Reviews Methods Primers*, 1(1), p. 18.

[8] Saxena, P., Goyal, A., Bivi, M.A., Singh, S.K., and Rashid, M., 2023. Segmentation of nucleus and cytoplasm from H&E-stained follicular lymphoma. *Electronics*, 12(3), p. 651.

[9] Hesamian, M.H., Jia, W., He, X., and Kennedy, P., 2019. Deep learning techniques for medical image segmentation: achievements and challenges. *Journal of Digital Imaging*, 32, pp. 582–596.

[10] Zhang, J., Xie, Y., Wu, Q., and Xia, Y., 2019. Medical image classification using synergic deep learning. *Medical Image Analysis*, 54, pp. 10–19.

[11] Ahmed, I., Jeon, G., and Piccialli, F., 2022. From artificial intelligence to explainable artificial intelligence in industry 4.0: a survey on what, how, and where. *IEEE Transactions on Industrial Informatics*, 18(8), pp. 5031–5042.

[12] Secinaro, S., Calandra, D., Secinaro, A., Muthurangu, V., and Biancone, P., 2021. The role of artificial intelligence in healthcare: a structured literature review. *BMC Medical Informatics and Decision Making*, 21, pp.1–23.

[13] Rashid, M., Singh, H., and Goyal, V., 2020. The use of machine learning and deep learning algorithms in functional magnetic resonance imaging—a systematic review. *Expert Systems*, 37(6), p. e12644.

[14] Rajpurkar, P., Chen, E., Banerjee, O., and Topol, E.J., 2022. AI in health and medicine. *Nature Medicine*, 28(1), pp. 31–38.

[15] Lv, W., Meng, F., Zhang, C., Lv, Y., Cao, N., and Jiang, J., 2017. A general architecture of IoT system. In: *2017 IEEE International Conference on Computational Science and Engineering (CSE) and IEEE International Conference on Embedded and Ubiquitous Computing (EUC)* (vol. 1, pp. 659–664). IEEE.

[16] Tresanchez, M., Pujol, A., Pallejà, T., Martínez, D., Clotet, E., and Palacín, J., 2018. A proposal of low-cost and low-power embedded wireless image sensor node for IoT applications. *Procedia Computer Science*, 134, pp. 99–106.

[17] Chandy, A., 2019. A review on IoT based medical imaging technology for healthcare applications. *Journal of Innovative Image Processing (JIIP)*, 1 (01), pp. 51–60.

[18] Kumar, A., Rawat, J., Kumar, I., *et al.*, 2022. Computer-aided deep learning model for identification of lymphoblast cell using microscopic leukocyte images. *Expert Systems*, 39(4), p. e12894.

[19] Jan, A., Parah, S.A., Malik, B.A., and Rashid, M., 2021. Secure data transmission in IoTs based on CLoG edge detection. *Future Generation Computer Systems*, 121, pp. 59–73.

[20] Reshma, V.K., Khan, I.R., Niranjanamurthy, M., *et al.*, 2022. Hybrid block-based lightweight machine learning-based predictive models for quality preserving in the Internet of Things-(IoT-) based medical images with diagnostic applications. *Computational Intelligence and Neuroscience*, 2022. https://doi.org/10.1155/2022/8173372

[21] Aslam, B., Javed, A.R., Chakraborty, C., Nebhen, J., Raqib, S., and Rizwan, M., 2021. Blockchain and ANFIS empowered IoMT application for privacy preserved contact tracing in COVID-19 pandemic. *Personal and Ubiquitous Computing*, 4, pp. 1–17.

[22] Elangovan, A., and Jeyaseelan, T., 2016. Medical imaging modalities: a survey. In: *2016 International Conference on Emerging Trends in Engineering, Technology and Science (ICETETS)* (pp. 1–4). IEEE.

[23] Rashid, M., Singh, H., and Goyal, V., 2021. Efficient feature selection technique based on fast Fourier transform with PSO-GA for functional magnetic resonance imaging. In: *2021 2nd International Conference on Computation, Automation and Knowledge Management (ICCAKM)* (pp. 238–242). IEEE.

[24] Chatterjee, P., Cymberknop, L.J., and Armentano, R.L., 2017. IoT-based decision support system for intelligent healthcare—applied to cardiovascular diseases. In: *2017 7th International Conference on Communication Systems and Network Technologies (CSNT)* (pp. 362–366). IEEE.

[25] Fahmy, K.A., Yahya, A., and Zorkany, M., 2022. A decision support healthcare system based on IoT and neural network technique. *Journal of Engineering, Design and Technology*, 20(3), pp. 727–748.

[26] Lin, X., Wu, J., Bashir, A.K., Yang, W., Singh, A., and AlZubi, A.A., 2022. FairHealth: long-term proportional fairness-driven 5G edge healthcare in Internet of medical things. *IEEE Transactions on Industrial Informatics*, 18 (12), pp. 8905–8915.

[27] Chang, L., Wu, J., Moustafa, N., Bashir, A.K., and Yu, K., 2021. AI-driven synthetic biology for non-small cell lung cancer drug effectiveness-cost analysis in intelligent assisted medical systems. *IEEE Journal of Biomedical and Health Informatics*, 26(10), pp. 5055–5066.

[28] Alharbe, N., and Atkins, A., 2014. A study of the application of automatic healthcare tracking and monitoring system in Saudi Arabia. *International Journal of Pervasive Computing and Communications*, 10(2), pp. 183–195.

[29] Li, J., Wu, J., Li, C., *et al.*, 2021. Information-centric wireless sensor networking scheme with water-depth-awareness content caching for underwater IoT. *IEEE Internet of Things Journal*, 9(2), pp. 858–867.

[30] Adcock, I.M., Caramori, G., and Barnes, P.J., 2011. Chronic obstructive pulmonary disease and lung cancer: new molecular insights. *Respiration*, 81 (4), pp. 265–284.

[31] Belhe, A.S., Pagariya, J.A., Ganthade, V.V., Rashid, M., and Uravane, P.S., 2022. An efficient deep learning based approach for the detection of brain tumors. In: *2022 5th International Conference on Contemporary Computing and Informatics (IC3I)* (pp. 417–421). IEEE.

[32] Madan, P., Singh, V., Chaudhari, V., *et al.*, 2022. An optimization-based diabetes prediction model using CNN and Bi-directional LSTM in real-time environment. *Applied Sciences*, 12(8), p. 3989.

[33] Markan, A., Agarwal, A., Arora, A., Bazgain, K., Rana, V., and Gupta, V., 2020. Novel imaging biomarkers in diabetic retinopathy and diabetic macular edema. *Therapeutic Advances in Ophthalmology*, 12, 2515841420950513.

[34] Kiran, P.S., Vangala, S.R., and Rashid, M., 2021. Efficient approach for measuring heart pulse from real time facial RGB color videos. In: *2021 2nd International Conference on Intelligent Engineering and Management (ICIEM)* (pp. 412–416). IEEE.

[35] Tang, N., Zhang, R., Zheng, Y., *et al.*, 2022. Highly efficient self-healing multifunctional dressing with antibacterial activity for sutureless wound closure and infected wound monitoring. *Advanced Materials*, 34(3), p. 2106842.

[36] Vamathevan, J., Clark, D., Czodrowski, P., *et al.*, 2019. Applications of machine learning in drug discovery and development. *Nature Reviews Drug Discovery*, 18(6), pp. 463–477.

[37] Mondal, S., Agarwal, K., and Rashid, M., 2019, November. Deep learning approach for automatic classification of x-ray images using convolutional neural network. In: *2019 Fifth International Conference on Image Information Processing (ICIIP)* (pp. 326–331). IEEE.

[38] Saghaleini, S.H., Dehghan, K., Shadvar, K., Mahmoodpoor, A., Sanaie, S., and Ostadi, Z., 2016. Bedsore: epidemiology; risk factors; classification; assessment scales and management. *Archives of Anesthesiology and Critical Care*, 2(3), pp. 226–230.

[39] Bertsimas, D., Masiakos, P.T., Mylonas, K.S., and Wiberg, H., 2019. Prediction of cervical spine injury in young pediatric patients: an optimal trees artificial intelligence approach. *Journal of Pediatric Surgery*, 54(11), pp. 2353–2357.

[40] Ushimaru, Y., Takahashi, T., Souma, Y., *et al.*, 2019. Innovation in surgery/ operating room driven by Internet of Things on medical devices. *Surgical Endoscopy*, 33, pp. 3469–3477.

Chapter 10

Internet of Things and medical imaging AI systems

Rajakumar Arul[1], Kalaipriyan Thirugnanasambandam[1] and M. Kiruthigga[2]

In recent years, the application of Artificial Intelligence (AI) in radiography has received a great attention. The technique's unique capacity presumably lies somewhere in the middle, and AI will play a vital part in the future of radiomics. Due to the computer's endless potential, AI is an attractive candidate for delivering the optimization, predictability, and dependability required to aid radiologists in their quest to provide exceptional patient care. With the computerization and resource optimization made possible by Internet of Things (IoT) systems in health application fields, the healthcare sector can increase treatment quality while reducing expenses.

Technologies including IoT, cloud computing, big data, and 5G mobile networks have arisen, and the use of AI systems in the medical business has become highly widespread. Furthermore, the deep integration of AI and IoT technology allows for the steady enhancement of medical diagnostic and treatment capacities, allowing for a more sustainable health sector. However, substantial barriers are presently preventing this field of medical imaging from enlarging. AI and IoT are now major entities; hence, AI integration with IoT is becoming mainstream. This chapter's overview outlines the important prospects for greater integration of these new technical AIoT into healthcare and radiology, as well as their boundaries, radiologic applications, and ongoing obstacles. It also includes a review of several AI, machine learning (ML) as well as deep learning (DL)-based strategies for diagnosing illnesses earlier in the medical field.

10.1 Introduction

Radiologists are dealing with a slew of technological advances that have the potential to provide a big influence on their field. Artificial Intelligence (AI) for automated

[1]Centre for Smart Grid Technologies/School of Computer Science Engineering, Vellore Institute of Technology, Chennai, India
[2]Research Division, Redfowl Infotech, Bengaluru, India

medical image processing is generating a lot of buzz in the healthcare industry, putting pressure on radiologists to reconsider the value and sustainability of their profession. From their perspective, radiologists appear to be hesitant to accept and exploit these new technology options [1]. But there will be a fundamental issue if they can be ready to abandon their old operating procedures in pursuit of a gradual shift to a digital environment based on AIoT technologies. Medical informatics, on the other hand, is required in radiology to improve information flow, image interpretation, clinical judgment, and connectivity with physicians and patients [2].

The multidisciplinary study of the design, development, integration, and use of information technology (IT)-based advances in healthcare service delivery, management, and planning is known as medical informatics. Medical image informatics, often known as radiology informatics, is a branch of information technology that strives to enhance the efficiency in interpreting the information that lies within medical images [3]. Medical informatics integrates two medical data sources behind doing field research. They are physiological records and radiological data with various morphologies. The differences in physiological records and imaging data necessitate different methodologies and techniques to investigate them. Biomedical records alternatively are made up of records from patient medical testing [4]. In general, imaging methods generate medical image information. Medical image information is made up of pixels that represent a physical item and is caused by imaging modalities. Exploration of medical image information approaches is difficult in view of determining their worth in terms of understanding, analysis, and illness diagnosis [5]. Furthermore, image classification is a significant difficulty in image analysis jobs and plays a vital part in computer-aided diagnosis. In image analysis applications, visual categorization is a major difficulty. The dilemma in the diagnostic imaging domain is learning how to extract images and categorize the extraction results into a similar pattern and then analyze and understand which sections of the human body are impacted based on the image classification results [6]. An accurate diagnosis of diseased areas in the human body is the major focus of medical image categorization. As a result of imaging methods, pixels that correspond to a component of a real object produce digital image data [7]. The problem concerned the medical informatics use of methodologies and strategies for leveraging computer vision techniques, ML, and classification models, as well as the validation of image prediction accuracy into medical expert knowledge [8]. For improved clinical treatment in the future, an automated diagnosis approach using image data will be required.

This chapter study focused only on a detailed review of drilling AI-enabled automatic image classification with the state of the art that addresses challenges and AI applications in radiology. The chapter's goal is to provide the reader with a comprehensive overview of AIoT in healthcare systems, including ML and DL strategies in radiology applications and healthcare benefits.

10.1.1   *What are the implications of amalgamating IoT with AI?*

It reinforces the view that IoT and AI are mutually beneficial. The IoT entails dealing with huge data that must be examined and used [9]. Consequently, IoT operations are made more efficient with the help of AI algorithms, which allow for the delivery of relevant answers to the problems faced by both developers and end users. So, what benefit does AI provide to the IoT?

Though IoT is an emerging concept that links billions of smart devices, it has flaws. Such requirements as to speed and accuracy of IoT data transfer, in an instance, have still to be addressed. Additionally, an AI system learns from the patterns it establishes while also mimicking human job performance. This technique for self-improvement is crucial to AI. Evolutionary algorithms are another subpart of AI where in the field of optimization such as mathematical benchmark functions [10], environmental [11], and in combinatorial optimization problems [12], it plays a vital role. The IoT can benefit more generally from AI. In an abstract sense, it is used as AI software that is included in IoT devices to supplement fog or peripheral computing solutions and provide IoT intelligence. As a result, smart gadgets create such a large volume of swiftly evaluated sensor data that automation can support the intelligence underlying IoT devices. Although it applies to amalgamating AI and IoT in the healthcare system, there is a good probability that they will boost efficiency and productivity. The important phases for the smart and effective deployment of AI techniques in IoT devices are predicting, constantly checking, supervision, refining, and automating (modeling, forecasting). They can minimize the administrative strain on healthcare practitioners by working together. With enhanced clinical protocols, radiographers will be free to focus on patients, and quality healthcare delivery will inevitably become more patient-centric.

10.1.2   IoMT becomes AI-IoMT

Though the healthcare system impacts everyone, mastering how to navigate it is crucial for everyone. However, remembering all of the specifics is a difficult process. Human mental and physical performance have limits. As a result, technologies like the IoT and AI must be limited to pushing beyond one's maximum [13]. Implementing new solutions in healthcare is always a good idea, and IoT and AI, regardless of the area in which the technologies are used, are powerful drivers of digital transformation. The entire digital ecosphere, an IoT ecosphere of smart devices, has been created and is steadily rising with each approaching day [14]. The city's connectivity encompasses various sectors, including industrial production, home automation, schooling, distribution networks, retail outlets, medical services, and bioinformatics. The entire digital ecosystem, an IoT sphere comprising internet-enabled devices, continues to grow stronger. IoT, powered by AI and ML, among other factors, is employed to provide intelligent assistance to individuals. It is gradually assuming control of both small and significant processes in a variety of businesses. Healthcare is not exceptional.

10.2   ML and deep learning in AI

AI is a branch of computer science concerned with the innovation and implementation of machine intelligence [15]. It is concerned with the use of computers to replicate human decision-making and carry out intelligent activities based on approaches, such as learning through experience, adapting to new input data, and executing humanoid tasks [16]. The instructional element of information processing is focused on ML, which is a subfield of AI. It involves creating computer programs that can monitor and improve without being distinctively programmed. This differs from typical computer algorithms, which contain explicit information that clarifies each step the process must take. Today, we virtually exclusively think of ML and its variants when we talk of AI [17]. Artificial neural networks (ANNs), which have been structures of elements termed artificial neurons structured into layers, continue to be used as an influence in ML approaches [18]. The ML technique necessitates the direct measurement of a collection of characteristics from the data like the size of breast lesions in computer tomography (CT) scans [19]. A deep neural network (DNN) is a type of ANN that has more layers (typically more than five) and can make better prognostications from data. DNNs have the benefit of constantly improving their performance as the amount of the trained dataset grows. So multiple factors have since come together to enable the rapid advancement of AI in medicine [20].

10.2.1   AI–IoMT radiology applications

With the emergence of magnetic resonance imaging (MRI), positron emission tomography (PET), ultrasound, and computed tomography (CT) scanning technologies, radiology has made remarkable progress. Additionally, the next breakthrough will come from AI exploiting visual information currently accessible from imaging modalities such as ultrasound, CT, MRI, and PET, rather than from new scanning technology [21]. The use of AI in medical imaging is expected to develop gradually, with the first stages already apparent. In this initial step, CT and MR pictures are scanned into AI systems, and then the systems do autonomous segmentation of the different structures within the images [22]. This will help researchers locate and categorize pathologic lesions, conserving radiologists' time. As a result, the following are the significant key AI-enabled IoT application cases in Figure 10.1.

Both radiology and histopathology are benefiting from AI's and notably ML's ability to analyze huge datasets and retrieve valuable insights. Images from MRI scanners, CT scans, and X-rays can include vast volumes of complicated information that is challenging and time-consuming to assess by humans. The integration of AI technologies into everyday clinical imaging is set to revolutionize

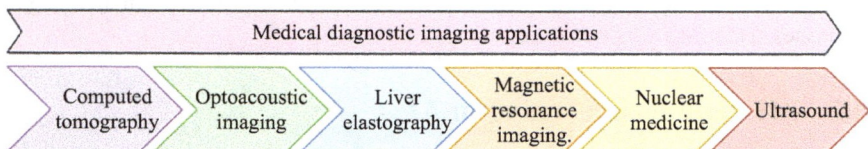

Figure 10.1   Medical diagnostic imaging systems

radiology [23]. Radiologists can benefit from AI's clinical decision assistance and improved patient care. AI algorithms may assist in the selection and extraction of features from medical imaging, along with the discovery of new specifications [24].

10.2.2 AIoT-enabled CT

Owing to the unavailability of overlapped tissues, CT scans focus on providing a more thorough view of the interior anatomy of the lung parenchyma than X-ray imaging. Although visual data image collection is simple and quick, interpretations can be difficult and time-consuming, particularly for unskilled or particularized medical personnel. So, the intelligence community has shifted its attention to the development of automated tomographic data analysis techniques [25]. Various AI techniques have been introduced in CT to screen disease projections and preparatory severity evaluation [26], which are illustrated in Figure 10.2.

When reconstructing a sequence of pictures from obtained projection data, the screening operator must give careful consideration to a number of parameters that will greatly impact the image's decisional and predictive qualities, including spatial resolution, the amount of overlap between successive frames, the thickness of anatomy represented in the image, the image noise level, and the magnification of the anatomy within the rebuilt image [27]. CNN-based deep learning to minimize image noise is an interesting application of AI in CT [28] (i.e. denoising). Missert *et al.* (2020) created a CT image denoising method that removes noise from source pictures to increase image quality and minimize radiation exposure. Developments in the area of deep learning suggest that multiple Deep CNN architectures would be used [29]. Individual CNN baseline models have been thoroughly tested models. VGG, Inception, ResNet, DenseNet, and DenseNet are among the baseline models [30]. In accordance with baseline models, the image reconstruction results can be converged and predictions on positive/negative can be diagnosed. Consequently, contemporary studies have concentrated on formulating suitable AI systems based on CT scans. From 3D CT scans, Li *et al.* established a 3D CNN for predicting COVID-19. Their model achieved a sensitivity (SN) of 90%, a specificity (SPC) of

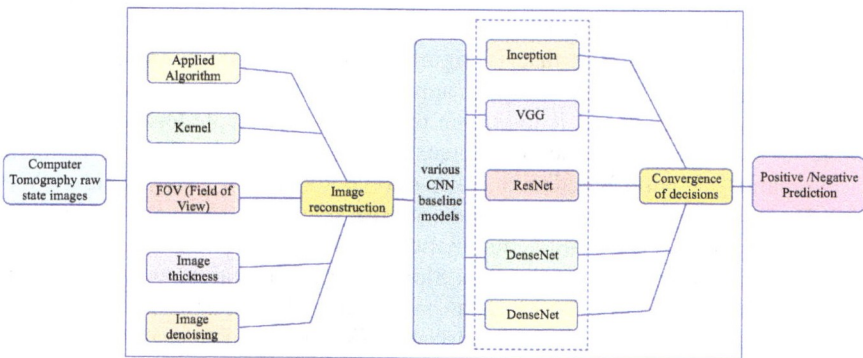

Figure 10.2   CNN-based diagnosing infection from CT images

96%, and appropriate use criteria (AUC) of 95% for the COVID-19 class. Each CT image data is represented by an identical ResNet50 model in their suggested model [31]. From Trivizakis *et al.* study, a comprehensive pipeline for automatic COVID-19 screening against different kinds of pneumonia (viral and bacterial) using CT images has been proposed, with lung segmentation used to improve accuracy. The advancement of a deep learning lung segmentation technique for multiple CT screen settings, and subsequently the modernization of a deep learning model to distinguish COVID-19 from CAP are some of the study's key innovations [32]. Additionally for lung diagnostics, a wearable belt-type electrical impedance tomography (EIT) system has been designed. A mobile software application on smart devices, such as tablet computers, and smartphones, can screen the visuals rebuilt by an EIT system. Under this research, researchers acquire visuals using a similar methodology to this reconstruction and then evaluate them using a CNN [33]. Singh and Ramandeep have proposed that lung cancer screening (LCS) with low-dose computed tomography (LDCT) contributes to the earlier lung cancer diagnosis, which typically manifests as microscopic hamartomas (lung nodules) [34]. The AI-based vessel suppression (AI-VS) and automated detection (AI-AD) algorithms can help in LDCT SSN (SubSolid Nodule) detection. They examined how AI-VS and AI-AD affected LDCT for LCS in terms of detecting and classifying SSN's ground-glass nodules (GGNs) and part-solid nodules (PSNs). AI approaches may be incorporated across every phase of a CT scan to improve screen resolution, enhance the workflows more efficiently for the operator and radiologist, minimize image noise, and also lower the radiation dosage delivered to the patient during data capture.

10.2.3 AI-enabled optoacoustic imaging

Optical imaging is extremely important in cancer research and diagnosis. Through a variety of genetic and environmental contrast sources, optical strategies are applied in the research center to uncover complicated physiological mechanisms driving cancer [35]. Opto endoscopes and laparoscopy, on the other hand, are commonly used for early diagnosis, clinical diagnosis in screening, and preventative procedures. Optoacoustic imaging incorporates optical technologies associated with ultrasonic imaging's sharpness [36]. Thereby, it can include more optical visibility of cancer that is significantly deeper in tissue than optical microscopy or other optical imaging approaches. To diagnose conditions with dermatological symptoms, it is important to identify the morphological features of skin lesions. Depending on the pixel intensity, it is frequently conducted manually or automatically. Ultra-broadband raster-scan optoacoustic mesoscopic (UWB-RSOM) was recently created to provide unique skin cross-sectional optical imaging. An ML technique enables automatic skin layer detection in UWB-RSOM data. The suggested technique is called SkinSeg in this research, and it is a multi-step methodology that includes data processing and transformations, feature selection, feature extraction, and categorization [37]. Image data characteristics and training models, including classic ML and more advanced deep learning algorithms, were reviewed for suitability in differentiating skin layers. To improve the

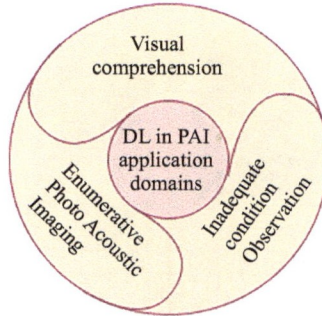

Figure 10.3   Framework of the DL in PAI application

classification results, a support vector machine-based postprocessing strategy was used. Changchun Yang has investigated that deep learning has notably been enabled throughout the photoacoustic imaging ecology chain, from picture reconstruction to illness detection. In his study, deep learning and photoacoustic imaging (PAI) are reviewed [38]. PA is also known as optoacoustic, which is a fusion imaging system that employs optical stimulation to create ultrasonic waves. Biological tissues undergo thermoelastic extension when exposed to pulsing laser light, resulting in the PA effect [39]. The creation of acoustic waves due to light absorption in a media is known as the photoacoustic effect. The framework of the DL in PAI application areas is represented in Figure 10.3, which also shows visual comprehension, inadequate condition absorption, and enumerative photoacoustic imaging.

Basic visual comprehension tasks include image categorization and segmentation. DL also contributed significantly to PA picture segmentation, which may be viewed as a unique reconstruction challenge. PAI is sure to capture flexibility and adaptability and opportunities as a result of DL's unrivaled capacity in information extraction, fusion, and high-speed processing. As a result, it is expected that unique PAI devices may be built to fulfill the demands of diverse applications when paired with DL.

10.2.4   AIoT operated liver elastography

Hepatitis B virus (HBV) infection in liver fibrosis stage-affected patients can lead to a serious health condition. So, it is vital to screen utilizing non-invasive ultrasonic liver stiffness measurement (LSM), which is suggested by numerous recommendations owing to its effectiveness and convenience in evaluating liver fibrosis. Hence with the deep learning radiomic algorithms may automatically learn features from image data that are incorporated in neural nets' hidden layers, eliminating the requirement for object segmentation and hard-coded feature extraction. Elastography is a non-invasive medical imaging technique used to examine the stiffness of organs and other internal parts [40]. The most typical application is to evaluate the liver. Low-frequency (LF) vibrations are sent into the liver without

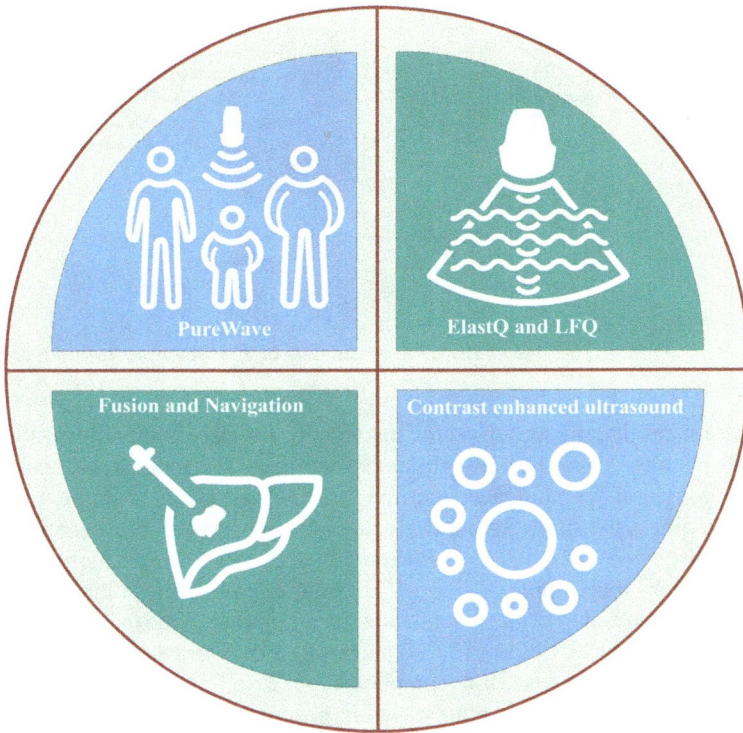

Figure 10.4   Liver elastography system

causing discomfort. In Figure 10.4, it is explained that the liver elastography system with steps followed in testing.

AI-assisted elastography has been examined in Pakanat Decharatanachart's work. Under his supervision, the diagnostic accuracy of the AI-assisted system was determined using a summary receiver operating characteristic (ROC) curve and the area under the curve (AUC) which enables the model to show predictions. Subgroup analyses were conducted based on diagnostic modalities, population, and AI classifiers. The proposed research evaluated AI-integrated non-invasive diagnostics for diagnosing and staging liver fibrosis and steatosis. Also, in this study, real-time elastography was used instead of transient elastography to diagnose liver cirrhosis, advanced fibrosis, and substantial fibrosis, with AUCs of 0.72, 0.86, and 0.69, respectively. For the diagnosis of all phases of liver fibrosis, AUCs were greater for AI-assisted elastography than real-time. AI-assisted elastography had a lower AUC for identifying liver cirrhosis but a higher AUC for diagnosing advanced fibrosis. Wang *et al.*'s work has reviewed the automated analysis of two dimensional-shear wave elastography (2D-SWE) photos under LSM methods, deep learning radiomics of elastography (DLRE) used the CNN method, which is one of the deep learning radiomic approaches. It can be employed with the three basic operations of CNN, which are convolution, activation, and pooling. The entire process methods separation is included with the forward computing and backpropagation [41]. Different liver elastography methods were discussed in the Li-Qiang Zhou study, which has been discussed above, along with ML system that quantifies color information from ultrasonic shear wave elastography (SWE) pictures and differentiates CLD from healthy instances. The SVM model correctly identified CLD patients 87.3% of the time with 93.5% sensitivity and 81.2% specificity, respectively. His study utilized SWE photos to provide objective CLD diagnostic measures. A two-stage multi-view AI learning system based on contrast-enhanced ultrasonography (CEUS) can discriminate benign from malignant liver tumors. Deep canonical correlation analysis (DCCA) was used on three picture pairings to create a total of six-view features. A multi-view features diagnosis result was then obtained using multiple kernel learning (MKL) classification techniques. For liver cancers, the DCCA-MKL framework based on hepatic CEUS has a high assessment and prediction performance [42].

10.2.5   AIoT in MRI

Internal anatomical structures may be analyzed with the use of a strong magnet and radio waves in an MRI scan. Medical professionals rely on MRI scans to diagnose anything from cancers to connective-tissue injuries. The spleen, heart, biliary tract system, kidneys, heart, colon, pancreas, and adrenals of the body are all evaluated using MRI. The bladder, as well as the reproductive system including the uterus and ovaries in females and the prostate gland in males, covering the pelvic organs, are also examined. The diagnosis of suspected lesions is still improving, with computer-extracted MRI characteristics increasingly being used to predict tumor subtypes and tumor recurrence [43]. Newer imaging tools, sophisticated treatment protocols, and multidisciplinary management strategies are all part of breast cancer care's evolution. AI has the potential to simplify and optimize radiologist diagnostic expertise, such as the recognition and stratification of intricate patterns in magnetic resonance images, associated with clinical malignant cells phenotype to genotype, and outcome prediction in relation to curative and predictive plans. Because of the extensive interactions between these numerous sectors, as well as the intrinsic tumor characteristics, radiogenomics is increasingly being used in all aspects of clinical decision-making [44]. The utilization of newer computer-aided diagnostic (CAD) systems that depend on early-phase kinetics resulting from high-temporal resolution MRI methods allows for the identification of worrisome lesions in a multimodality format [45]. The use of AI in breast imaging might lead to the development of imaging biomarkers that take into account both patient and tumor-specific features, allowing patients to be risk-stratified using individualized imaging criteria. To precisely estimate the detected radioactive tissue content, PET pictures must be adjusted for photon attenuation [46]. A gradient map for attenuation correction (AC) must be extracted from the MRI in a dual modalities PET and MRI scanner. This was not feasible at first, which limited the use of PET/MRI scanners in clinical and research settings, particularly for brain investigations. The contribution of this project was to develop a deep learning CNN for clinical MR-AC application, as well as to explore the influence of training group size and MRI input on computational accuracy and clinical interpretation of PET scans. The revival of AI, DNNs, and compressed sensing (CS) algorithms are being merged to redefine the state of the art of rapid MRI, according to a study by Yutong Chen *et al*. The systematic DL-based CS approaches for rapid MRI were reviewed in that meta-study [47]. Breakthroughs are emphasized and key model designs are explained. The deep learning in CS-based MRI acceleration has been assessed using a complete analytic methodology and a classification system. ANN learning in deep learning may be used to rebuild pictures under the CS, resulting in greater quality reconstruction. Similarly, in the evaluation of breast cancers with MRI, CAD systems are used. Breast tumors can be detected and diagnosed using CAD systems as a "second opinion" evaluation in addition to the radiologist's assessment [48]. Many typical components of CAD systems, including image pre-processing, tumor feature extraction, and data classification, are based on ML approaches. So, according to Anke Meyer-Base *et al*. research study, the ML technique is used in the identification of diagnostically problematic breast lesions such as non-mass enhancing (NME) lesions using ML-based CAD systems in MRI. It also covers how multiparametric MRI and radiomics may be used to research NME, including predicting neoadjuvant chemotherapy response (NAC) [49]. NAC is a treatment used to reduce a tumor before it is treated with the primary treatment. Thereby, NME is an augmenting abnormality that is not linked to a mass's three-dimensional volume, form, or outline. Especially when compared to dynamic breast MRI, it is distinguished from the enhancement of normal fibro glandular tissue.

10.2.6   AI-enabled ultrasound

Ultrasound scans, often known as sonograms, employ ultrasonic waves of a certain frequency to provide a picture of the body's internal structures. An ultrasound may monitor a fetus, identify a disease, or guide a surgeon during surgery. Many believe ultrasound imaging to be a robust imaging technology, but the study by Wang *et al*. in the current issue of investigational radiology shows the numerous improvements that show it is far from stagnant. Although ultrasonic imaging has its roots in radiology and continues to be used in that field, experiments with ultrasound for heart imaging, dubbed echocardiography, may have driven the method to its current status as a critical patient care tool. Portable ultrasound systems have emerged as a result of advancements in transducers and quick imaging technologies, as well as condensed computing and image processing capabilities (PoUSs). These PoUSs have become available globally for a lesser price than a typical scanner, either for directing needle positioning, giving ultrasound stimulation treatment, or enabling critical care diagnostic data. In addition to mammography, AI-US is used for breast cancer screening. AI-US has been used to classify benign and malignant breast tumors. Han *et al*. taught CNN to differentiate benign and malignant breast tumors. The CNN-based Inception model performed as well or better than radiologists. Byra *et al*. created a matching layer to convert grayscale US pictures to RGB for CNN's discrimination. Antropova *et al*. employed VGG and SVM to classify CNN and CAD features. The Breast Imaging Reporting and Data System (BI-RADS) provides recommendations and criteria for classifying breast tumors using imaging. Zhang *et al.* created a network that includes BI-RADS features in task-oriented semi-supervised deep learning for diagnosing US pictures with a restricted training dataset. US imaging suggests using a CNN with a spatially constrained layer to identify papillary thyroid cancer. In US images, inception distinguished papillary thyroid carcinomas from benign tumors. It may assist physicians detect 0.5–1.0 cm microcalcified nodules with a higher shape. A ResNet-based fine-tuning method improved thyroid nodule classification accuracy over VGG. Li *et al.* used CNNs to classify thyroid lesions. Their model has the same sensitivity and specificity as expert radiologists in diagnosing thyroid cancer. US imaging analysis using CNN ensemble models categorized ovarian tumors similar to human experts. Feng *et al.* used 3D CNN to detect prostate cancer in sequential CEUS imaging. During transrectal US identity chronic prostate brachytherapy, a CTV segmentation strategy was provided. To generate the CTV form in advance using automatically sampled pseudo-landmarks, a CNN was used, as well as an encoder-decoder CNN architecture for low-level feature extraction.

10.2.7   AI in nuclear medicine

Nuclear medicine examines the functioning of organs and tissue within the body with radioactive material to identify and eliminate damaged or diseased organs and tissue. The main distinction between nuclear medicine and radiology is that nuclear medicine uses internal radiation waves from within the body to make pictures, whereas radiology uses external energy waves to create images. With a vast quantity of training data, AI can learn the mapping connection between sinogram data and reconstructed pictures. It is made up of millions of parameters and gathers information for a rough answer to the inverse issue. Thereby, AI can help to prevent incorrect assumption patterns. However, after the training process, direct AI reconstruction is performed efficiently and computed reconstruction from the ground up. It is no wonder that PET and single-photon emission computerized tomography (SPECT) imaging involves enhancement. Although anatomical image-guided PET/SPECT reconstruction has not been commonly employed in all clinical applications, with the introduction of hybrid imaging systems under anatomical picture-directed nuclear medicine image reconstruction, incorporating anatomical information can increase picture quality. The implementation of the sparse signal recognition algorithm relies on dictionary learning and could further enhance its understanding of the dictionary through correlating anatomical images. These images are utilized to construct a preliminary signal in the picture reconstruction process, effectively addressing the issue encountered in typical cases. In conventional scenarios, where smoothing is applied before reconstruction, the automated system often results in excessive smoothing in the reconstructed image. Attenuation maps and scatters correction are still used in nuclear medicine. Reconstruction was reencoded as a data-directed supervised training job using manifolds approximation automated transformation (AUTOMAP) by Zhu *et al.* AUTOMAP can train a reconstruction function for sinogram data from noisy and under-sampled acquisitions to increase artifact elimination and reconstruction accuracy.

To improve the clarity and low-level noise of PET scanner images, Hong *et al.* developed a deep residual CNN. According to Kim *et al.*, the picture quality was enhanced by recursive PET reconstruction utilizing a denoising CNN with local linear fitting. Using CNN or GAN, many companies have successfully generated full-dose PET images from low-dose scans, which represents a decrease in administered radioactivity.

Using CNN, Berg and Cherry were able to improve timing resolution by 20% compared to leading-edge and 23% compared to a constant fraction by predicting time-off light from digitalized detector waveforms for simultaneous occurrences. The methodology that Choi *et al.* used was novel. The amount of amyloid in the brain's cortex was measured using synthetic MR images generated from florbetapir PET scans by use of GANs. Radiology scans in nuclear medicine are time consuming and expensive. The prediction of drug–target interactions (DTIs) has long been done with computer help; AI-based techniques are increasingly used.

10.3   Discussion

Radiology is integrating AI for numerous reasons. First, radiology physicians are scarcer than diagnostic imaging demand in many nations. This increases productivity and efficiency requirements. Between the years 2012 and 2015, CT and MR scans in England climbed by 29 and 26 percentage points, whereas radiology experts (consultant workforce) increased by 5%. Scotland's deficit grew (The Royal College of Radiologists 2016). Radiologists now assess images every 3–4 s, 8 h a day [50].

Second, scanner picture resolution is increasing, creating more data. Radiologists need automated digital processing to make effective use of medical data, which doubles every 3 years. Medical imaging has always used ML, but today's algorithms are far more sophisticated [51]. DL-based ANNs contain numerous functional layers, often over 100, with thousands of neurons and millions of connections. "Shallow" ANNs have just one intermediate layer. During ANN training, weights are gradually changed to modify all of these connections. Deep networks can simulate complicated, non-linear environments and process information in practically infinite ways. With each layer of training, an ANN abstractly structures the incoming data.

10.4   Future directions

In the future, AI advancement will be inextricably tied to medical labor, and physician work will be tightly related to AI. Medical services that are helped by machines will be the best option for future medical treatment. It is figured out with the specific radiology activities that are most likely to benefit from the deep learning algorithm. Physicians must stay up with the times and apply technology systematically to become a technic driver and ultimately benefit patients in the context of the rapid growth of AI in medical informatics. AI derives computational methods of tasks from information and algorithms that are frequently as good as people. AI is now a reality and is a significant source of healthcare innovation, assisting in the advancement of new medications, medical decision assistance, and quality assurance. Deep learning is particularly good at visual pattern identification, and solutions based on this method can help healthcare professionals like radiographers, pathologists, and sonologists who rely largely on information derived from images. Furthermore, doing a medical comprehensive study in this medical imaging domain is essential, which focuses on AI-enabled radiology with enormous studies that have evaluated clinical imaging applications. Better imaging increases in radiology, and adherence to guidelines and standards of care have all contributed to developments in medical image informatics. AI allows a third person to be introduced into the patient-care interaction who may contribute to healthcare. Improved picture quality by automatic classification or interpretation, as well as ensuring that images are suited for the purpose, can boost trust in imaging-based diagnoses. This might help to enhance healthcare efficiency and screening workflow in early tumor diagnosis. Simultaneously, clinicians should have a better knowledge of how AI approaches function to appropriate screening AI solutions. Billions of connected gadgets produce health sensor data. Improve data organizing strategies. Powerful prediction algorithms and AI will result in smarter settings with more efficient and safer human–machine interaction. IoT is becoming part of healthcare firms' daily operations.

References

[1] https://www.researchgate.net/publication/330722193_Introduction_Game_Changers_in_Radiology_Opportunities_Applications_and_Risks

[2] Rundo, L., R. Pirrone, S. Vitabile, E. Sala, and O. Gambino. "Recent advances of HCI in decision-making tasks for optimized clinical workflows and precision medicine." *Journal of Biomedical Informatics* 108 (2020): 103479.

[3] Ranschaert, E.R., S. Morozov, and P.R. Algra, eds. *Artificial Intelligence in Medical Imaging: Opportunities, Applications and Risks.* Springer, 2019.

[4] Miranda, E., M. Aryuni, and E. Irwansyah. "A survey of medical image classification techniques." In *2016 International Conference on Information Management and Technology (ICIMTech)*, pp. 56–61. IEEE, 2016.

[5] Sarvamangala, D.R. and R.V. Kulkarni. "Convolutional neural networks in medical image understanding: a survey." *Evolutionary Intelligence* 15 (2021): 1–22.

[6] Bezdek, J.C., L. O. Hall, and L.P. Clarke. "Review of MR image segmentation techniques using pattern recognition." *Medical Physics-LANCASTER PA-*20 (1993): 1033–1033.

[7] Razzak, M.I., S. Naz, and A. Zaib. "Deep learning for medical image processing: overview, challenges and the future." *Classification in BioApps* (2018): 323–350.

[8] Cai, L., J. Gao, and D. Zhao. "A review of the application of deep learning in medical image classification and segmentation." *Annals of Translational Medicine* 8(11) (2020).

[9]   Mohamed, E.. "The relation of artificial intelligence with internet of things: a survey." *Journal of Cybersecurity and Information Management* 1 (2020): 30–24.

[10] Singh, R., A. Gehlot, M. Rashid, R. Saxena, S.V. Akram, S.S. Alshamrani, and A.S. AlGhamdi. "Cloud server and internet of things assisted system for stress monitoring." *Electronics* 10(24) (2021): 3133.

[11] Thirugnanasambandam, K., S.V. Sudha, D. Saravanan, R.V. Ravi, D.K. Anguraj, R.S. Raghav. "Reinforced Cuckoo Search based fugitive landfill methane emission estimation." *Environmental Technology & Innovation* 21 (2020): 101207.

[12] Thirugnanasambandam, K., M. Rajeswari, D. Bhattacharyya, and J-y. Kim. "Directed Artificial Bee Colony algorithm with revamped search strategy to solve global numerical optimization problems." *Automated Software Engineering* 29(13) (2022). https://doi.org/10.1007/s10515-021-00306-w

[13] Bohr, A. and K. Memarzadeh. "The rise of artificial intelligence in health-care applications." In *Artificial Intelligence in Healthcare*, pp. 25–60. Academic Press, 2020.

[14] Akram, S. Vaseem, R. Singh, M.A. AlZain, A. Gehlot, M. Rashid, O.S. Faragallah, W. El-Shafai, and D. Prashar. "Performance analysis of iot and long-range radio-based sensor node and gateway architecture for solid waste management." *Sensors* 21(8) (2021): 2774.

[15] Bashir, A.K., R. Arul, S. Basheer, G. Raja, R. Jayaraman, and N.M.F. Qureshi. "An optimal multitier resource allocation of cloud RAN in 5G using machine learning." *Transactions on Emerging Telecommunications Technologies* 30(8) (2019): e3627.

[16] Salehi, H. and R. Burgueño. "Emerging artificial intelligence methods in structural engineering." *Engineering Structures* 171 (2018): 170–189.

[17] Wuest, T., D. Weimer, C. Irgens, and K.-D. Thoben. "Machine learning in manufacturing: advantages, challenges, and applications." *Production & Manufacturing Research* 4(1) (2016): 23–45.

[18] Arul, R., G. Raja, A.O. Almagrabi, M.S. Alkatheiri, S.H. Chauhdary, and A. K. Bashir. "A quantum-safe key hierarchy and dynamic security association for LTE/SAE in 5G scenario." *IEEE Transactions on Industrial Informatics* 16(1) (2019): 681–690.

[19] Gardezi, S.J.S., A. Elazab, B. Lei, and T. Wang. "Breast cancer detection and diagnosis using mammographic data: systematic review." *Journal of Medical Internet Research* 21(7) (2019): e14464.

[20] Rathour, N., S.S. Alshamrani, R. Singh, *et al.* "IoMT based facial emotion recognition system using deep convolution neural networks." *Electronics* 10 (11) (2021): 1289.

[21] Ahuja, A.S. "The impact of artificial intelligence in medicine on the future role of the physician." *PeerJ* 7 (2019): e7702.

[22] Pesapane, F., M. Codari, and F. Sardanelli. "Artificial intelligence in medical imaging: threat or opportunity? Radiologists again at the forefront of innovation in medicine." *European Radiology Experimental* 2(1) (2018): 1–10.

[23] Serag, A., A. Ion-Margineanu, H. Qureshi, *et al.* "Translational AI and deep learning in diagnostic pathology." *Frontiers in Medicine* 6 (2019): 185.

[24] Arul, R., R. Alroobaea, U. Tariq, A.H. Almulihi, F.S. Alharithi, and U. Shoaib. "IoT-enabled healthcare systems using block chain-dependent adaptable services." *Personal and Ubiquitous Computing*, 2 (2021): 1–15.

[25] Waite, S., A. Grigorian, R.G. Alexander, *et al.* "Analysis of perceptual expertise in radiology–Current knowledge and a new perspective." *Frontiers in Human Neuroscience* 13 (2019): 213.

[26] Sarker, I.H. "Machine learning: algorithms, real-world applications and research directions." *SN Computer Science* 2(3) (2021): 1–21.

[27] Thandapani, S., M.I. Mahaboob, C. Iwendi, *et al.* "IoMT with deep CNN: AI-based intelligent support system for pandemic diseases." *Electronics* 12 (2) (2023): 424.

[28] Yang, Q., P. Yan, Y. Zhang, *et al.* "Low-dose CT image denoising using a generative adversarial network with Wasserstein distance and perceptual loss." *IEEE Transactions on Medical Imaging* 37(6) (2018): 1348–1357.

[29] Missert, A.D., L. Yu, S. Leng, J.G. Fletcher, and C.H. McCollough. "Synthesizing images from multiple kernels using a deep convolutional neural network." *Medical Physics* 47(2) (2020): 422–430.

[30] Mishra, A. K., S.K. Das, P. Roy, and S. Bandyopadhyay. "Identifying COVID19 from chest CT images: a deep convolutional neural networks based approach." *Journal of Healthcare Engineering* 2020 (2020).

[31] Li, L., L. Qin, Z. Xu, *et al.* "Using artificial intelligence to detect COVID-19 and community-acquired pneumonia based on pulmonary CT: evaluation of the diagnostic accuracy." *Radiology* 296(2) (2020): E65–E71.

[32] Trivizakis, E., N. Tsiknakis, E.E. Vassalou, *et al.* "Advancing COVID-19 differentiation with a robust preprocessing and integration of multi-institutional open-repository computer tomography datasets for deep learning analysis." *Experimental and Therapeutic Medicine* 20(5) (2020): 1–1.

[33] Thirugnansambandam, K., D. Bhattacharyya, J. Frnda, D.K. Anguraj, and J. Nedoma. "Augmented node placement model in t-WSN through multi-objective approach." *CMC-Computers, Materials & Continua* 69(3) (2021): 3629–3644.

[34] Singh, R., K.K. Mannudeep, F. Homayounieh, *et al.* "Artificial intelligence-based vessel suppression for detection of sub-solid nodules in lung cancer screening computed tomography." *Quantitative Imaging in Medicine and Surgery* 11(4) (2021): 1134.

[35] Raghav, R.S., K. Thirugnanasambandam, V. Varadarajan, S. Vairavasundaram, and L. Ravi. "Artificial bee colony reinforced extended Kalman Filter Localization Algorithm in Internet of Things with big data blending technique for finding the accurate position of reference nodes." *Big Data.* 2021 Nov 5. doi:10.1089/big.2020.0203. Epub ahead of print. PMID: 34747652.

[36] Yang, C., H. Lan, F. Gao, and F. Gao. "Review of deep learning for photoacoustic imaging." *Photoacoustics* 21 (2021): 100215.

[37]   Moustakidis, S., M. Omar, J. Aguirre, P. Mohajerani, and V. Ntziachristos. "Fully automated identification of skin morphology in raster-scan optoacoustic mesoscopy using artificial intelligence." *Medical Physics* 46(9) (2019): 4046–4056.

[38]   Bechelli, S. and J. Delhommelle. "Machine learning and deep learning algorithms for skin cancer classification from dermoscopic images." *Bioengineering* 9(3) (2022): 97.

[39]   Han, S.H.. "Review of photoacoustic imaging for imaging-guided spinal surgery." *Neurospine* 15(4) (2018): 306.

[40]   Mueller, S. and L. Sandrin. "Liver stiffness: a novel parameter for the diagnosis of liver disease." *Hepatic Medicine: Evidence and Research* 2 (2010): 49.

[41]   Wang, K., X. Lu, H. Zhou, *et al.* "Deep learning radiomics of shear wave elastography significantly improved diagnostic performance for assessing liver fibrosis in chronic hepatitis B: a prospective multicentre study." *Gut* 68 (4) (2019): 729–741.

[42]   Zhou, L.-Q., J.-Y. Wang, S.-Y. Yu, *et al.* "Artificial intelligence in medical imaging of the liver." *World journal of gastroenterology* 25(6) (2019): 672.

[43]   Soto, J.A. and W.A. Stephan. "Multidetector CT of blunt abdominal trauma." *Radiology* 265(3) (2012): 678–693.

[44]   Yankeelov, T.E., G.A. Richard, and C.C. Quarles "Quantitative multi-modality imaging in cancer research and therapy." *Nature Reviews Clinical Oncology* 11(11) (2014): 670–680.

[45]   Sheth, D. and M.L. Giger. "Artificial intelligence in the interpretation of breast cancer on MRI." *Journal of Magnetic Resonance Imaging* 51(5) (2020): 1310–1324.

[46]   Andersen, F.L., S.H. Keller, A.E. Hansen, *et al.* "Bone attenuation in brain-PET/MR imaging should be accounted for during attenuation correction and PET reconstruction." *European Journal of Nuclear Medicine and Molecular Imaging* 39 (2012): S174–S174. 233 SPRING ST, NEW YORK, NY 10013 USA: SPRINGER.

[47]   Chen, Y., C.-B. Schönlieb, P. Liò, *et al.* "AI-based reconstruction for fast MRI—a systematic review and meta-analysis." *Proceedings of the IEEE 110*, 2 (2022): 224–245.

[48]   Jiménez-Gaona, Y., M.J. Rodríguez-Álvarez, and V. Lakshminarayanan. "Deep-learning-based computer-aided systems for breast cancer imaging: a critical review." *Applied Sciences* 10(22) (2020): 8298.

[49]   Shen, D., G. Wu, and H.-Il Suk. "Deep learning in medical image analysis." *Annual Review of Biomedical Engineering* 19 (2017): 221–248.

[50]   Abbara, S., P. Blanke, C.D. Maroules, *et al.* "SCCT guidelines for the performance and acquisition of coronary computed tomographic angiography: a report of the society of Cardiovascular Computed Tomography Guidelines Committee: endorsed by the North American Society for Cardiovascular Imaging (NASCI)." *Journal of Cardiovascular Computed Tomography* 10(6) (2016): 435–449.

[51]   Litjens, G., T. Kooi, B.E. Bejnordi, *et al.* "A survey on deep learning in medical image analysis." *Medical Image Analysis* 42 (2017): 60–88.

Chapter 11
Role of artificial intelligence in medical IoT devices

Ankita Wadhawan[1], Nagnath Aherwadi[1] and Usha Mittal[1]

Artificial intelligence (AI) and Internet of Things (IoT) advancements are assisting the medical industry and allowing hospitals to utilize the data provided. Doctors are discovering AI applications all over the medical field. They may now simply monitor patients and keep track of them without having to be present. Because of medical developments and AI contributions to medical IoT devices, they will know which patients require rapid attention. Medical IoT devices are increasing the quality of care as well as monitoring and advising patients on the side effects of certain medical procedures. This chapter investigated the impact of AI and its advancement in medical IoT, as well as its contribution.

11.1 Introduction

11.1.1 Artificial Intelligence

AI is now allowing doctors and medical professionals for making faster and more accurate diagnoses with the help of IoT devices. Mathematical algorithms and human body data science are used by AI in medicine. It makes accurate diagnoses than doctors and health specialists or doctors can take proper decisions and immediate action for that disease before it becomes severe [1,2].

AI stores the patient's details along with his medical condition which means what disease he/she had and suffering through which disease now and family information. That saved data becomes a primary source across the globe anywhere if that patient's treatment is going on the doctors can get all the history of that patient within time. AI is used in human disease analysis by identifying the internal human body part damage using X-rays, electrocardiography, and another different type of scans. Advancement in technology allows doctors to human body parts interaction and allows them to compare the findings to previous instances to determine efficacy [3].

This lowers the number of times patients have to wait for treatment and they will get the proper treatment and compare the findings to previous instances to

---

[1]Department of Computer Science and Engineering, Lovely Professional University, Punjab, India

determine efficacy. This lowers the number of times patients have to wait for treatment and they will get the proper treatment for their disease in desired time [4].

11.1.2   IoT devices

IoT referred to as the IoT, these devices use wireless connectivity networks to transfer data from one place to another. The IoT entails expanding Internet connectivity beyond typical devices such as personal computers, and tablets along with phones and laptops. We can connect them to the Internet and can be easily operated remotely [5,6].

In the smart hospital, medical IoT devices are arranged in a particular manner for sensing and responding to a patient's movement. If the patient requires help or any serious condition occurs, the doctors or medical staff will come to know through these devices. Advancement in technology is helping the medical field with accurate prediction and fast diagnosis. Technology is giving the right to use advanced medical devices and get benefits from them. Nowadays advanced machinery is developed for a hospital that can make operations without taking any help from a human being [7,8].

11.1.3   IoT devices used in the healthcare monitoring of patients

There are many medical IoT devices available for the healthcare monitoring of patients. Some of them are included in Figure 11.1.

Five examples of AI-powered IoT are:

i. WALMART: To improve retails it uses a facial recognition system and IoT tags.
ii. INTEL: For remote patient monitoring Icon uses Intel's AI-driven technology.

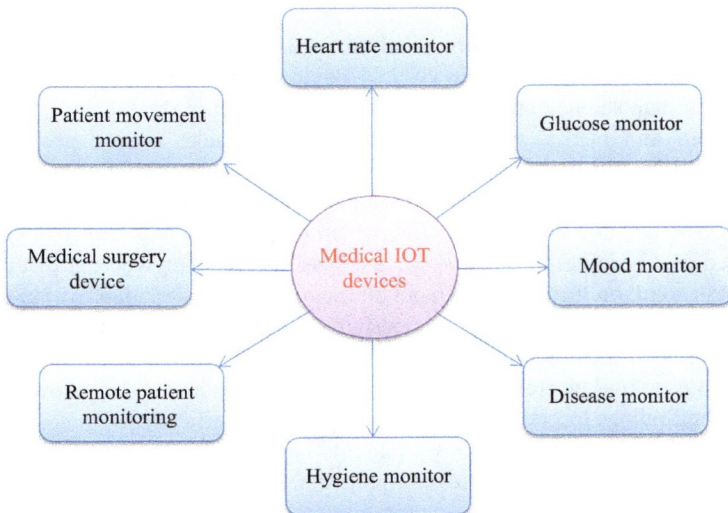

Figure 11.1   IoT devices used in the medical field

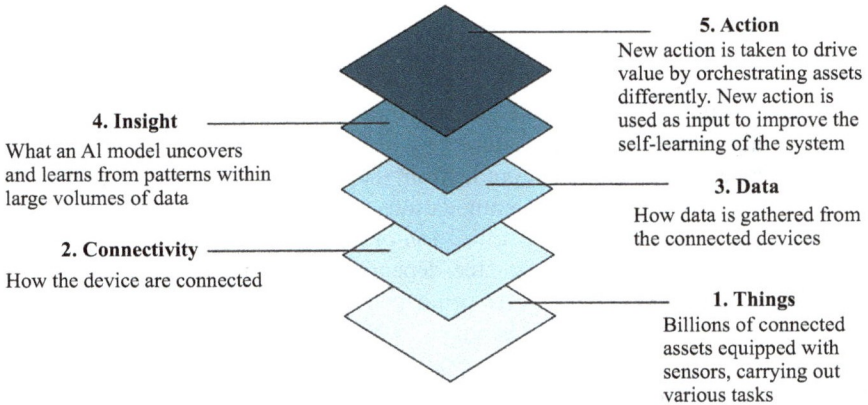

4. Insight
What an AI model uncovers
and learns from patterns within
large volumes of data

2. Connectivity
How the device are connected

5. Action
New action is taken to drive
value by orchestrating assets
differently. New action is
used as input to improve the
self-learning of the system

3. Data
How data is gathered from
the connected devices

1. Things
Billions of connected
assets equipped with
sensors, carrying out
various tasks

Figure 11.2   AI in IoT device

iii. LOGISTICS: Along with AI-powered IoT uses better transit monitoring.
iv. CARFORCE: For better predictive maintenance, it takes advantage of industrial AI software.
v. SHELL: The power of AI and IoT is tapped to save millions of dollars.

11.1.4   AI in the IoT

When AI is merged with IoT, these connected devices gather, analyze, and act on sensor data where human involvement is not there, and adapt to the current environment around them [9]. The broad outline of AI used in the IoT is shown in Figure 11.2.

11.2   Literature review

Van Leeuwen *et al.* [10] presented the role of AI in radiology. AI's promise of whether it could improve healthcare and reduce cost or not was explained here. They described that AI support six main clinical objectives: the first is effective workflow, the second is earlier detection of disease, the third is dose decrement, the fourth is diagnosis accuracy improvement, the fifth is the private diagnosis, and the last is shortened reading time. They provided impact-based hierarchical model efficacy example use cases with medical shreds of evidence. They also told that the market is maturing and slowly knowing about AI but definitely, everyone is soon going to know the value and contribution of AI in clinical practice, making informed development, procurement, and reimbursement decisions. They concluded that after properly assessing and observing the results and impact of clinical experiments on AI products. The contribution of AI in the improvement of health care and cost reduction was also given.

Beckers *et al.* [11] presented their perspective regarding the New European Medical Device Regulation (EU MDR). A medical device manufacturing company making advancements in products to improve patient health. They were supported by health institutions that were developing their own algorithms. After the development of algorithms, they were addressing requirements. The creators introduced how to execute an administrative guide, from the beginning phase through plan and advancement, administrative accommodation, and post-market observation. They had additionally incorporated a clarification of how to set up an agreeable quality administration framework to guarantee dependable and steady item quality. The author made the conclusion that AI could make the reduction in requirement of physicists. More authority would be given to other medical specialists.

Ghosh *et al.* [12] proposed a developmental disorder that impedes a person's growth is autism. Autistic people struggle to keep up with the pace of the world, are unable to communicate effectively, and do not properly express feelings. AI, ML, and the IoT are used for a variety of medical equipment, and who is an autistic person can benefit from an automatic system. Research efforts of different applications are given in this chapter. A total of 58 articles with important contributions in this field were chosen. The research papers that were chosen were evaluated, represented, and contrasted. Finally, the inclusion of a smart city autistic facility setting was discussed, certain time gaps and obstacles were identified, and recommendations were offered for future study. This study described 58 research papers on the usage of ML, AI, and the IoT in the detection of autism, and guidance.

Muehlematter *et al.* [13] explained that since 2015, the number of AI and ML devices had grown significantly, with many of them approved by them for usage in radiotherapy. Only a minimum number of gadgets were designated as high-risk gadgets. Eighty of the 184 products that are routinely authorized in the United States and Europe were initially certified in Europe. One possible explanation for European approval ahead of the United States might be Europe's perhaps less stringent assessment of medical devices. A large number of authorized devices emphasize the importance of stringent control of these devices. There is currently no particular regulatory process in the United States or Europe for AI-ML-based medical devices. More openness on how devices are regulated and authorized is recommended to allow and increase the quality, public confidence, efficiency, and safety of AI-ML-based medical devices. A database available publically having details of FDA-approved devices in the United States is required.

Rastogi *et al.* [14] described that AI technologies are becoming more widespread in a variety of areas throughout the world, including banking, healthcare, agriculture, and automobile transport. ML is a sophisticated technical technique that uses AI to consider vulnerable regions of different models. Diabetes is a serious medical problem. When body cells fail to absorb energy from meals, particularly glucose then, illness occurs. People with diabetes are more likely to have lifelong issues such as hypertension, other diseases, and eye problems. People who suffer from tension headaches typically increase blood pressure (BP). Six out of eight individuals possess hypertension with tension-type headaches, and more than 75% had a tension-type headache. From this, we can say that hypertension is linked directly to headaches. Tension-type headache occurs when the person is having diabetes and mostly occurs in men.

Raj *et al.* [15] compared cloud computing to this system and stated that cloud computing is more complex due to resource constraints, transmission efficiency, functionality, and other edge network-based contextual variables. Instability arises during edge device collaboration that cannot be disregarded. This study proposed a unique paradigm for optimizing the edge cooperative network. This contributed to the increased efficiency of edge computing jobs. The measures for evaluating collaboration were specified at the outset. Furthermore, by improving edge network collaboration, specific task performance was improved. For illustrating the performance of the proposed architecture, real datasets acquired from old individuals and their wearable sensors were used. Extensive testing also aided in confirming the efficacy of the suggested optimization technique. The framework's efficiency was demonstrated in the experimental part using a dataset of wearable medical sensors. A case study was used to validate the viability of the edge cooperative optimization technique. The future scope was focused on increasing the datasets and fine-tuning the framework's efficiency.

Badnjević *et al.* [16] explained that medical field IoT devices are using AI. Nowadays owing to design diversity, and ethical issues, there is a continuing requirement to assess the performance and use of the system. The authors are providing an artificial neural network (ANN) and machine learning applications. This study was focused on identification challenges along with issues connected to the use of AI in medical IoT devices. From medical equipment to the engineering of the clinic, AI was transformed. Fulfilling its full potential, ethical problems were provided solutions and use controlled for privacy and access.

Abir *et al.* [17] explained that Corona (COVID-19) had a huge influence around the globe today. Various governments had taken a variety of steps to create resilience against this potentially fatal illness. The extremely infectious nature of this epidemic, on the other hand, had called into question established healthcare and treatment approaches. AI and ML provide new avenues for effective treatment throughout this epidemic. AI and ML can help with medical development by creating efficient diagnosis techniques and forecasting illness spread. These applications rely heavily on real-time observing of the patients and good information coordination, which is where the IoT comes in. IoT may also aid with applications like automated medicine distribution, responding to patient inquiries, and tracking illness transmission reasons. This article provided a thorough examination of all technologies for combating the corona pandemic.

Iskanderani *et al.* [18] described that since December 2019, the globe had been dealing with the COVID-19 epidemic. The timely and accurate identification of COVID-19-suspected patients was critical in medical therapy. To combat the COVID-19 epidemic, a deep transfer learning (DL)-based automatic corona (COVID-19) diagnosis X-ray was necessary. Using ensemble learning, this study gave a real-time IoT framework for the early detection of probable COVID-19 patients. The proposed system allowed for real-time requirement meetings and diagnosis of suspected COVID-19 instances. The IoT framework consisted of four DL models: Inception-ResNet-V2, ResNet-152-V2, VGG-16, and DenseNet-201. Using the deep ensembling approach saved on the cloud server, the sensors were used to get X-ray modalities and identify the illness. According to the comparative study, the suggested model could assist radiologists in efficiently and quickly diagnosing COVID-19 suspicious patients.

Ahmad *et al.* [19] presented that some medical professions, such as radiotherapy, were very quick to adjust to AI like pathologists are just now started to use AI. AI has the capacity to significantly improve cancer diagnosis, prognosis, and treatment. The broad concepts of AI were outlined first in this chapter, a thorough description of the current functions in medicine. AI used in the past, present, and future in surgical-pathology was explored to length in the second part of this study. Also, it considered the practical challenges involved in it. Computer algorithms were replaced by pathologist requirements.

Fouad Mansour *et al.* [20] used AI and IoT convergence approaches to create an illness diagnostic system for diabetes and heart disease patients. The model described includes several phases, including data gathering, pre-processing, classification, and parameter deciding. IoT devices like wearables and sensors enabled continuous data collecting, while AI algorithms used the data to diagnose diseases. Crow search optimization (CSO) was used for fine-tuning biases and weights of the cascaded long short-term memory (CSLTM) algorithm to obtain better classifying of medical data. Furthermore, the isolated forest approach was used in this study to eliminate outliers. The use of CSO significantly improved the test results of the CSLTM algorithm. The healthcare data was used to validate CSO–CSLTM model performance. At the time of testing, the given CSO–CSLTM model got the highest accuracies which are 96.16% and 97.26% for detecting diabetes and heart disease. As a result, the suggested CSO–CSLTM approach might be used as the best disease-detection device for smart healthcare facilities.

Ibraheem Abdullah *et al.* [21] presented computer power and storage capacity growth of medical big data aided the AI deployment boom in health care and research. Ophthalmology is a prominent medical profession that uses AI for diagnosis as well as therapy. The first FDA-approved autonomous diagnostic device was used to diagnose and categorize diabetic retinopathy. AI has also been used to treat various ocular diseases such as age-related eye problems, hypertension, retinal detachment, and infantile cataract. To assess the existing literature on the medical ethics challenges posed by AI in medicine and optometry, categorize ethical issues in medical AI, and propose appropriate standards of ethical frameworks for AI performance. The findings were examined, cross-referenced, and reported. There are several parties involved in the ethical concerns regarding AI in medicine and optometry.

VikramPuri *et al.* [22] explained about several parties involved in the ethical concerns regarding AI in medicine and ophthalmology. It is quite difficult to look at the different elements of AI ethics, especially as technology advances. A cloud-based healthcare system offers a variety of methods for gathering patient data as well as on-demand, well-managed reporting of patients and health professionals.

To address these problems, the given study offered decentralized AI-enabled health architecture that accessed and stopped IoT devices while also increasing the surety and transparency of inpatient healthcare information (PHR). The method was based on AI-enabled smart contracts and the design of a public network. In addition, the framework detected malicious IoT nodes in the system. The practical evaluations were carried out in a real-time test environment, and considerable improvements in device energy usage, date, time, throughput, packet delay, and switching costs were proposed.

Yoo *et al.* [23] explained that health big data gathering and the advancement of ML, the healthcare industry had experienced fast changes. The data complexity of medicine was the necessity of knowledge, and the confidentiality of personal information distinguishes research in the field of data mining in healthcare from studies. To solve these difficulties, many approaches had been adopted, including the cloud platform and machine learning method. They offered a cloud-based health platform. The data processing system decreased medical data management expenses while improving safety. They also proposed a mining method for health risk identification, which is at the heart of health. At last, they suggested research utilizing explaining AI to improve the dependability and accuracy of the decision-making system, which they named the black-box model due to its lack of transparent entity.

Amit *et al.* [24] presented that early illness forecasts assisted doctors in making early decisions to save patients' lives. The IoT was acting as a trigger to increase the effectiveness of AI applications in medicine. The main goal of the research was to offer an ML-based healthcare model that could detect various illnesses early and correctly. Different ML classification techniques were used: decision tree (DT), support vector machine (SVM), naive Bayes, adaptive boosting, and k-means clustering. Heart disease, diabetes, breast cancer, liver issue, surgical data, and thyroid are among nine deadly illnesses predicted by random forest (RF), ANN, and K-nearest neighbors (k-NN). For various illnesses, the RF classifier achieved high accuracy of 97.62%, and this system aided clinicians in early illness detection.

Komal *et al.* [25] described that various regulatory cycles and patient ideas could be aided by the application of AI in healthcare services through service providers of healthcare. Mostly AI and IoT medical service innovations have significant implications for the medical field. However, the techniques they supported could shift significantly, and keep in mind that AI in healthcare recommended that utilizing AI in healthcare could perform as same as other techniques, for example, disease diagnosis. The employment of AI mimics human mental powers and limitations. It is getting a new viewpoint to restrict by increasing access to medical services, service knowledge, and the rapid advancement of research methods. Significant disease areas where AI approaches are used include neurology, cardiology, and cancer. They covered the ethical issues in the use of AI in healthcare.

Barnawi *et al.* [26] explained about how the IoT improved the existing healthcare practicals by bringing together social, economic, and technological perspectives. The global spread of COVID-19 from December 2019 had a bad effect economy of the globe. IoT technology combined with AI could aids in the resolution of COVID-19. IoT sensors collected source data that was needed for computation and analyzed it to make smart decisions where no need for people interaction. In this work, they presented an IoT, UAV-based strategy for collecting the source data utilizing temperature sensors to reduce the influence of COVID-19. The temperature was measured using the thermal picture taken by the thermal camera. It was used to identify prospective persons in the photo (of a huge metropolis crowd) who suffering from COVID-19. For face recognition, an effective hybrid technique was presented. A face-mask identification system was included, which identified whether a person was wearing a mask or not on their face.

Oniani *et al.* [27] presented big data, AI, and the IoT that have a significant influence on the development of improved customized healthcare systems. The author covered the evaluation of AI for IoT and healthcare systems, as well as the use and application of AI technology in many sectors of healthcare. According to the literature study, four major fields in medicine employ AI techniques, including heart disease diagnostics, prediction methods, robotic surgery, and customized therapy. The findings showed that the leading AI approaches include k-NN, SVM, support vector regression (SVR), naive Bayes, linear regression (LR), regression tree, classification tree, and RF. These approaches were mostly used to analyze patient data to improve the conditions of patient health. Automatic surgery technologies had numerous benefits, including minimum violent treatment and getting good results in terms of speedier recovery of patients. The Internet of Medical Things covered a wide range of health issues.

Yu *et al.* [28] proposed the cloud fusion healthcare IoT architecture. In this study, bidirectional data collection of healthcare IoT network layers, spiritual perspective, and psychic interaction in healthcare IoT were explained. The cloud connection healthcare IoT structure was designed to connect the cloud platform of healthcare. Finally, decision layer fusion for mood categorization prediction was used. This article explained the fundamental hypothesis and key points of multisensory data collection, as well as the structure and production of a healthcare monitoring Cloud platform. An industrial automation platform, robot-based multidimensional data assessing and grouping, and high convenience particular data collection premised on smart dresses. Simulation models were used to validate the usefulness and fulfillment of the framework. This paper showed how learning of migration was utilized to construct data labeling of emotion, as well as continuous artificial potential fields to detect emotions using data gathered from cellphones and smart clothing.

Mao *et al.* [29] described that AI-assisted diagnostic systems were quickly evolving, yet doctors were currently unaware of their existence. They showed how doctors accepted and used AI healthcare professional diagnosis system apps that might help to boost their deployment. With the existing challenges in IoT from medical consulting services, this article offered a commercial operating approach on the basis of different party involvement and source-splitting inpatient treatment. An enhanced new learning algorithm was presented on the basis of the problems in medical investigation. The technique penalized risky sample loss such that the CNN gave attention to harmful samples and learning in an effective way. This article modified the topology of the CNN and considered the eight physiological features of information available.

Ardito *et al.* [30] presented that every day, new, and constantly developing dangers arose in the E-Health arena. The security of E-Health telemonitoring models was no longer an afterthought. The author presented a cyber-attack detection system (CADS) model in this work that used AI approaches to identify abnormalities without the need for security analysis, described spiteful activities, and displayed specific data attacks to healthcare staff for a response. The description of the system was tailored to the hacked remote patients' medical tele-monitoring scenario. The approach focused on the challenge of detecting cyber-attacks, in this case, exploiting a compromised remote patient tele-monitoring system. A specific running case, namely heartbeat tele-monitoring, had been taken into account.

Makridis *et al.* [31] investigated the recently discovered concepts of dependable AI, and easy implementation to disadvantaged populations. They investigate the concepts of dependable AI that were of special relevance to increasing populations. They were guided by three principles first one was creating, developing, purchasing, and employing AI. The advantages and problems were analyzed and controlled. The second one was confirming that AI applications were applied in proper areas and that they were effective, reliable, and a perfect fit for something like the required purposes. The last one was making sure the processes and results of AI technologies were properly considerable and excusable by all senior persons in the field, end-users, and all people.

Sestino *et al.* [32] described in the academic and professional literature that concept of AI for business technology had emerged in a disorganized and unstructured manner. This research sheds light on the phenomena of AI business development through a complete and systematic literature analysis. The research examined a set of 3,780 works using an innovative mixture of two well-known ML techniques (LDA and hierarchical clustering). This work generated a systematic grouping of existing research branches as well as a list of prospective new topics. The findings focused on six subjects related to three distinct topics namely implications, applications, and methods (IAM model).

Ilhan *et al.* [33] explained that even though early identification and rapid treatment provided the best results for patients, the maximum oral cancer (OC) lesions were identified at the last stage, with a 45% persistence rate for 2 years. The major reason for bad OC resulted in a lack of accessible or effective sensing and monitoring at the local point of care level, which caused late expert referral treatment. Less appropriate knowledge of OC in the general public and experts, as well as impediments, to prompt access to healthcare resources, all caused a delay in diagnosis. Image analysis and diagnosis technology advances, various machine intelligence techniques, specialized algorithms, and predictive analytics were beginning to have a significant influence on increasing OC diagnostic accuracy.

Gunasekeran *et al.* [34] described that the COVID-19 pandemic had overburdened healthcare facilities, which were confronted with the dual task of fulfilling the medical requirements of COVID-19 patients while providing critical services for non-COVID-19 diseases. As nations that managed early epidemics begin to suffer resurgences, the need to re-invention, reorganization, and change health care, as well as manage medical services at the community place, became critical. A wide number of digital health solutions had been offered, but for actual-world these technologies applied were unknown. The purpose of this research was to examine the use of AI, tele-health, and different related digital healthcare technologies for people, who were in the hospital operational domain during the COVID-19 epidemic. Recognizing digital public health limitations and possibilities, the efficiency of the digital health-care method for applications such as occupiers tracking and access viewpoints were not thoroughly assessed.

Babic *et al.* [35] presented about smart medical applications that are rapidly being utilized in a range of diagnostic evaluations, and during the COVID-19 pandemic, the focus on tele-medicine and household healthcare may expand their use even more. Technology was made for use with the help of an expert and individuals used it on their own. Because of the nature of consumer users, who were statistically and medically illiterate and risk cautious about their health outcomes, primary applications presented distinct problems. While comparable problems occurred in other areas of the medical field, the simplicity and regularity with which AI–ML applications might be utilized, as well as their rising popularity in the consumer market, necessitates serious consideration of how to properly govern them. They believed that experts should work for a good understanding of how customers engaged with direct-to-consumer medical (AI–ML) applications, specifically diagnosis apps, and that was needed more than a focus on the system specs. They also suggested that the ideal continuous assessment would take into account the societal costs of such technologies in broad usage.

Fu *et al.* [36] proposed a mobile-based automated system to increase patients' cardiovascular health management abilities while also lowering physicians' burden. Based on current improvements in IoT and AI technology, their model combined cloud software with hardware devices. Electrocardiogram (ECG) information could be collected from the human body by using a hardware device. For accurate diagnosis of cardiovascular disease, a unique automated DL-based cloud service was implemented. The experimental findings demonstrated the efficacy of their method. With a 0.9011 ROC–AUC score, their model could ensure the best quality ECG information by eliminating high-frequency as well as low-frequency compressions and reversal identification.

Susy Mathew *et al.* [37] explained that the data included in the EHR was used by analytics principals and ML algorithms. The work in the backend of a clinical environment made treatment choices and outcomes more accurate and reliable than previously. Google had created an ML system to aid in the detection of malignant tumors on mammograms. To enhance radiation therapy DeepMind Health, a division of Google, and University College London Hospital (UCLH) collaborated to make ML algorithms reliable in differentiating between healthy and malignant cells. Stanford is employing a deep learning system to detect skin cancer. The goal of the author is to give useful information on DL techniques applied in healthcare settings. DL framework approaches, and tools, along with their limits and potential were given.

Saif *et al.* [38] presented how the concept of IoT came from the plan of linking numerous physical items and gadgets to the internet. Heating, ventilation, and air conditioning (HVAC) observation and control was a simple example of such an object and equipment that enabled a smart house. There were several more sectors in which IoT had a significant part in increasing our life quality. These technologies had been widely used in recent years in healthcare, transportation, and agriculture. IoT allowed us to look, listen, and do particular tasks on the physical object, making them smart. Many residential and commercial applications would be on the basis of IoT throughout time, which will increase the quality of life and the global economy.

Anceschi *et al.* [39] demonstrated a hypothetical functioning scenario for such an alert. Each of the "SaveMeNow.AI" gadgets constantly observed their states and assessed whether the alarm should be sent or not. It was made for the detection of the fall at the working place. The machine learning core (MLC) component of a "SaveMeNow.AI" device detected a fall then it sent an alarm to the other gadgets which were in the range of the fallen gadget and called them for help. If any device was there not in range, then it would send an alarm to the catalyst device. They were set in such a place that they would occupy the total working area. The one which was at the gateway will continuously receive signals. Whenever it got an alarm, it started a timer for 30 s. If there was no "SaveMeNow.AI" gadget, after that time span it activated the rescue efforts.

Pradhan *et al.* [40] compared and contrasted multiple machine learning methods that could be used to identify lung cancer using IoT devices. Chawla *et al.* [41] explained that healthcare was driven by technology more than any other force, and it would continue to evolve in spectacular ways in the future. AI, IoT, big data, cloud computing, smart wearables, and other cutting-edge healthcare technologies had transformed traditional healthcare into smart healthcare. Technology had allowed us to keep a close eye on health in recent years. Cabitza *et al.* [42] introduced evaluation metrics, including accuracy score, sensitivity, and other error-based measurements, to assess the validity of AI systems in the medical field. This type of validity required that a numerical, statistical threshold be proven valid under well-defined experimental conditions. Unfortunately, there was a lot of terminological ambiguity in AI research, and the concept of validation was no exception. There were two simple ways to assess a computational system. One was objectivistic, which focused on technology as an active actor, and the second was consequentialist, which focused on technology's impacts in a specific circumstance. The former imputed to AI systems the character of things with features like accuracy score and reliability.

Tran *et al.* [43] described about wearable biometric monitoring devices (BMDs) and AI which made it possible to capture and analyze patient data remotely and in real-time. The application of AI to screen for skin cancer, remote monitoring of chronic illnesses to forecast exacerbations, smart garments to guide physical treatment, and AI chatbots to handle emergency calls were among the topics discussed in the vignettes. From May to June 2018, 1,183 patients enrolled at that time. Overall, 20% of respondents believed that the benefits of technology (such as improved reactivity in care and reduced treatment burden) outweighed the risks. Davenport *et al.* [44] explained that because of the rising complexity and volume of data in healthcare, AI would be used more frequently. Payers and

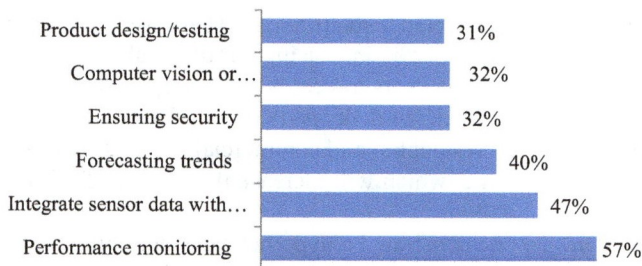

Figure 11.3   Use cases for AI/ML in IoT deployments

providers of care, as well as life sciences corporations, were already using AI in various forms. Diagnoses and treatment recommendations, patient involvement and adherence, and administrative duties were among the most common types of applications. Although AI could execute healthcare duties as well as or better than humans in many cases, implementation issues might delay large-scale automation of healthcare professional occupations for a long time. Ethical concerns around the use of AI in healthcare were also highlighted.

11.3   Use of AI in IoT deployments

The majority of respondents (69%) are using AI/ML in their IoT deployments as shown in Figure 11.3. Most are likely to use it for performance monitoring (56%), followed by integrating sensor data with other business data (47%), and forecasting trends (41%).

11.4   Conclusion

In this chapter, 45 publications on AI's contribution to medical IoT devices are reviewed. According to the present research, AI's contribution to medical IoT devices has successfully assisted needy people. As new technologies emerge, medical IoT is becoming more complex, and AI is the primary pillar of a medical IoT device for healthcare automation.

References

[1]   Holzinger, A., Langs, G., Denk, H., Zatloukal, K., and Müller, H. "Causability and explainability of artificial intelligence in medicine", *Wiley Interdisciplinary Reviews: Data Mining and Knowledge Discovery*, vol. 9, no. 4, p. e1312, 2019.

[2]   Sethi, G.K., Ahmad, N., Rehman, M.B., Dafallaa, H.M.E.I., and Rashid, M., "Use of artificial intelligence in healthcare systems: state-of-the-art survey",

In *2021 2nd International* Conference *on* Intelligent Engineering *and* Management *(ICIEM)* (pp. 243–248), 2021, IEEE.

[3] Rashid, M., Singh, H., and Goyal, V., "The use of machine learning and deep learning algorithms in functional magnetic resonance imaging—a systematic review", *Expert Systems*, vol. 37, no. 6, p. e12644, 2020.

[4] Zhang, B., Zhu, J., and Su, H. "Toward the third generation artificial intelligence", *Science China Information Sciences,* vol. 66, no. 2, pp. 1–19, 2023.

[5] Kumar, S., Tiwari, P., and Zymbler, M. "Internet of Things is a revolutionary approach for future technology enhancement: a review", *Journal of Big Data*, vol. 6, no. 1, pp.1–21, 2019.

[6] Kumar, V., Tripathi, V., Pant, B., *et al.* "Hybrid spatiotemporal contrastive representation learning for content-based surgical video retrieval", *Electronics*, vol. 11, no. 9, p.1353, 2022.

[7] Habibzadeh, H., Dinesh, K., Shishvan, O.R., Boggio-Dandry, A., Sharma, G., and Soyata, T., "A survey of healthcare Internet of Things (HioT): a clinical perspective", *IEEE Internet of Things Journal*, vol. 7, no. 1, pp. 53–71, 2019.

[8] Jan, A., Parah, S.A., Malik, B.A., and Rashid, M. "Secure data transmission in IoTs based on CloG edge detection", *Future Generation Computer Systems*, vol. 121, pp. 59–73, 2021.

[9] Nord, J.H., Koohang, A., and Paliszkiewicz, J. "The Internet of Things: review and theoretical framework", *Expert Systems with Applications*, vol. 133, pp. 97–108, 2019.

[10] Van Leeuwen, K.G., de Rooij, M., Schalekamp, S., van Ginneken, B., and Rutten, J.C.M., "How does artificial intelligence in radiology improve efficiency and health outcomes?", *Pediatric Radiology*, vol. 52, pp. 2087–2093, 2022, https://doi.org/10.1007/s00247-021-05114-8.

[11] Beckers, R., Kwade, Z., and Zanca, F., "The EU medical device regulation: Implications for artificial intelligence-based medical device software in medical physics", *Physica Medica*, vol. 83, pp. 1–8, 2021, https://doi.org/10.1016/j.ejmp.2021.02.011.

[12] Ghosh, T., Al Banna, Md.H., Rahman, Md.S., *et al.*, "Artificial intelligence and internet of things in screening and management of autism spectrum disorder", *Sustainable Cities and Society*, vol. 74, 103189, 2021, https://doi.org/10.1016/j.scs.2021.103189.

[13] Muehlematter, U.J, Daniore, P., and Vokinger, K.N., "Approval of artificial intelligence and machine learning-based medical devices in the USA and Europe (2015–20): a comparative analysis", *The Lancet Digital Health*, vol. 3, no. 3, pp. e195–e203, 2021, doi:10.1016/S2589-7500(20)30292-2.

[14] Rastogi, R., Singhal, P., Chaturvedi, D.K., and Gupta, M. "Investigating correlation of tension-type headache and diabetes: IoT perspective in health care", in: Chakraborty, C., Banerjee, A., Kolekar, M., Garg, L., Chakraborty, B. (eds), *Internet of Things for Healthcare Technologies. Studies in Big Data*, vol. 73. Springer, Singapore.

[15] Raj, J.S., "Optimized mobile edge computing framework for IoT based medical sensor network nodes", *Journal of Ubiquitous Computing and*

Communication Technologies, vol. 3, no. 1, pp. 33–42, 2021, https://doi.org/ 10.36548/jucct.2021.1.004.

[16]   Badnjević, A., Avdihodžić, H., and Gurbeta Pokvić, L., "Artificial intelligence in medical devices: past, present and future", *Psychiatr Danub*, vol. 33 (Suppl 3), pp. S336–S341, 2021, PMID: 34010259.

[17]   Abir, S.M.A.A., Islam, S.N., Anwar, A., Mahmood, A.N., and Oo, A.M.T, "Building resilience against COVID-19 pandemic using artificial intelligence, machine learning, and IoT: a survey of recent progress", *IoT*, vol. 1, no.2, pp. 506–528, 2020, https://doi.org/10.3390/IoT1020028.

[18]   Iskanderani, A.I., Mehedi, I.M., Jeza Aljohani, A., *et al.*, "Artificial intelligence and medical Internet of Things framework for diagnosis of coronavirus suspected cases", *Journal of Healthcare Engineering*, vol. 2021, 3277988, 2021, https://doi.org/10.1155/2021/3277988.

[19]   Ahmad, Z., Rahim, S., Zubair, M., and Abdul-Ghafar, J., "Artificial intelligence (AI) in medicine, current applications and future role with special emphasis on its potential and promise in pathology: present and future impact, obstacles including costs and acceptance among pathologists, practical and philosophical considerations. A comprehensive review", *Diagnostic Pathology*, vol. 16, 24, 2021, https://doi.org/10.1186/s13000-021-01085-4.

[20]   Fouad Mansour, R., El Amraoui, A., Nouaouri, I., García Díaz, V., Gupta, D., and Kumar, S., "Artificial intelligence and Internet of Things enabled disease diagnosis model for smart healthcare systems", *IEEE Access,* vol. 9, pp. 45137–45146, 2021.

[21]   Abdullah, Y.I., Schuman, J.S., Shabsigh, R., Caplan, A., and Al-Aswad, L. A., "Ethics of artificial intelligence in medicine and ophthalmology", *Asia-Pacific Journal of Ophthalmology*, vol. 10, no. 3, pp. 289–298, 2021, https:// doi.org/10.1097/APO.0000000000000397.

[22]   VikramPuri, A.K. and Sharma, V., "Artificial intelligence-powered decentralized framework for Internet of Things in healthcare 4.0", *Transactions on Emerging Telecommunications Technologies*, e4245, 2021, doi:10.1002/ett.4245.

[23]   Yoo, H., Park, R.C., and Chung, K., "IoT-based health big-data process technologies: a survey", *KSII Transactions on Internet and Information Systems*, vol. 15, no. 3, pp. 974–992, 2021, https://doi.org/10.3837/tiis.2021. 03.009.

[24]   Amit, K., and Chakraborty, C., "Artificial Intelligence and Internet of Things based healthcare 4.0 monitoring system", *Wireless Personal Communications*, vol. 127, pp. 1615–1631, 2022, https://doi.org/10.1007/s11277-021-08708-5.

[25]   Komal, Sethi, G.K., Ahmad, N., *et al.*, "Use of artificial intelligence in healthcare systems:state-of-the-art survey", In *2021 2nd International Conference on Intelligent Engineering and Management (ICIEM).*, pp. 243–248, 2021.

[26]   Barnawi, A., Chhikara, P., Tekchandani, R., Kumar, N., and Alzahrani, B. "Artificial intelligence-enabled Internet of Things-based system for COVID-19 screening using aerial thermal imaging", *Future Generation Computer Systems*, vol. 124, pp. 119–132, 2021, https://doi.org/10.1016/j.future.2021.05.019.

[27] Oniani, S., Marques, G., Barnovi, S., Miguel Pires, I., and Kumar Bhoi, A., "Artificial intelligence for Internet of Things and enhanced medical systems", in *Advances in Intelligent Systems and Computing*, vol. 1227, pp. 29–45, 2021, https://doi.org/10.1007/978-981-15-5495-7_3.

[28] Yu, H. and Zhou, Z., "Optimization of IoT-based artificial intelligence assisted telemedicine health analysis system?", *IEEE Access*, vol. 9, pp. 118521–118529, 2021, https://doi.org/10.1109/ACCESS.2021.3088262.

[29] Mao, Y. and Zhang, L., "Optimization of the medical service consultation system based on the artificial intelligence of the Internet of Things", IEEE Access, vol. 9, pp. 134722–134730, 2021, https://doi.org/10.1109/ACCESS.2021.3096188.

[30] Ardito, C., Di Noia, T., Di Sciascio, E., Lofù, D., Pazienza, A., and Vitulano, F., "An artificial intelligence cyberattack detection system to improve threat reaction in e-Health", ITASEC21: Italian Conference on Cybersecurity, 2021, doi:10.5772/intechopen.97196.

[31] Makridis, C., Hurley, S., Klote, M., and Alterovitz, G., "Ethical applications of artificial intelligence: evidence from health research on veterans", *JMIR Medical Informatics*, vol. 9, no. 6, p. e28921, 2021, https://medinform.jmir.org/2021/6/e28921.

[32] Sestino, A. and De Mauro, A., "Leveraging artificial intelligence in business: implications, applications and methods", *Technology Analysis & Strategic Management*, vol. 34, no. 1, pp. 16–29, 2022, https://doi.org/10.1080/09537325.2021.1883583.

[33] Ilhan, B., Guneri, P., and Wilder-Smith, P., "The contribution of artificial intelligence to reducing the diagnostic delay in oral cancer", *Oral Oncology*, vol. 116, 105254, 2021, https://doi.org/10.1016/j.oraloncology.2021.105254.

[34] Gunasekeran, D.V., Wei Wen Tseng, R.M., Tham, Y.-C., and Yin Wong, T., "Applications of digital health for public health responses to COVID-19: a systematic scoping review of artificial intelligence, telehealth and related technologies", *npj Digital Medicine*, vol. 4, 40, 2021, https://doi.org/10.1038/s41746-021-00412-9.

[35] Babic, B., Gerke, S., Evgeniou, T., and Cohen, I.G., "Direct-to-consumer medical machine learning and artificial intelligence applications", *Nature Machine Intelligence*, vol. 3, pp. 283–287, 2021, https://doi.org/10.1038/s42256-021-00331-0.

[36] Fu, Z., Hong, S., Zhang, R., and Du, S., "Artificial-intelligence-enhanced mobile system for cardiovascular health management", *Sensors*, vol. 21, no. 3, 773, 2021, https://doi.org/10.3390/s21030773.

[37] Mathew, P.S. and Pillai, A.S., "Boosting traditional healthcare-analytics with deep learning AI: techniques, frameworks and challenges", in: Hassanien, AE., Taha, M.H.N., Khalifa, N.E.M. (eds), *Enabling AI Applications in Data Science. Studies in Computational Intelligence*, vol. 911. Springer, Cham, pp. 335–365, 2021, https://doi.org/10.1007/978-3-030-52067-0_15.

[38]   Saif, S., Datta, D., Saha, A., Biswas, A., and Chowdhury, C. "Data science and AI in IoT based smart healthcare: issues, challenges and case study", in: Hassanien, AE., Taha, M.H.N., Khalifa, N.E.M. (eds), *Enabling AI Applications in Data Science*. Studies in Computational Intelligence, vol. 911. Springer, Cham, pp. 415–439, 2021, https://doi.org/10.1007/978-3-030-52067-0_19.

[39]   Anceschi, E., Bonifazi, G., Callisto De Donato, M., Corradini, E., Ursino, D., and Virgili, L., "SaveMeNow.AI: a machine learning based wearable device for fall detection in a workplace", in: Hassanien, AE., Taha, M.H.N., Khalifa, N.E.M. (eds), *Enabling AI Applications in Data Science*. Studies in Computational Intelligence, vol. 911. Springer, Cham, pp. 493–514, 2021, https://doi.org/10.1007/978-3-030-52067-0_22.

[40]   Pradhan, K. and Chawla, P., "Medical Internet of things using machine learning algorithms for lung cancer detection", *Journal of Management Analytics*, vol. 7, no. 4, pp. 591–623, 2020, doi:10.1080/23270012.2020.1811789.

[41]   Chawla, N., "AI, IOT and wearable technology for smart healthcare – a review", *International Journal of Recent Research Aspects*, vol. 7, no. 1, pp. 9–13, 2020.

[42]   Cabitza, F. and Zeitoun, J.-D., "The proof of the pudding: in praise of a culture of real-world validation for medical artificial intelligence", *Annals of Translational Medicine*, vol. 7, no. 8, p. 161, 2019, http://dx.doi.org/10.21037/atm.2019.04.07.

[43]   Tran, V.-T., Riveros, C., and Ravaud, P., "Patients' views of wearable devices and AI in healthcare: findings from the ComPaRe e-cohort", *npj Digital Medicine*, vol. 2, 53, 2019, https://doi.org/10.1038/s41746-019-0132-y.

[44]   Davenport, T. and Kalakota, R., "The potential for artificial intelligence in healthcare", *Future Healthcare Journal*, vol. 6, no. 2, pp. 94–98, 2019, https://www.ncbi.nlm.nih.gov/pmc/articles/PMC6616181/.

Section 3

Applications of artificial intelligence in healthcare

Chapter 12

Internet automation indulgence of virtual reality in psychiatric health disorder

Shweta Pandey[1], Samta Kathuria[1], Rajesh Singh[2] and Anita Gehlot[2]

As a therapeutic technique in psychology and psychiatry, virtual reality (VR) has been utilized increasingly often. VR therapies have become more widely used in recent years in diseases like anxiety, panic, and phobias. To determine future directions to develop the science in this area, a thorough synthesis and critical assessment of the literature have not yet been conducted. To carry out a comprehensive analysis of reviews to expansively characterize the articles to date concerning the use of VR in treating psychiatric conditions, categorize the same research limitations that have already been done, recommend future study directions to identify the gaps, and offer helpful advice for integrating VR into treatments for mental disorders. The primary aim of this paper is to evaluate the research on the practice of VR in the behavior of a diverse range of psychiatric diseases, with an emphasis on visibility interventions for mental illnesses. To find research using VR-based therapy for depression or other mental diseases, a thorough literature search was carried out. With respect to the study region, the influence is defined variously. Therefore, given the ongoing advancements in VR technology and software, it is indeed crucial to give additional recommendations concerning how to integrate VR into mental healthcare as well as for the future trends of VR-based medical research and therapy.

12.1 Introduction

There are still a lot of people who struggle with this kind of issue, with advances in our understanding of the causes of mental diseases as well as more accessibility to professionals who deal with their therapy and treatment needs. The total incidence rate of a common mental condition (anxiety attack, mental issue, chronic depression, or drug use illnesses) was calculated to be 29.2% [1] in the comprehensive

[1]Law College of Dehradun, Uttaranchal University, Dehradun, India
[2]Uttaranchal Institute of Technology, Uttaranchal University, Dehradun, India

study and meta-analysis released in 2014 by Steel *et al.* Several somatic disorders are accompanied by depression disorder, being both the root and the result of such ailments. This dilemma has an impact on a variety of chronic medical illnesses that call for protracted therapy or a permanent lifestyle change, including cardiovascular disease [2], insulin [3], and obesity, among others. Psychological problems interfere with the implementation of lifestyle adjustments aimed at improving one's health [4]. Psychotherapy of individuals with disabilities, like stroke rehabilitation, may reveal a similar dependence. Physical treatment is substantially less effective when there are behavioral disturbances present, which frequently leads to long-term incapacity and dependency on others (family or institutions).

In the initial mental health use, VR technology has swiftly improved. The speed of digital hardware has dramatically increased, along with the accuracy of head-mounted displays. Rather more crucially, the technologies are now much more affordable, which has led to the creation of application areas. Considering interactivity is the core goal of VR, it stands to reason it as technology advances and allows for more interaction, the medicinal values of VR should likewise grow even "low tech" settings (such as VR-based computer games) have had positive outcomes [5]. Though they are aware that the settings are not genuine, subjects are already feeling their effects [6].

VR is a technical interface that enables people to interact with device surroundings in a secure environment. In medical research as well as in the setting of psychological health therapy, technological method has become more prevalent. This chapter's main objective is to examine the data on VR's efficacy in psychiatric therapy, with a focus on mental illnesses in particular. Due to its ability to provide users with a sensation of participation and engrossment in the dreaded environment, VR is highly suited to be utilized in visibility therapy for mental illnesses. We will also go through the possible benefits and drawbacks of employing VR in mental research and therapy, along with offering helpful suggestions for integrating VR within psychotherapy. An effective virtual experience gives the consumer a feeling of presence, like they are literally submerged in the digital world. To create this impression, "realistic" sensations are blocked, leaving only device sensations visible and audible. Technology provides sensory feedback using data gloves or other input methods. Sound, touch, and aroma are just a few of the several sensory perceptions that add to the realism of the sensation.

12.2   Benefits of VR in psychiatric treatment and research

The ability of patients to successfully visualize particular fearful sensations is a prerequisite for imaginable exposures in conventional exposure treatment. Patients who have trouble visualizing or envisioning things are no longer at risk because of virtual reality. In contrast to VR techniques, in vivo acquaintances could be classy like a real flight) or prohibitive to carry out (which includes warfare in Iraq or Afghanistan), it is also possible to create exposures that might be challenging to apply in vivo. With VR-based exposure therapy (VRE), experiences could be deployed in ways that may not be practical in material life, by repeatedly simulating a fly landing. A therapist can promise no turbulence, as one, if a sufferer with a phobia of flies is not prepared for it. In performing exposures, secrecy may be maintained using VR methods, which might not be possible with in vivo risks.

Patient satisfaction using VR-based therapy has been shown to be high, but some patients might also find it more agreeable than conventional methods. An early chapter on VRE for people who post-traumatic disorder (PTSD) brought on by auto accidents found that patients had a really positive attitude about the therapy [7]. Its refusal incidence for VR exposure (3%) is much lower than it is in exposure (27%) in a cohort of 150 patients having particular phobias [8], suggesting that patients may find VR-based exposure relatively tolerable. One research in a PTSD population revealed that VRE and imaginal exposure were equally satisfying, but another indicated that VRE was more satisfying. A majority of the 352 US troops who participated in the study after 9/11 said they would be prepared to adopt the majority of the digital techniques for mental health care that were examined (e.g., VR) [9]. There are VR methods for getting mental health care, indicating that VR could be able to remove certain treatment-related obstacles.

If individuals can be very present in circumstances that distress them, VR offers incredible potential to assist in overcoming mental health issues shown in Figure 12.1 that what are the barriers and benefits of adopting VR in mental health. The core of mental health problems is difficulty in direct interaction with the outside world [e.g., becoming arachnophobia causes great anxiety among animals, post-traumatic stress disorder (PTSD) causes powerful flashes with recollections of previous trauma, hallucinations cause living in dread of assault from everyone, and

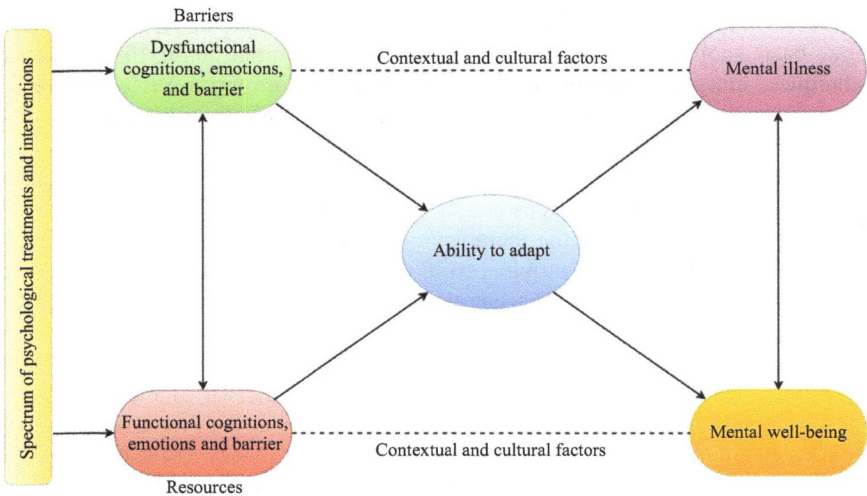

Figure 12.1   Ability to adopt VR in psychiatric treatment

alcoholic problems cause denying the need to take extra]. Rehabilitation consequently focuses on responding, perceiving, and looking different in these circumstances. Therapies that empower individuals to implement these adjustments in actual circumstances are the most beneficial. Using VR, people may experience realistic simulations of challenging circumstances and receive coaching on how to respond appropriately based on the most end theories of the particular disease. The simulations may be played again with varying degrees of difficulty until the desired learning is achieved. With the flip of a switch, unpleasant scenarios that are difficult to identify in real life might become a reality. The benefit of VR is that even when people are aware that their surroundings is digital and not realistic, their minds and bodies feel it as existing in the real world. Like a result, patients may experiment with novel therapy techniques also deal with challenging circumstances far more readily in VR than that in real life. The knowledge may subsequently be applied in real-world situations. For some diseases, it could be conceivable to do away with the requirement for any therapy, yet for other disorders; the amount of time necessary for experienced therapists might be significantly cut back. VR might therefore facilitate better access to the best psychiatric therapies. With its settee gone, headsets could soon be the preferred way of psychological therapy.

12.3   Treatment method for VRE

By replacing VR with all other exposures or activities, VR-based cognitive therapy basically follows the same path as standard therapies. VRE usually starts with two to three first sessions that go over the following topics: psycho-education on the individual disease, psychosocial history, a summary of resistance or the case for exposure, or the procedure for VR-based risks. Many VRE therapies also incorporate basic soothing or coping techniques during the initial phase, like relaxation techniques, muscle relaxation, or psychotherapy. Performing a VR exposure for each session after that usually involves the patient moving through a sequence of graded exposures at their own speed.

The patient-specific nature of quality VRE provide solutions to complex cases. For instance, the hierarchy's steps can be carried out repeatedly until the patient's subjective distress level and the therapist's own observations show a considerable reduction in anxiety. Before moving on to the next phase in the graded exposure, the therapist should talk with the patient about each step as they go through the hierarchy. Since customized VR system material is created for various illnesses and special emotional trauma or phobias, material content that is accessible for a phobia hierarchy is frequently chosen for VR exposures. In advance of the exposure, a comprehensive examination of the patient's anxiety or unique traumatic event is necessary to individualize how they move through the hierarchy's levels or the duration of time they spend with various content. For example, the hierarchy of fly phobias has eight phases, from strolling through the departure lounge to taking off during a turbulence-filled rainstorm.

Taxiing and take-off could be a key area of treatment for a client with panic and agoraphobia, including an emphasis on certain triggers connected to these disorders (e.g., the sound of the cabin door closing). In fact, traveling during a hurricane or turbulence might be a central priority for a patient with a particular anxiety about flying which is brought on by an inherent dread of the plane hitting. A detailed evaluation of the patient's baseline trauma enables the psychotherapist to create in advance the exact VR application (like Virtual Iraq) or the precise location and stimulation (such as the time of day or certain weapon sounds) to be utilized with PTSD patients.

The patient will be actively involved in triggering the fear structure during a high-quality VR exposure by the therapist. Therapists should encourage and facilitate feelings in VR or, as necessary, talk about ways to get past any unsafe or unpleasant behavior. Precisely, the psychologist should evaluate the justification for exposed, emphasize the value of not engaging in such behaviors, and assist the patient to psychologically engage even during overexposure because patients may attempt to take part in safety behaviors (e.g., reiterating a particular catchphrase all through take-off in simulated flight), loss of concentration, or energetic cognitive therapy during VR-based risks.

12.4   Methodology

We will now examine the research on the use of VR in the therapy of different psychiatric diseases, with an emphasis on W3exposure-based interventions for mental illnesses. PsycINFO, MDPI, MEDLINE, SCIENCE DIRECT, and Google Scholar were all used for systematic searches. Virtual reality, VR-based exposure therapy, device exposure, virtual reality with mental health therapy, behavioral, depression, neurological condition, phobias, chronic anxiety, post-traumatic stress disorder fear, social phobia, altitude fear, obsessive–compulsive disorder mood disorders, schizophrenia, delusions, pain, alcoholism, binge eating, lack of appetite, and autism were among the relevant keywords used. Studies with references to VR-based psychiatric therapy in the title, abstract, or keywords were found. Psychiatric patients who got VR-based treatment were included in the chapter that we reviewed. Studies that do not provide assessments of treatment outcomes were disregarded. We did not demand randomized (or semi) nor controlled experiments because many VR-based technologies are still in the early stages of development.

12.5   Results

12.5.1   Anxiety disorder

A patient with social anxiety disorder (SAD) feels anxious while engaging in social engagements (such as discussions, interacting with new people, or public speeches) in which they could be assessed or socially appraised by others [10]. VR-based therapies for SAD frequently employ device social contexts with virtual audiences, such as schools, auditoriums, and meeting rooms. Two RCTs that looked at generalized SAD discovered that VR-based CBT was more efficacious than the normal control and on par with standard CBT [11]. VR-based CBT for stage fright has produced results comparable to standard CBT and superior than controls [12], as benefits persisted a year after therapy. Lastly, preliminary studies indicate that VR can effectively cure anxiety levels and other types of anxiety that are related to education. The structure is shown in Figure 12.2 as how VR helps to remove generalized anxiety disorders.

But generally speaking, VR therapies appear to be equally as effective as their face-to-face equivalents. The order to improve its performance has been demonstrated in conceptual to be high, providing evidence that the therapeutic benefits transcend to the real life, with the caveat about the quality of the findings [13]. Treatment benefits for these brief interventions have impressively been demonstrated to last for several years when lengthy follow-ups were added. There are signs that drop-out statistics may be reduced with VR therapies, but this might just be a production control issue with the implementation of face-to-face therapies. The variety of VR-like techniques that have been employed is broad, ranging from big projects ranging to the computer-assisted research environment (CAREN)

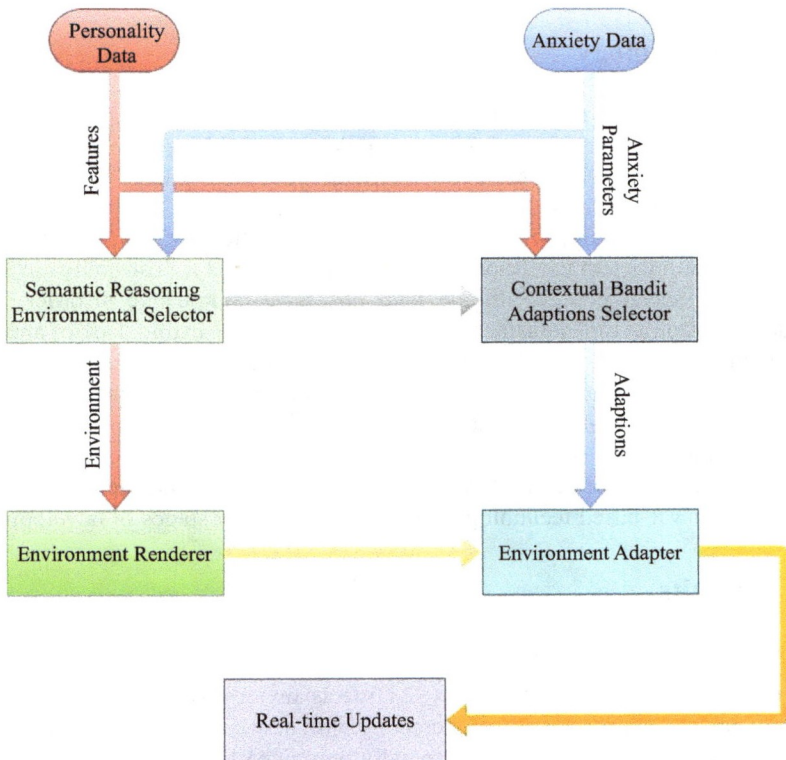

Figure 12.2   Structure of VR in helping to treat generalized anxiety disorder

system, where the user does have a moving platform encircled by a 360° monitor, to CAVEs, training missions, or HMDs. Some publications would not specify the sensitive to the specific techniques that were applied. Anxiety seems to be more likely to arise the stronger the experience of participation in VR that is attained [14]. It is crucial to remember the role that hearing plays in creating a sense of existence in virtual reality. Though they are necessary, in-depth research on the optimal ways to display information in VR is far too seldom, in our perspective.

12.5.2 Fear of height

In the middle to late 1990s, experiments using VR on people with height anxiety were done [15]. These were the initial proof that by utilizing VR, one may lessen their fear of heights. Rothbaum *et al*. carried out the initial randomized investigation in 1995 [16]. In this study, 20 undergrads that fulfilled the DSM-IV diagnostic for a phobia of heights were randomized to either a waitlist control healthy controls or a VR technology-graded psychosocial intervention. The participants who were part of the therapy group went to seven weekly VR immersion sessions. Increased levels of difficulty were offered for three separate scenarios (a footbridge, an outdoor balcony, and a glass elevator) (e.g., balcony on the ground, 10th, and 12th floors). The VR procedure was completed by 10 individuals. Compared to the seven participants from the surviving waiting list group, they displayed vast improvements in anxiousness, aversion, beliefs, and distress related to exposure to altitudes. It is uncertain if these outcomes were entirely attributable to the VR exposure because 7 out of the 10 students who recently achieved the psychotherapy also engaged in self-directed in vivo conditions at that time.

12.5.3 Panic disorder and agoraphobia

A rapid surge of anxiety, such as that experienced by people with panic disorder and agoraphobia (PDA), is characterized by physical (like chest pains, sweating, and choking feelings) plus mental (like overthinking, worry of death) experiences. These symptoms cause individuals who suffer from or be afraid of particular locations or circumstances [17]. VRE for PDA simulates scenarios including tunnels, parking spaces, meeting places, and motorways that frequently cause anxiety episodes. Early data from various baseline designs indicated some preliminary evidence in favor of using VR to treat PDA. While RCTs have typically concluded that VRE for PDA is effective, research on the similarities between VRE and conventional exposure treatment has been inconsistent. For treating PDA symptoms, the majority of studies have demonstrated that VRE is just as effective as conventional exposure treatment. The results of certain studies point to the possibility that VRE is comparable to standard exposure therapy, especially when looking at lengthy outcomes, and could even lead to greater therapeutic responses with fewer therapeutic options being necessary. The conclusion is that any progressively superior outcomes could show up at an early stage of treatment. For 3, 6, 9, and 12 months [18,19], the comparable, relatively long therapy effect of VRE vs. conventional methods have held constant. The effectiveness of these techniques for treating PDA has been confirmed by the research on VR-based exposures for PDA utilizing a strict study approach and methods. Additionally, VR-based CBT for PDA offers a number of benefits, along with a better therapeutic efficacy as well as a shorter treatment period.

12.5.4   Obsessive–compulsive disorder

Obsessive–compulsive disorder (OCD) is distinguished by anxious thoughts, ideas, or emotions that induce discomfort (e.g., a desire for harmony, a dread of contagion), or corrective repeated activities that relieve anxiety (e.g., obsessive cleaning, precise arrangement of objects). While two studies look at the capacity of VR to evoke unpleasant responses in OCD patients, no RCTs have yet evaluated the effectiveness of VR in curing OCD [20]. According to the results of those experiments, OCD sufferers were more likely than controls to experience anxiety when exposed to VRE versions of the triggers they dreaded (as no diagnosis). Second, the degree of participants' immersion in their perception of how much individuals were visible in the virtual environment was strongly correlated to their level of anxiety.

This finding implies that VR situations must be plausible and pertinent to the patient's worries. Like GAD, different individuals experience compulsions and addictions for different reasons, which makes it challenging to create all-inclusive VR programs that cater to the requirements of every sufferer. The challenges are increased by the fact that several individuals have such a variety of phobias and related comprehension. VR may not be required for OCD, though, as many of the dreaded stressors may be easily available in the surroundings (such as lavatories) or patient's thoughts of making mistakes. Facing major challenges, OCD patients who have preoccupations that are too challenging or inappropriate for standard psychotherapy may benefit from adopting VR during treatments (e.g., exposure to restrooms). Continued study in this area is necessary given the modest but encouraging evidence regarding VR-based CBT treating OCD.

12.5.5   Body image disturbance

The 28 obese females receiving permanent weight management therapy were selected at random to one of the VR psychotherapy or the "psychonutritional" groupings using a positivist paradigm in a controlled trials experiment [21]. All of the patients were following a calorie-restricted fitness regime. Participants in the VR indicate that positive more than those in the "psychonutritional" category in terms of body pleasure, consciousness, and motivation for change. There was no follow-up therefore in trial, thus it was impossible to determine if improvements persisted.

In a companion trial, Riva *et al.* [22] selected randomly 20 obsessive disorder sufferers to groups that either received VR-based treatment or CBT-based psychonutritional interventions. Even while VR-based psychotherapy was more successful in enhancing physical health satisfaction, consciousness, as facilitate change, it exhibited no additional success at curbing emotional eating.

The most randomized placebo-controlled study to date, involving 211 patients who were morbidly obese, was just completed by Riva *et al.* [23]. According to past investigations, this experiment evaluated cognitive-behavioral (CBT), nutritional, and experiential cognitive therapy (ECT) methods with housing list controls. Dietician-led dietary groups were held five times a week for patients in the NT class. The NT group received so same care as the CBT patients, plus 15 more treatments spread across 6 weeks. The CT team received the same care as the NT side in additional to 15 extra meetings, including ten 60-minute, twice-weekly virtual reality sessions. Two physical health comparison regions and scenarios relevant to processes for maintaining and relapsing from obesity were provided in the VR settings. There was absolutely no variation in either losing weight and the key psychological characteristics between the waiting list individuals or any of the three groups, which all lost weight considerably more than the standby list people did anxiety & body satisfaction. Contrary to other treatments, interactive CT led to gains in identity and body image contentment at the 6-month follow-up.

12.5.6 Acute and chronic pain

Cognitive diversion is frequently used as a component of pain therapy in an effort to divert attention and concentrate it aside from uncomfortable medical interventions since the feeling of pain necessitates full attention. VR has been investigated as a means of facilitating neuropathic diversion during uncomfortable treatments, like burn-related discomfort or physiotherapy. As patients are all in VR while in occupational therapy, their subjective stress ratings were decreased, according to a preliminary experiment utilizing a small group of four burn victims [24]. More evidence suggesting VR distractions may be helpful in reducing pain during grueling surgical treatments was revealed by a scenario study that followed in a young terminally ill patient [25]. In a within-subjects randomized experiment comparing standard analgesia with standard analgesia plus a VR game, it was discovered the former was much more effective at lowering reaction in children receiving burnt rehabilitation. In a controlled study equating virtual reality to all other deflection methods, it was discovered that while VR seemed to be considerably more effective at minimizing interpretive pain severity compared to other diversion methods (such as music, childcare workers, and TV with headphones), it was neither infinitely greater to television viewing. Patients in fMRI research studying the effect of VR on pain-related neural activity reportedly reported less energy wondering about pain but less pain intensity, as their brain's activity in areas that deal with both psychological and sensory pain was massively reduced [26]. These results do provide positivist and interpretive evidence that VR methods could help people feel less pain.

In complement to cognitive or behavioral therapies that are already in place, VR has been utilized to assist people suffering from chronic pain in studying and practicing pain-management skills. This is because VR may indeed be able to assist those who have not responded to conventional treatments or can offer the opportunity to standardize directions and stimulation. Preliminary data reveal that such a system is far more successful than non-VR contemplation in lowering subjectively pain. A VR approach for chronic back pain patients has already been created in which sufferers undergo a simulated meditation stroll to acquire mindfulness-based reducing stress. In a study of fibromyalgia patients, this was discovered that using VR in conjunction with activity-management therapy, which would include VR-based meetings incorporating action guidelines, motivation augmentation, struggling to overcome exercise barriers, and acknowledging individual skills is significantly more successful than standard care at reducing functional deficits.

In summary, studies suggest that VR combined with conventional pharmaceutical pain treatment can be more successful than conventional analgesics alone in lowering perceived symptom severity particularly quick, intense pain during medical procedures. Even though the method underlying this finding is not yet known [27], it is likely linked to cognitive distractions. Proposed experiments may look into the molecular mechanisms underlying that result. As per the initial study, VR may also be useful in teaching and practicing particular anguish approaches, of that kind insight of meditation or activity control, for those who have chronic pain.

12.5.7 Schizophrenia

Though the majority of studies examining the use of virtual reality in psychiatric treatment have concentrated on anxiety disorders, such a therapeutic strategy has shown promise in the therapy for other diseases. Schizophrenia is a serious mental disorder that involves psychotic symptoms (such as psychotic episodes), disturbances to regular anxiety and depression behavior (such as flat emotion, less pleasurable experiences, solitude), as problems with mental abilities [17]. There is little research on VR as a therapeutic component in these demographic, but early results are encouraging.

VR treatment for schizophrenia has featured social environments where patients might proactive basis techniques and learn coping mechanisms for societal suffering brought on by erroneous beliefs. Inside a short RCT, it was discovered that integrating exposure and cognitive treatment and VR-based social situations reduced either hallucination delusions and suffering during in-person socializing [28]. Two of the three research that employed VR as a supplement to social skills training (SST) for individuals with schizophrenia were uncontained pilot studies that offer early evidence of the effectiveness of this strategy in encouraging social skills & interaction [29]. The RCT of 91 patients with schizophrenia discovered that SST with VR elements boosted interest in SST, generalized treatment-related abilities, as improved patients' capacity for conversation and assertiveness, even if conventional SST patients had higher gestural social skills [30]. Despite the small amount of available data and the aforementioned obstacles to social communication exposure, these early findings are encouraging.

12.5.8 Eating pathology

VR techniques have been utilized to manage body-image issues as well as eating, posture, and weight concerns in various kinds of eating disorders. VR has been utilized to investigate and confront body part aberrations, to expose people to food signals in a way to discover and address eating, shaping, and weight issues, and to practice more successful eating behaviors. An early study explored patient eating, form, and weight opinions and worries using various distinct VR settings, comprising domestic rooms with food products, and also employed pictures of diverse body kinds to settle disparities in patients' impressions of their own bodies [31]. The findings provided early evidence that these techniques increased body consciousness in obese and binge-eating syndrome individuals.

A regulated follow-up study of 28 obese persons randomly assigned to VR therapy or organizations that use CBT discovered that VR therapy caused much higher incremental enhancements in physique comfort, concern degree, and troublesome consumption [21]. There were no substantial distinctions in self-identity or phases of improvement in psycho-therapy between the two different groups. A clinical study includes a total of 13 eating disorders clients trying to compare body physique CBT using virtual reality disruptions to conventional CBT found that VR-based CBT resulted in substantially having greater advancement in body-image perturbations; no distinctions in eating-disorder symptomatology were found between the two sets [21]. In a careful experiment comparing CBT for unhealthy eating containing and without a component of VR-based methods focus, the VR group exhibited greater improvement at intervention period or one adopt; however, it is worth noting that the VR group might well have received greater diversified treatments. Similarly, the present research provides little proof of the usefulness of adding VR into therapy for different disorders connected with disordered eating and overweight concerns; results imply that VR may simply result in restoration responses equivalent to standard CBT procedures or may lead to higher recovery for some particular outcomes.

12.5.9   Posttraumatic stress disorder

PTSD is characterized by a record of encounters with a harrowing incident as well as signs of interference, denial, negative changes in thought patterns and emotions, and changes in attention and responsiveness [17]. Numerous studies show that VRE for PTSD offers a format rehabilitative effect size and produces improved treatment outcomes over the waiting list control system, and results equivalent to conventional exposure therapy. Initial case studies [32] and open-trial layouts spanning a wide spectrum of traumatic situations [33] showed that this therapy method might be effective in treating PTSD. Early research comparing VR-based psychosocial interventions for PTSD after the World Trade Center attacks discovered that the VR group showed a substantial decrease in PTSD ratings relative to the wait-list group, and that the recovery was sustained at a six-month follow-up evaluation [34].

The results demonstrated both statistical and clinical significance. Baseline ratings in both categories were in the serious range, however, the average post-treatment score for the VR group fell within the moderate range. Moreover, seven out of the ten participants in the VR group confirmed that they no longer met the conditions for PTSD investigation. Although no substantial effect was seen for depressing signs or overall distress, both groups' starting ratings were quite low. The sample used for this study was not truly demographically representative, mainly consisting of mid-aged individuals, however, respondents' awareness of attack vectors varied among groups such as fire crews, disaster laborers, and citizens. This suggests that the standardized virtual stimulation was effective in engaging people with a diverse range of potentially traumatic personal experiences.

12.5.10   Autism

Autism spectrum disorder (ASD) is a neurological disease characterized by repetitive or limiting behavioral patterns, along with difficulties involving social interactions and engagement. The research on the effectiveness of VR in the rehabilitation of ASD provides just a small amount of assistance for social development. Lahiri *et al.* [35] revealed data supporting the use of a VR-based device exercise to improve social graces in autistic youth.

Moreover, the significance of the findings is put into question due to the chapter limited sample size or confirmation technique. The study sample was modest, and the degree of ASD was restricted. So, because the activity used a menu-driven communications network that needed a specific degree of reading skills, the investigators only included autistic teens with medium or above-average intelligence, restricting the sample's generalizability. Interference research has shown relative gains in a theorem of mind, emotion detection, and effective communication [36]. All of the research described show low drop-out rates and indicates that VR is widely accepted [35–37]. Ultimately, preliminary research suggests that VR might be safely and efficiently included in ASD psychiatric therapy.

12.6   Recommendations for integrating VR into psychiatric care

- VR is used at the point of therapy where in utero exposure would normally be used. A common VR prescription for the phobia of flying, for instance, teaches stress management approaches in the initial four meetings, and integrates VR experience to a simulated airport and aeroplane during the final four meetings. To properly incorporate VR into mental therapy, certain technology and training are required. AVR systems generally involve a head-mounted device and a podium (for the sufferers), as well as a laptop with two monitoring devices for the supplier's interface, within which he or she produces the dosage in a timely manner, one for the supplier's initiates of the person's placement in the VR configuration exposure, and a third for the supplier's perspective of the patient's movement in the virtual space.
- It has been advised that sensitivity management initiatives for patients and VR comprise (a) testing processes to identify individuals who may pose significant hazards, (b) methods for regulating patient access to VR apps, and (c) processes for detecting unforeseen adverse effects. If sufferers get

overloaded and are not able to continue, therapeutic interventions should include mechanisms for temporarily discontinuing VR exposure. Likewise, protocols for determining if, how, and when they ought to be reinstated into the virtual experience must be devised.

- VR-specific teaching is a crucial factor for incorporating VR into psychiatric practice. VR providers offer both Internet-based VR treatment training classes and onsite, scheduled VR treatment training. Prior to employing VR modern technologies with patients, practitioners should be appropriately trained, especially via role acting. Provider education must include knowledge and practice on debugging difficulties inside sessions, as well as contact details for personnel from the VR supplier who might be able to assist with troubleshooting. Furthermore, providers should be adequately trained on the logic for introducing VR into psychiatric care, so that they can successfully convey that rationalization hence the legitimacy of the therapeutic strategy to patients.

- Because VR is most commonly utilized during exposure treatment for anxiety disorders, adequate exposure treatment training should indeed be viewed as a precondition for incorporating VR into patient care. There must also be ongoing monitoring and assistance for exposure treatment. Poor VR treatment is still poor therapy.

12.7   Recommendations for integrating VR into psychiatric care

As the experiments described this chapter demonstrates how VR technology may assist in the understanding, evaluation, and therapy of a wide range of clinical diseases. The possible advantages of virtual reality are numerous: virtual worlds are adaptable and configurable, and their application fits very well-known cognitive theory and practice. Patients are usually tolerant of the device, and there is solid evidence that individuals behave in virtual surroundings as when they are genuine.

According to traditional belief, it takes roughly 20 decades from the moment the original study is published for it to become popular usage. The first research employing virtual reality to treat a psychiatric condition was conducted in 1995, and now we are 20 years later! VR had already become an effective tool to aid in the treatment of a variety of abnormalities, with the strongest evidence supporting its use in exposure based for patients with borderline personality disorder, cue behavioral therapies for sick people with stimulant use disorders, and diversionary tactic for those suffering from acute pain needing invasive surgery. Generally, meta-analyses have shown that virtual reality is an effective tool that measures up to available therapies and has long-term benefits that generalize to the actual world. Furthermore, problems with previous studies have indeed been identified, such as limited sample numbers, a limitation of methodological quality, and a shortage of comparator groups. With the decreasing cost of head-mounted screens and the development of compact mobile apps, it is probable that VR tools will spread. It is critical that they are recognized as tools and that counselors are provided with training in their use.

References

[1]   Steel, Z., Marnane, C., Iranpour, C., *et al.* (2014). The global prevalence of common mental disorders: a systematic review and meta-analysis 1980–2013. *International Journal of Epidemiology*, 43(2), 476–493.

[2]   Dhar, A. K. and Barton, D. A. (2016). Depression and the link with cardiovascular disease. *Frontiers in Psychiatry*, 7, 33.

[3]   Sweileh, W. M. (2018). Analysis of global research output on diabetes depression and suicide. *Annals of General Psychiatry*, 17(1), 1–13.

[4]   Gilman, S. E., Sucha, E., Kingsbury, M., Horton, N. J., Murphy, J. M., and Colman, I. (2017). Depression and mortality in a longitudinal study: 1952–2011. *Cmaj*, 189(42), E1304–E1310.

[5]   Emmelkamp, P. M., Krijn, M., Hulsbosch, A. M., De Vries, S., Schuemie, M. J., and van der Mast, C. A. (2002). Virtual reality treatment versus exposure in vivo: a comparative evaluation in acrophobia. *Behaviour Research and Therapy*, 40(5), 509–516.

[6]   Walshe, D., Lewis, E., O'Sullivan, K., and Kim, S. I. (2005). Virtually driving: are the driving environments "real enough" for exposure therapy with accident victims? An explorative study. *CyberPsychology & Behavior*, 8(6), 532–537.

[7]   Beck, J. G., Palyo, S. A., Winer, E. H., Schwagler, B. E., and Ang, E. J. (2007). Virtual reality exposure therapy for PTSD symptoms after a road accident: an uncontrolled case series. *Behavior Therapy*, 38(1), 39–48.

[8]   Garcia-Palacios, A., Botella, C., Hoffman, H., and Fabregat, S. (2007). Comparing acceptance and refusal rates of virtual reality exposure vs. in vivo exposure by patients with specific phobias. *Cyberpsychology & Behavior*, 10(5), 722–724.

[9]   Wilson, J. A., Onorati, K., Mishkind, M., Reger, M. A., and Gahm, G. A. (2008). Soldier attitudes about technology-based approaches to mental health care. *CyberPsychology & Behavior*, 11(6), 767–769.

[10] Caponnetto, P., Triscari, S., Maglia, M., and Quattropani, M. C. (2021). The simulation game—virtual reality therapy for the treatment of social anxiety disorder: a systematic review. *International Journal of Environmental Research and Public Health*, 18(24), 13209.

[11] Klinger, E., Bouchard, S., Légeron, P., *et al.* (2005). Virtual reality therapy versus cognitive behavior therapy for social phobia: a preliminary controlled study. *Cyberpsychology & Behavior*, 8(1), 76–88.

[12] Anderson, P. L., Price, M., Edwards, S. M., *et al.* (2013). Virtual reality exposure therapy for social anxiety disorder: a randomized controlled trial. *Journal of Consulting and Clinical Psychology*, 81(5), 751.

[13] Ghayvat, H., Awais, M., Bashir, A. K., *et al.* (2022). AI-enabled radiologist in the loop: novel AI-based framework to augment radiologist performance for COVID-19 chest CT medical image annotation and classification from pneumonia. *Neural Computing and Applications*, 35, 1–19.

[14] Ling, Y., Nefs, H. T., Morina, N., Heynderickx, I., and Brinkman, W. P. (2014). A meta-analysis on the relationship between self-reported presence and anxiety in virtual reality exposure therapy for anxiety disorders. *PLoS One*, 9(5), e96144.

[15] Hodges, L. F., Kooper, R., Meyer, T. C., *et al.* (1995). Virtual environments for treating the fear of heights. *IEEE Computer*, 28(7), 27–34.

[16] Rothbaum, B. O., Hodges, L. F., Kooper, R., Opdyke, D., Williford, J. S., and North, M. (1995). Virtual reality graded exposure in the treatment of acrophobia: a case report. *Behavior Therapy*, 26(3), 547–554.

[17] American Psychiatric Association. (2013). Diagnostic c and Statistical Manual of Mental Disorders, *Arlington:* American Psychiatric Association.

[18] Peñate, W., Pitti, C. T., Bethencourt, J. M., de la Fuente, J., and Gracia, R. (2008). The effects of a treatment based on the use of virtual reality exposure and cognitive-behavioral therapy applied to patients with agoraphobia. *International Journal of Clinical and Health Psychology*, 8(1), 5–22.

[19] Choi, Y. H., Vincelli, F., Riva, G., *et al.* (2005). Effects of group experiential cognitive therapy for the treatment of panic disorder with agoraphobia. *CyberPsychology & Behavior*, 8(4), 387–393.

[20] Belloch, A., Cabedo, E., Carrió, C., *et al.* (2014). Virtual reality exposure for OCD: is it feasible?. *Revista de Psicopatología y Psicología Clínica*, 19(1), 37–44.

[21] Riva, G., Bacchetta, M., Baruffi, M., and Molinari, E. (2001). Virtual reality–based multidimensional therapy for the treatment of body image disturbances in obesity: a controlled study. *Cyberpsychology & Behavior*, 4(4), 511–526.

[22] Riva, G., Bacchetta, M., Baruffi, M., and Molinari, E. (2002). Virtual-reality-based multidimensional therapy for the treatment of body image disturbances in binge eating disorders: a preliminary controlled study. *IEEE Transactions on Information Technology in Biomedicine*, 6(3), 224–234.

[23] Riva, G., Bacchetta, M., Cesa, G., *et al.* (2006). Is severe obesity a form of addiction?: Rationale, clinical approach, and controlled clinical trial. *Cyberpsychology & Behavior*, 9(4), 457–479.

[24] Hoffman, H. G., Patterson, D. R., Carrougher, G. J., and Sharar, S. R. (2001). Effectiveness of virtual reality-based pain control with multiple treatments. *The Clinical Journal of Pain*, 17(3), 229–235.

[25] Rashid, M., Singh, H., and Goyal, V. (2023). FFTPSOGA: fast Fourier Transform with particle swarm optimization and genetic algorithm approach for pattern identification of brain responses in multi subject fMRI data. *Multimedia Tools and Applications*, 1–20.

[26] Hoffman, H. G., Richards, T. L., Coda, B., *et al.* (2004). Modulation of thermal pain-related brain activity with virtual reality: evidence from fMRI. *Neuroreport*, 15(8), 1245–1248.

[27] Sharar, S. R., Miller, W., Teeley, A., *et al.* (2008). Applications of virtual reality for pain management in burn-injured patients. *Expert Review of Neurotherapeutics*, 8(11), 1667–1674.

[28] Freeman, D., Bradley, J., Antley, A., *et al.* (2016). Virtual reality in the treatment of persecutory delusions: randomised controlled experimental

study testing how to reduce delusional conviction. *The British Journal of Psychiatry*, 209(1), 62–67.

[29]   Rus-Calafell, M., Gutiérrez-Maldonado, J., and Ribas-Sabaté, J. (2014). A virtual reality-integrated program for improving social skills in patients with schizophrenia: a pilot study. *Journal of Behavior Therapy and Experimental Psychiatry*, 45(1), 81–89.

[30]   Park, K. M., Ku, J., Choi, S. H., *et al.* (2011). A virtual reality application in role-plays of social skills training for schizophrenia: a randomized, controlled trial. *Psychiatry Research*, 189(2), 166–172.

[31]   Riva, G., Bacchetta, M., Baruffi, M., Rinaldi, S., Vincelli, F., and Molinari, E. (2000). Virtual reality–based experiential cognitive treatment of obesity and binge-eating disorders. *Clinical Psychology & Psychotherapy*, 7, 209–219.

[32]   Freedman, S. A., Hoffman, H. G., Garcia-Palacios, A., Weiss, P. L., Avitzour, S., and Josman, N. (2010). Prolonged exposure and virtual reality-enhanced imaginal exposure for PTSD following a terrorist bulldozer attack: a case study. *Cyberpsychology, Behavior, and Social Networking*, 13(1), 95–101.

[33]   Walshe, D. G., Lewis, E. J., Kim, S. I., O'Sullivan, K., and Wiederhold, B. K. (2003). Exploring the use of computer games and virtual reality in exposure therapy for fear of driving following a motor vehicle accident. *CyberPsychology & Behavior*, 6(3), 329–334.

[34]   Difede, J., Cukor, J., Jayasinghe, N., *et al.* (2007). Virtual reality exposure therapy for the treatment of posttraumatic stress disorder following September 11, 2001. *Journal of Clinical Psychiatry*, 68(11), 1639.

[35]   Rashid, M., Singh, H., and Goyal, V. (2020). The use of machine learning and deep learning algorithms in functional magnetic resonance imaging—a systematic review. *Expert Systems*, 37(6), e12644.

[36]   Kandalaft, M. R., Didehbani, N., Krawczyk, D. C., Allen, T. T., and Chapman, S. B. (2013). Virtual reality social cognition training for young adults with high-functioning autism. *Journal of Autism and Developmental Disorders*, 43(1), 34–44.

[37]   Mitchell, P., Parsons, S., and Leonard, A. (2007). Using virtual environments for teaching social understanding to 6 adolescents with autistic spectrum disorders. *Journal of Autism and Developmental Disorders*, 37(3), 589–600.

Chapter 13
Role of big data analytics in healthcare systems

Prathamesh Suhas Uravane[1], Vedant Vinay Ganthade[1], Adityaraj Sanjay Belhe[1], Abhiraj Sandeep Gadade[1] and Mamoon Rashid[1]

Generating data at an abundant scale has become a boon nowadays, as we see the shining side of its features and practicality but, data quality, integrating it with other physical, cloud systems, or storing this data could be impenetrable. Every sector including finance, retail, government, and technology produces giant lofts of data every year. But the data produced by the healthcare sector is very important and diverse as compared to other sectors. The records in the healthcare industry start from electronic health records, list of medications provided to a patient, clinical trials, insurance claims, etc. Just imagine the amount of data produced by every multinational hospital present on this planet! It would be unimaginably huge. And this data obviously could not be handled by traditional data processing systems, as this type of data is real-time continuous and data storage along with analysis could be a big issue with it, hence the big data approach is beneficial when dealing with healthcare data or any type of complex and unstructured data types which is abundant in scale and is not easy to handle. Big data practices would lead to better data handling, storing, and analyzing it in many cost-efficient ways.

13.1 Introduction

The total population of humans on Earth has recently crossed an unbelievable number of 8 billion [1]. It is a big number and with increasing population, the resources required by this number are steadily increasing. But, with the expanding technological and scientific advancements, the global life expectancy index has risen in the past 65 years according to the World Economic Forum [2]. Also, according to an article published in the National Library of Medicine, due to the medical advancements in the healthcare industry in the past few decades, the situation now has completely changed in terms of the expectancy index and this study of medicine has impacted people on a greater scale to live longer [3]. One more factor which

[1]Research Center of Excellence for Health Informatics, Vishwakarma University, Pune, India

affected this number is urbanization, and an example of improving the healthcare sector can be seen as a rise in fertility rates, as the maternal risks during pregnancy can be reduced due to these medical and technological advancements.

The other thing that has been evolving for the past few decades apart from the healthcare industry is the technical sector. The last century resulted in starting technological advancements and improvements in petroleum, atomic energy, textile industries, agriculture, and healthcare [4]. This century has already started the technical revolution in the computer industry and the concept of the digital world has taken a boom. Today, almost every urban household has a personal computer and an active internet connection. According to an article by Forbes, the world generates nearly 2.5 quintillion bytes of data every day, which may be about 1,000 Petabytes every day [5]. The importance of data has frequently been increasing for the past few decades and nowadays, and people have been trusting it more than anybody else. Every sector generates a large amount of data and the most important three factors are very necessary to prove its worth. These are storage of data, preprocessing, and analyzing the patterns present within the data to investigate, discover, and predict various possible events required to take probable business decisions, make a pivot in an existing business crisis or finding which gene can be used to make a vaccine against a virus.

Every sector makes use of data and generates a huge amount of data every year. Some of these sectors are retail, government, banking, and the huge amount of data generated by any sector is healthcare. If we take an idea of the Indian healthcare sector, it has become one of the biggest sectors to influence the Indian economy [6]. The market size of the healthcare sector in India is predicted to outstretch at about 553.80 million us dollars in 2023 [7]. Now we can roughly make an idea of how much of the data is generated by every country, depending upon their economic and technological stability. According to the article of Capital Markets, almost 30% of the world's total data is generated by the healthcare sector, and in the upcoming couple of years, it is going to break this threshold by a bigger margin [8].

The healthcare industry generates large amounts of data from a variety of sources, including EHRs, medical devices, clinical trials, insurance claims, and more. This information can be used to improve patient care, reduce costs, and advance clinical research.

According to the Health Science Library from the University of Washington [9], some examples of records created by the healthcare industry are:

1. Electronic Health Records (EHR): EHRs contain the patient's medical history, including diagnoses, treatments, medications, and test results. This information is created when a patient visits a hospital or clinic.
2. Medical devices: Data generated by medical devices such as blood pressure monitors, blood glucose monitors, and heart rate monitors can be used to track a patient's time.
3. Clinical trials: Clinical trials produce information about the safety and efficiency of a new drug or treatment. This information can help researchers identify new therapies and treatments for a variety of diseases.

4. Insurance claims: Insurance claims data includes information about medical services and procedures provided to patients. This information is used to control medical costs and improve the quality of care.
5. Other types of data generated by the medical industry include genomic data, patient-generated data, and public health data.

The challenge for the healthcare industry is not just collecting data, but making sense of it. Using advanced analytics and artificial intelligence, doctors can extract insights from big data to improve patient outcomes and make informed decisions. This type of data generated at a huge scale continuously is termed as big data and storing, processing, and making inferences out of it is very necessary.

13.2 Literature review

The authors of [9] have prepared a systematic review of literature on the study of BDA in the healthcare domain. Based on SLR, it gives 41 studies' outcomes and the application of BDA in healthcare that they have noticed from five perspectives. The authors in [10] have concluded that there is an increasing rate of the information technology sector as well as development also. Because of this, varieties of data are generated and it is a large amount of data. They have prepared the issues, challenges, and difficulties in big data analytics [10].

The author of [11] has suggested that a very huge amount of real-time data is generated by healthcare as well as government agencies. Also, Hadoop plays an important and effective role in this field. It can handle the data very easily and predicts the critical situation before it happens. The authors have prepared how big data will help in the healthcare and government sectors. Research in [12] states that the data is growing at a high rate with the use of some advanced techniques. For these new analytical techniques are needed so it can effectively work. They have discussed various factors that may help individual health. It will also help in analyzing facts and can also improve healthcare. With the use of big data analytics, it will also assist in fact analysis and may even enhance global healthcare.

The authors of the survey in [13] have mentioned how they had used the practices of big data in healthcare. The authors have claimed that this research was carried out at 2017 medical facilities in Poland. They have also mentioned issues of structured and unstructured data from various healthcare teams. Their survey concludes that the healthcare sector and their facilities are moving towards data-driven decisions. The authors in [14] have presented that data is currently increasing at a rapid pace in all domains with the availability of high end, huge as well as diverse datasets. The authors have discussed the overview of big data analytics along with benefits of using big data analytics, opportunities as well as challenges.

The author of the survey in [15] has stated that there are different analytical techniques that are involved nowadays. There are big data tools that can be used synch as Hadoop. They have explained how it will help in pandemic conditions and in the future. In research work [16], the authors have stated the importance of big data.

Also, they have covered advantages, challenges of using big data analytics in the healthcare domain. They also have explored various real-time applications.

13.3   Big data analytics

Big data refers to large, complex data that cannot be efficiently managed or analyzed using traditional data processing techniques. This information can come from many sources, including social media, sensors, financial markets, and more. It is characterized by its size, speed, and diversity and is often referred to as the three V. Big data refers to a huge amount of data created and collected, often reaching TB level or even PB level data volume. The speed of big data refers to the amount of data produced and needs to be processed in real time or near real time. The difference between big data refers to different types and types of data, including structured data like numbers, dates), unstructured data (like text, images), and partial data (like files). The sources of real-time data generation are shown Figure 13.1.

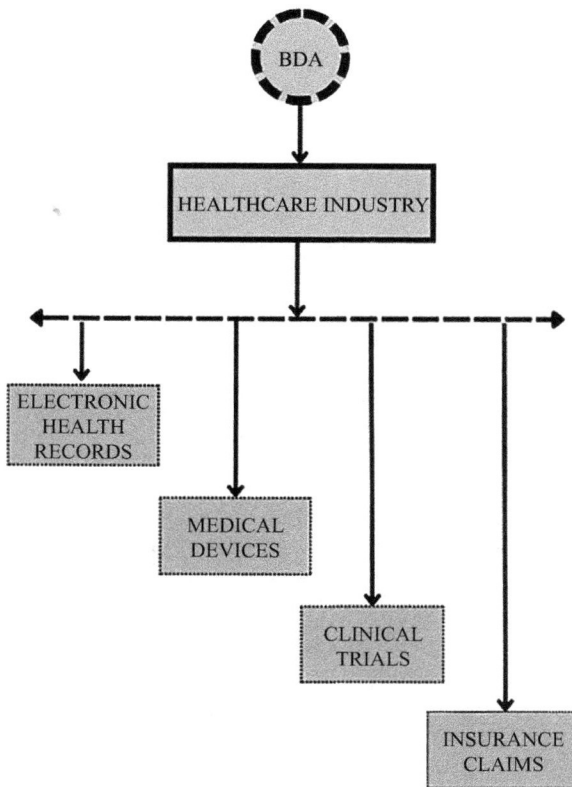

Figure 13.1   Sources of data generation

As was already mentioned, huge data cannot be handled by conventional data processing and storage methods. To address these drawbacks, big data analytics approaches are applied. According to the global giant IBM [17], big data practices have developed and become more potent and scalable in every way feasible in today's growing science and technology. Some of the techniques and terminologies of big data analytics are the following.

13.3.1 Clustering

According to an article by Nvidia [18], in big data, a cluster of computers refers to a group of interconnected computers or servers that work together to process and store large amounts of data. A team usually has one owner and several employees, and each employee is responsible for a portion of the document. The master node manages the cluster and assigns the jobs to the workers' workers and the jobs' workers to work for them. The cluster allows the partitioning of large files, which means that data can be split into smaller chunks and processed simultaneously by different nodes in the cluster. This can be faster and more efficient, making it possible to process larger files from a single machine. Additionally, the integration provides security because data is replicated across multiple nodes, reducing the risk of data loss in case of hardware failure or other issues. The need for clustering in big data analytics is listed in Table 13.1. Overall, clustering is an important initial phase of applying big data analytics in real life and dealing with complex data to improve business decisions and data handling.

13.3.2 Hadoop

Hadoop is increasingly used in the healthcare industry to store, process, and analyze large and complex data. Here are some ways Hadoop can be used in healthcare [19]:

1. Electronic Health Record (EHR) Management: Hadoop can be used to store and manage EHR data, including patient information, treatment history, and

Table 13.1 Need for clustering

Features	Significance
Dimensionality reduction	Clustering can help reduce the dimensionality of big data by identifying clusters of similar data points. This can simplify data analysis and make it easier to find patterns and insights
Anomaly detection	Clustering can help identify anomalies or outliers in the data that do not fit into any cluster. This can help in detecting fraud, errors, or other unexpected events
Data segmentation	Clustering can be used to segment large datasets into smaller subsets based on certain characteristics, such as demographics or user behavior. This can help in targeted marketing, personalization, and customer segmentation
Resource optimization	Clustering can help optimize resource utilization by distributing processing tasks among different clusters, improving processing speed and efficiency

diagnostic results. Hadoop's distributed architecture and scalability make it a hypothetical solution for the distribution of large and growing EHR data.

2. Clinical analytics: It can be used to process and analyze clinical data such as patient demographics, diagnostic codes, and clinical outcomes. This information can be used to spot trends and unseen patterns in patient's healthcare data, which improve clinical performance and improve health outcomes.

3. Medical imaging: Hadoop can be used to store and process large medical images such as X-rays and MRIs. This enables doctors to identify and share medical images across multiple departments and locations, increasing diagnostic accuracy and reducing treatment times.

4. Predictive analytics: Hadoop can be used for predictive analytics in healthcare, such as predicting patient readings, identifying patients at risk for certain conditions, or predicting the effects of certain treatments' outcomes.

5. Precision medicine: Hadoop can be used to store and process genomic data that can be used in precision medicine to create personalized treatment plans based on a person's genetic makeup.

Overall, Hadoop's scalability, fault tolerance, and processing power make it an ideal solution for processing large and complex datasets in the healthcare industry. Hadoop also enables healthcare providers to better use data to improve patient outcomes and deliver better and more efficient healthcare [20].

13.3.3   MapReduce

MapReduce is a powerful and scalable tool used to analyze complex datasets of almost any sector, with high probability to give efficient results and improve business outcomes. There are several approaches to use MapReduce to analyze medical data, including [21]:

1. Data preprocessing: Before evaluating massive amounts of medical data, MapReduce can be used to preprocess and clean the data. Data normalization, cleansing, and transformation are all included here. Data can be divided into manageable parts, parallelized, and then combined using MapReduce.

2. Data gathering: MapReduce can be used to combine clinical data to get insightful results. It can be used, for instance, to estimate the typical length of stay in a hospital or the typical cost of care.

3. MapReduce can be used for data mining to examine medical data and look for unseen patterns. It can be used, for instance, to determine how certain diseases and lifestyle choices are related, or to pinpoint drug usage patterns.

4. Predictive modeling: Based on clinical data, MapReduce can be used to create prediction models. It can be used, for instance, to forecast readmission rates or patient outcomes based on a variety of variables.

5. Analytics in real time: MapReduce can be used to analyze medical data in real time. It can be used, for instance, to instantly analyze a patient's vital signs and notify medical professionals when specific thresholds are surpassed.

The role of big data analytics is a never-ending story as the need to store and analyze data is increasing day by day. From Figure 13.2, we can take a look at how big data methods could influence the healthcare industry in every way possible.

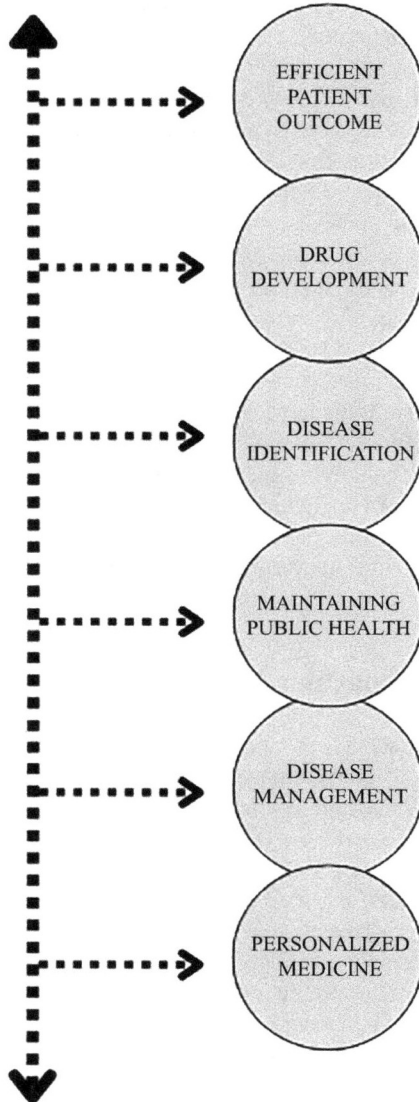

Figure 13.2   Big data analytics influencing healthcare industry

Implementing big data techniques at the local level in a hospital may be resilient, but keeping in mind some concepts and important steps, this could be possible [22]. Identification of the goal is crucial. We must determine the precise objectives that we hope to accomplish before putting any big data analytics' techniques into practice. Some of the primary objectives of the healthcare business in terms of big data are thought to be improved patient outcomes, decreased costs, and increased operational efficiency. Once our objectives have been established, it is crucial to choose the categories of data to gather and examine [23].

The gathering and management of the data comes next. Every data analyst needs access to enormous data sets to employ big data analysis methods. This could entail compiling information from patient satisfaction surveys, billing software, electronic health records, and other sources. Also, ensuring the way of organizing data is crucial as the analysis phase is completely dependent on it. The appropriate tool selection is equally crucial. Big data analysis uses a variety of techniques and technologies, and analysts must select those that best match the objectives of the institution. From a managerial standpoint, this can entail making software purchases or hiring data analytics specialists [24].

Analysis of computed analytics data; once the data has been gathered, organized, and the appropriate tools have been chosen, we can start analyzing our data to find patterns and trends. Techniques like machine learning, natural language processing, and predictive analytics may be employed in this. To create predictions, address a specific problem, or conduct research, we next take action using the insights we learned from our data analysis. This could entail introducing new treatment regimens, altering organizational procedures, or acquiring new technologies. There is very much more to offer for BDA in the healthcare sector [25].

13.4   Big data and machine learning in healthcare

Big data analytics with machine learning can be used to improve patient outcomes and reduce healthcare costs. By analyzing patient data such as medical history, lab results, and genetic information, machine learning algorithms can identify patterns that indicate a patient is at risk for a particular disease or condition and recommend appropriate interventions. Machine learning and big data analytics both employ technologies to draw conclusions from data, but they do it in different ways [26]. To find patterns, trends, and links among enormous amounts of data, big data analytics is used. On the other hand, machine learning entails creating algorithms that can absorb knowledge from data and base choices or predictions on that knowledge [27].

Machine learning and big data analytics can be combined to improve both technologies' precision and efficacy. The data can be preprocessed to enable this integration [28]. Before data is used for machine learning, it can be cleaned up and prepared using big data analytics. This may entail eliminating outliers, filling in blanks, and altering the data to make machine learning algorithms more effective. Engineering features are the following phase. From the data, pertinent features and trends can be found and extracted using BDA. Then, machine learning algorithms

Table 13.2   Big data analytics tools

Cloud	This platform/tool provides beneficial infrastructure for BDA applications
Apache Spark	It is a fast data processing engine that is primarily used for large datasets
Machine learning	It is a tool that can be trained on both structured and unstructured data
NoSQL	It is a fast data processing engine that is primarily used for large datasets
Natural language processing	Natural language processing is a branch of artificial intelligence that focuses on assisting computers in understanding human textual language with the help of natural language processing Toolkit (NLTK) and Spacy
Apache Kafka	Accurately helps process real-time data in a fault-tolerant way

can use these features as inputs. Model training is equally crucial since big data analytics-processed and analyzed massive datasets can be used to train machine learning algorithms. The performance of the machine learning models would improve as more data becomes available. According to the U.S. Food and Drug Administration [29], data can be analyzed in real-time and used as input by machine learning algorithms, thanks to the real-time analysis capability. Applications like fraud detection or predictive maintenance can really benefit from this.

Also, BDA and their methods could be integrated with many other feasible technologies like Cloud Computing, Tableau, Apache Spark, Kafka, etc. Table 13.2 provides a detailed explanation of the potential benefits that various BDA technologies, whether standalone or integrated with them, could offer to the healthcare sector.

13.5   Conclusion

In conclusion, the use of big data analytics in the healthcare industry has the potential to completely alter how care is provided, overseen, and managed. Healthcare professionals can learn important lessons about patient care, illness prevention, and community health by utilizing vast amounts of patient data. Big data analytics in healthcare can help with patient outcomes, healthcare cost reduction, and overall care quality. Concerns and challenges related to compliance, security, and privacy must also be addressed. Overall, big data analytics in healthcare has many advantages, and more study and funding are required to fully realize this technology's promise to enhance patient outcomes.

References

[1]   Sen, C. K. (2021). Human wound and its burden: updated 2020 compendium of estimates. *Advances in Wound Care*, 10(5), 281–292.

[2] Farjana, S. H., Huda, N., Mahmud, M. P., and Saidur, R. (2019). A review on the impact of mining and mineral processing industries through life cycle assessment. *Journal of Cleaner Production*, 231, 1200–1217.

[3] Sugimoto, C. R., Ahn, Y. Y., Smith, E., Macaluso, B., and Larivière, V. (2019). Factors affecting sex-related reporting in medical research: a cross-disciplinary bibliometric analysis. *The Lancet*, 393(10171), 550–559.

[4] Marr, B. How Much Data Do We Create Every Day? *The Mind-Blowing Stats Everyone Should Read*. https://www.forbes.com/sites/bernardmarr/2018/05/21/how-much-data-do-we-create-every-day-the-mind-blowing-stats-everyone-should-read/?sh=58c5c95d60ba.

[5] Ghayvat, H., Pandya, S., Bhattacharya, P., *et al.* (2021). CP-BDHCA: blockchain-based confidentiality-privacy preserving big data scheme for healthcare clouds and applications. *IEEE Journal of Biomedical and Health Informatics*, 26(5), 1937–1948.

[6] Pandey, A., Brauer, M., Cropper, M. L., *et al.* (2021). Health and economic impact of air pollution in the states of India: the Global Burden of Disease Study 2019. *The Lancet Planetary Health*, 5(1), e25–e38.

[7] Dhagarra, D., Goswami, M., and Kumar, G. (2020). Impact of trust and privacy concerns on technology acceptance in healthcare: an Indian perspective. *International Journal of Medical Informatics*, 141, 104164.

[8] Sethi, G. K., Ahmad, N., Rehman, M. B., Dafallaa, H. M. E. I., and Rashid, M. (2021). Use of artificial intelligence in healthcare systems: state-of-the-art survey. *In 2021 2nd International Conference on Intelligent Engineering and Management (ICIEM)* (pp. 243–248). IEEE.

[9] Khanra, S., Dhir, A., Najmul Islam, A. K. M., and Mäntymäki, M. (2020) Big data analytics in healthcare: a systematic literature review. *Enterprise Information Systems*, 14:7, 878–912.

[10] Vaidya, G. M. and Kshirsagar, M. M. (2020). A survey of algorithms, technologies and issues in big data analytics and applications. In *2020 4th International Conference on Intelligent Computing and Control Systems (ICICCS)* (pp. 347–350). IEEE.

[11] Lv, Z. and Qiao, L. (2020). Analysis of healthcare big data. *Future Generation Computer Systems*, 109, 103–110.

[12] Reddy, S. S. R. D. and Ramanadham, U. K. (2017). Big data analytics for healthcare organization, BDA process, benefits and challenges of BDA: a review. *Advances in Science Technology and Engineering Systems Journal*, 2(4), 189–196.

[13] Rashid, M., Singh, H., Goyal, V., Ahmad, N., and Mogla, N. (2022). Efficient big data-based storage and processing model in Internet of Things for improving accuracy fault detection in industrial processes. In *Research Anthology on Big Data Analytics, Architectures, and Applications* (pp. 945–957). IGI Global.

[14] Lalmi, F. and Adala, L. (2021). Big data for healthcare: opportunities and challenges. In *The Fourth Industrial Revolution: Implementation of Artificial Intelligence for Growing Business Success*, pp. 217–229.

[15] Putchala, B., Kanala, L. S., Donepudi, D. P., and Kondaveeti, H. K. (2023). Applications of big data analytics in healthcare informatics. In *Health Informatics and Patient Safety in Times of Crisis* (pp. 175–194). IGI Global.

[16] Rashid, M., Ahmad, A. J., and Prashar, D. (2023). Integration of IoT with big data analytics for the development of smart society. In *Artificial Intelligence and Machine Learning in Smart City Planning* (pp. 13–27). Elsevier.

[17] Jin, X., Wah, B. W., Cheng, X., and Wang, Y. (2015). Significance and challenges of big data research. *Big Data Research*, 2(2), 59–64.

[18] Chen, C., Li, K., Ouyang, A., Zeng, Z., and Li, K. (2018). GFlink: an in-memory computing architecture on heterogeneous CPU-GPU clusters for big data. *IEEE Transactions on Parallel and Distributed Systems*, 29(6), 1275–1288.

[19] Sharmila, K. and Vethamanickam, S. A. (2015). Survey on data mining algorithm and its application in healthcare sector using Hadoop platform. *International Journal of Emerging Technology and Advanced Engineering*, 5(1), 567–571.

[20] Harb, H., Mroue, H., Mansour, A., Nasser, A., and Motta Cruz, E. (2020). A Hadoop-based platform for patient classification and disease diagnosis in healthcare applications. *Sensors*, 20(7), 1931.

[21] Nishadi, T. (2019). AS: healthcare big data analysis using Hadoop MapReduce. *International Journal of Scientific and Research Publication*, 9(3), 87104.

[22] Brossard, P. Y., Minvielle, E., and Sicotte, C. (2022). The path from big data analytics capabilities to value in hospitals: a scoping review. *BMC Health Services Research*, 22(1), 134.

[23] Galetsi, P., Katsaliaki, K., and Kumar, S. (2020). Big data analytics in health sector: theoretical framework, techniques and prospects. *International Journal of Information Management*, 50, 206–216.

[24] Khanra, S., Dhir, A., Islam, A. N., and Mäntymäki, M. (2020). Big data analytics in healthcare: a systematic literature review. *Enterprise Information Systems*, 14(7), 878–912.

[25] Kumar, A., Kumar, A., Bashir, A. K., Rashid, M., Kumar, V. A., and Kharel, R. (2021). Distance based pattern driven mining for outlier detection in high dimensional big dataset. *ACM Transactions on Management Information System (TMIS)*, 13(1), 1–17.

[26] Athmaja, S., Hanumanthappa, M., and Kavitha, V. (2017). A survey of machine learning algorithms for big data analytics. In *2017 International Conference on Innovations in Information, Embedded and Communication Systems (ICIIECS)* (pp. 1–4). IEEE.

[27] Jan, B., Farman, H., Khan, M., *et al.* (2019). Deep learning in big data analytics: a comparative study. *Computers & Electrical Engineering*, 75, 275–287.

[28] Rashid, M., Yousuf, M. M., Ram, B., and Goyal, V. (2019). Novel big data approach for drug prediction in health care systems. In *2019 International conference on automation, computational and technology management (ICACTM)* (pp. 325–329). IEEE.

[29] Boudhaouia, A., and Wira, P. (2021). A real-time data analysis platform for short-term water consumption forecasting with machine learning. *Forecasting*, 3(4), 682–694.

Index

www.ingramcontent.com/pod-product-compliance
Lightning Source LLC
Chambersburg PA
CBHW050512190326
41458CB00005B/1510